"This fresh and innovative volume critically examines the history of bibliotherapy from the First World War to its modern use in mental health practice. Its chapters by leading scholars draw on rich veins of material from previously unexplored archival sources to contemporary digital texts to provide an interdisciplinary and fascinating survey of 'the healing book' and the transformative power of reading."

Dr Jane Potter, *Reader in Arts, Oxford Brookes University*

A Hundred Years of Bibliotherapy

The First World War gave new and vital impetus to the ancient idea that books could heal. This interdisciplinary collection provides a targeted survey of 100 years of historical and contemporary understandings and practices of 'the book as cure'.

The contributors explore the curative practices of wartime reading, how they were developed and institutionalised after the war, and the afterlives of these ideas and practices today. Divided into three parts, the first part of the book considers bibliotherapy during the First World War. It is rooted in the wartime cultures which ensured bibliotherapy became part of the active treatment of soldiers' damaged minds and bodies on both sides of the Atlantic after 1914. Parts II and III examine the expanding variety of critical contexts, both historical and more modern, in which reading and well-being continued to intersect. The chapters draw on a wide range of source materials from trench magazines to autograph books to e-novels, as well as on data and information drawn from practice-based encounters. They also provide the basis for further scholarly exploration of, for example, national traditions and the contexts and interdisciplinary relationships which they inspire.

A Hundred Years of Bibliotherapy: Healing through Books provides the first interdisciplinary dialogue on and account of bibliotherapy, addressing both historical and present-day modes of engaging with the ostensibly curative power of reading and reading cultures. It is an invaluable resource for scholars of literary studies, book history, and the medical humanities.

Siobhan Campbell is Senior Lecturer in the School of Arts at The Open University, UK. She researches the theory and applications of social literary practice. She has developed creative writing projects to be used therapeutically and for social reconstruction in pressurised environments, with partners like Combat Stress UK, NHS Trusts, NGOs, UNDP, and third-sector organisations. Her publications include *The Expressive Life Writing Handbook* (with Meg Jensen; 2017).

Sara Haslam is Professor of Twentieth-Century Literature at The Open University, UK. A scholar of modernism and First World War literature, her publications include 'Reading, Trauma and Literary Caregiving 1914–1918: Helen Mary Gaskell and the War Library', *Journal of Medical Humanities* (2018), and *Life Writing* (with Derek Neale; 2008).

Edmund G. C. King is Senior Lecturer in English Literature at The Open University, UK. A book historian with a particular focus on the history of reading, he is most recently the co-editor of *Memorialising Shakespeare: Commemoration and Collective Identity, 1916–2016* (with Monika Smialkowska; 2021).

A Hundred Years of Bibliotherapy

Healing through Books

Edited by Siobhan Campbell, Sara Haslam, and Edmund G. C. King

Routledge
Taylor & Francis Group
LONDON AND NEW YORK

First published 2025
by Routledge
4 Park Square, Milton Park, Abingdon, Oxon OX14 4RN

and by Routledge
605 Third Avenue, New York, NY 10158

Routledge is an imprint of the Taylor & Francis Group, an informa business

British Library Cataloguing-in-Publication Data
A catalogue record for this book is available from the British Library

Library of Congress Cataloging-in-Publication Data
Names: Campbell, Siobhán, 1962– editor. | Haslam, Sara, editor. |
King, Edmund G. C., editor.
Title: A hundred years of bibliotherapy : healing through books /
edited by Siobhan Campbell, Sara Haslam, and Edmund G.C. King.
Description: Abingdon, Oxon ; New York, NY : Routledge, 2025. |
Includes bibliographical references and index. |
Identifiers: LCCN 2024058703 (print) | LCCN 2024058704 (ebook) |
ISBN 9781032749297 (hardback) | ISBN 9781032749310 (paperback) |
ISBN 9781003471561 (ebook)
Subjects: LCSH: Books and reading–Psychological aspects. |
Bibliotherapy. | Well-being. | World War, 1914–1918–Literature and the war. |
Soldiers–Books and reading. | LCGFT: Essays.
Classification: LCC Z1003 .H897 2025 (print) | LCC Z1003 (ebook) |
DDC 940.4/75–dc23/eng/20250208
LC record available at https://lccn.loc.gov/2024058703
LC ebook record available at https://lccn.loc.gov/2024058704

ISBN: 978-1-032-74929-7 (hbk)
ISBN: 978-1-032-74931-0 (pbk)
ISBN: 978-1-003-47156-1 (ebk)

DOI: 10.4324/9781003471561

Typeset in Times New Roman
by Newgen Publishing UK

Contents

Figures

Contributors

Katarina Båth is Associate Professor in Literature at the Centre for Languages and Literature, Lund University, Sweden. Research areas include philosophical and literary Romanticism from gender and queer theoretical perspectives, literary trauma studies and bibliotherapy, literature didactics, and creative writing. A unifying research interest is the question of the healing and transformative potential of fiction and reading.

Laura Gray Blair is Research Manager (Postgraduate and Skills) for the Science Museum Group. She recently submitted her Wellcome Trust-funded doctoral thesis, examining the use of reading within the therapeutic regimes of nineteenth-century asylums.

Siobhan Campbell is Senior Lecturer in the School of Arts at The Open University, Milton Keynes, UK. She researches the theory and applications of social literary practice. She has developed creative writing projects to be used therapeutically and for social reconstruction in pressurised environments, with partners like Combat Stress UK, NHS Trusts, NGOs, UNDP, and third-sector organisations. Her publications include *The Expressive Life Writing Handbook* (with Meg Jensen; 2017).

Helen Chambers is Visiting Fellow in English at The Open University, Milton Keynes, UK. She is the author of *Conrad's Reading: Space, Time Networks* (Palgrave, 2018) and has recently contributed chapters to *Shipboard Literary Cultures* (Palgrave, 2022) and the *Routledge Companion to Joseph Conrad* (2024).

Lindsay Davies is Clinical Professor Emerita of Global Liberal Studies at New York University. She has taught in New York, London, Florence, and Tokyo. The interdisciplinary nature of her teaching led to publication on a wide range of subjects, including heritage cinema, international adoption memoir and fiction, and Romantic poetry.

Laura Dietz is Lecturer in Publishing at University College London. She speaks and publishes widely on reading, authorship, and digital literary culture. Her most recent book, *E-books and 'Real Books': Digital Reading and the Experience of Bookness*, was published by Cambridge University Press in 2025.

Véronique Duché is A.R. Chisholm Professor of French at the University of Melbourne. Her expertise lies in the history of translation during the Renaissance, comparative literature, and the history of the book. She also researches Australian soldiers during the First World War.

Danni Glover is an independent researcher from Glasgow publishing on eighteenth-century print culture, including in *Suicide and the Gothic, The Cambridge Guide to the Eighteenth Century Novel,* and *The Year's Work in English Studies*. As a bibliotherapy practitioner, her research appears in *Conversations: Lecture Notes in Computer Science*. Currently working in the public sector, she researches print culture, bibliotherapy, and queer cinema.

Sara Haslam is Professor of Twentieth-Century Literature at The Open University, Milton Keynes, UK. A scholar of modernism and First World War literature, her publications include 'Reading, Trauma and Literary Caregiving 1914–1918: Helen Mary Gaskell and the War Library', *Journal of Medical Humanities* (2018), and *Life Writing* (with Derek Neale; 2008).

Barbara Hochman is Professor Emerita at Ben-Gurion University. She is the author of *Getting at the Author: Reimagining Books and Reading in the Age of American Realism* and the prize-winning *Uncle Tom's Cabin and the Reading Revolution: Race, Literacy, Childhood, and Fiction 1852–1911*.

Edmund G. C. King is Senior Lecturer in English at The Open University, Milton Keynes, UK. An historian of reading, his recent published work can be found in *The Edinburgh Companion to First World War Periodicals* (2023) and in 'Bookshelves, Social Media and Gaming', a special issue of *English Studies* (2022).

Amanda Laugesen is a historian and lexicographer and is chief editor of the *Australian National Dictionary* at the Australian National University, Canberra. She has published extensively in the fields of book history, the social and cultural history of war, and the history of Australian English.

Mary Mahoney is a historian working at Trinity College in Hartford, Connecticut. Currently at work on a history of bibliotherapy in America, she is also the co-author of *Dolls of Our Lives: Why We Can't Quit American Girl*.

Jesse Miller is Site Director and Instructor for the Bard Prison Initiative programme at Albion Correctional Facility in Western New York. Recent publications can be found in *Modernism/Modernity*, *MFS: Modern Fiction Studies*, and *Mosaic: An Interdisciplinary Critical Journal*.

Vincent Trott is Senior Lecturer in History at The Open University, Milton Keynes, UK. His first book, *Publishers, Readers and the Great War: Literature and Memory Since 1918*, was published in 2017 (Bloomsbury Academic). His current research explores humour, propaganda, and political satire in the USA, 1914–1918.

Acknowledgements

This edited volume has its origins in 'The Book as Cure: Bibliotherapy and Literary Caregiving from the First World War to the Present', a one-day conference held at Senate House, University of London, on 14 September 2018 under the joint sponsorship of The Open University (OU) and the Institute of English Studies. Firstly, we would like to thank Jane Potter (Oxford Brookes University) and Peter Leese (University of Copenhagen) for generously agreeing to be our plenary speakers and for taking part in a thought-provoking roundtable on the legacies and futures of bibliotherapy, the implications of which fed directly into the thinking behind this volume. We would also like to acknowledge the assistance and support of academic and administrative staff at The Open University and the Institute of English Studies (particularly Maya Parmar, Tamanna Yasmin, and Katy Thompson). We owe a particular debt of thanks to our Open University colleague, Shafquat Towheed, for his generosity and collegiality throughout. We are also indebted to the OU's History of Books and Reading research group (HOBAR), a valued collaborative arena for our thinking and discussion which provided funding support and enabled us to award a small number of PhD travel bursaries to participants at the London conference. Many thanks, too, to all those who attended and presented at the conference, as well as to our conference reviewer, Jenny Cattier.

However, this volume is much more than a set of conference proceedings, and we would like to thank all our contributors for their hard work in developing their chapters, as well as for their patience and continued support during the volume's long period of incubation. We would like to thank our departmental colleagues in English and Creative Writing at the OU for their support and collegial presence, even in the midst of a global pandemic. For instrumental support in producing this volume, we would like to thank Nicola Watson and The Open University Arts & Humanities Research Centre (OpenARC). At Routledge, we would like to thank Karen Raith and Chris Ratcliffe, along with our anonymous readers.

Healing through Books

An Introduction

Edmund G. C. King, Sara Haslam, and Siobhan Campbell

In *A Hundred Years of Bibliotherapy: Healing through Books*, we bring together scholars and practitioners working in this diverse and growing field to provide, for the first time, an interdisciplinary account of bibliotherapy since the First World War, addressing both historical and present-day modes of engaging with the ostensibly curative power of reading. The chapters in this volume offer a targeted survey of 100 years of understandings and practices of 'the book as cure', intervening in the debates that have surrounded bibliotherapy and the therapeutic role of books and reading historically and which have come to underpin contemporary practice.

Even as writers on bibliotherapy acknowledge its ancient history (citing, for example, the inscription 'healing-place of the soul' placed above the portal of the library of the Egyptian pharaoh Ramesses II) and even as they debate the term, the story of its wartime coining by the American Unitarian minister Samuel McChord Crothers (1857–1927) is a frequent touchstone.[1] The word bibliotherapy, and the immediate contexts from which it emerged, accordingly determines our historical framing of this collection, but in *A Hundred Years of Bibliotherapy: Healing through Books* we look behind and beyond what was an unintentionally momentous intervention on the part of Crothers.[2] Across the Introduction and in three sections – Bibliotherapy and the First World War; Institutional Legacies from Libraries to Hospitals, 1919–1950; and Contemporary Critical Interventions – our aims in this volume are to question origin stories, develop and nuance the historiography, and examine and challenge existing narratives and practices, animating more completely the distinct and vital impetus war gave to the idea that books could heal.

In rendering more visible the variety of related debates about reading and reading cultures, and particularly the transatlantic conversation that turbo-charged the institutionalisation of 'bibliotherapy', the broad-based analysis gathered here allows the charting of related influences on contemporary practice in the United Kingdom and beyond. The volume's chapters, the result of archival and critical exploration, social policy research, and interviews by our contributors will, its three editors hope, provide the basis for further scholarly exploration of, for example, national traditions and contexts and the interdisciplinary relationships which they continue to inspire.

DOI: 10.4324/9781003471561-1

In our Introduction, we examine key terms and historic assumptions as we situate the collective contribution of these chapters in what is a fast-expanding field. Pandemic-era commentary on the benefits of reading was almost impossible to avoid, but frequently neglected to question its evidence or terms of reference.[3] In this volume, overall, we seek to expose and examine a range of related critical processes, central as they are to understanding the potent notion of 'the healing book'.

Healing through Books?

Reading and writing, like all cognitive technologies, may be understood as *pharmaka* – that is, as media phenomena that can simultaneously act as medicines and poisons, remedies and sources of harm.[4] In Plato's *Phaedrus*, Socrates recounts a myth describing how Theuth, the Egyptian god of knowledge, appeared before King Thamous to extol the benefits of his new invention, writing. Writing, Theuth announces, is a new 'science' that will 'increase the intelligence of the people of Egypt and improve their memories'. Thamous replies, however, that all of Theuth's many inventions must be assessed for the potential they have to do 'harm' as well as their intended 'benefit'. Rather than writing being a simple 'potion for memory and intelligence', it might prove instead to have precisely the opposite effect. If spread throughout the Kingdom of Egypt as a general practice, Thamous predicts, writing 'will atrophy people's memories', so that they will only be able to 'remember things by relying on marks made by others, from outside themselves, not on their own inner resources'.[5]

Commenting on the implications of the Theuth myth for understanding the nature of reading and writing, Jacques Derrida argues that it is (in part) writing's ability to 'penetrate' the interior world of the reader that makes it both poison and remedy. While writing confers on ideas and literary works the remedies of permanence and transmissibility, it also has the power to reorder the human psyche in unseen and unpredictable ways – to, as Derrida puts it, 'affect or infect what lies deepest inside' in ways that could be *both* beneficial *and* harmful.[6] In *Phaedrus*, this process of psychological reordering manifests itself as the loss of the capacity for memory. In a text like Johann Wolfgang von Goethe's *The Sorrows of Young Werther* (1774), it lies in reading's ability to create new forms of social and psychological affiliation. In *Werther*, it is Lotte's and Werther's discovery that they possess a shared repertoire of reading memories that creates their initial psychic bond. Gazing out a window at the summer rains, Lotte utters a single word, 'Klopstock!', suspecting that Werther will understand instantly what she means.[7] In the moment that follows, Lotte and Werther in effect enter the realm of Klopstock's poetry together, simultaneously experiencing the rainstorm through the same aesthetic frame. Yet, if the affiliative power of literature has a remedial quality in temporarily synchronising Lotte's and Werther's inner worlds, in its poisonous mode it leads Werther to inappropriately idealise and fixate on Lotte, to become depressed and ultimately to commit suicide. Werther's temptation to make real life conform to the ideals and plot structures he has encountered through reading fiction ultimately ends in tragedy.

'Even in the case of drugs used exclusively for therapeutic ends', Derrida writes, there is 'no such thing as a harmless remedy. The *pharmakon* can never be simply beneficial'.[8] The fundamental ambivalence of the written word has not deterred scholars and bibliotherapeutic practitioners from attempting to isolate the therapeutic or 'improving' potential within literature. Viewed through the interpretive lens of *pharmaka*, it is the pharmacological power that literature offers to *reshape the inner world of the reader* that makes it an appealing tool for therapeutic intervention. However, viewing bibliotherapy through the metaphorics of the *pharmakon* can also be revealing in other ways. Dominant modes of literary valuation – from canon formation to the identification of literary classics – have sought to distinguish between 'good' and 'bad' texts (or between the supposed 'defects' and 'beauties' within a single text).[9] As Anna Vaninskaya notes, nineteenth-century journalistic accounts of the supposed harms inflicted on working-class readers by cheap print and 'penny dreadfuls' typically prescribed the 'remedies' of 'good literature' inculcated through the medium of classroom instruction as their ideal antidote.[10]

Bibliotherapy has engaged in its own para-canonical forms of list making, although its criteria for selection have been *health* or *therapeutic* benefit, rather than 'beauty', 'excellence', or the aesthetic judgement of the literary critic. The so-called 'fever-chart' used by the Oxford don H. F. Brett-Smith to assess reading matter suitable for wounded British soldiers during the First World War illustrates this slippage from literary value to therapeutic value. According to the legend passed down in the 1980s by his former student, Martin Jarrett-Kerr, Brett-Smith 'was employed by hospitals to advise on reading matter for the war-wounded. His job was to grade novels and poetry according to the "fever-chart". For the severely shell-shocked he selected Jane Austen'.[11] Here, the selective and grading actions associated with literary criticism are superficially retained but are repurposed to create a new, therapeutic form of measurement – the degree to which a text could alleviate psychological trauma. In their handbook *Biblio/Poetry Therapy*, Arleen McCarty Hynes and Mary Hynes-Berry are similarly overt in juxtaposing literary and therapeutic value systems. It is not that 'bibliotherapeutic and literary criteria' are necessarily 'incompatible'. Instead, in selecting texts for use in sessions, the bibliotherapist needs to distinguish between poetry that is merely 'good' and the kind of writing that 'would be a good tool for therapeutic discussion'.[12] In bibliotherapeutic terms, they write, 'the value of literature depends strictly on its capacity to encourage a therapeutic (feeling) response from the participants'. Wider questions of aesthetics and 'meaning' are irrelevant to this process. Instead, a 'good' bibliotherapeutic text is implicitly 'pharmacological' – something capable of opening up the inner world of the reader to potential therapeutic transformation.[13]

Timelines, Origin Stories, and Definitions

The basic concept that books and reading can have a medicinal or therapeutic value has a long history, but it is difficult to attribute to it a single 'origin story', a problem exacerbated by the incommensurable distances separating historical reading and writing cultures across time and space. Moreover, while bibliotherapeutic approaches have many parallels with other traditions of literary study, they are also in many ways distinct from them. One way of grappling with this conceptual fuzziness is to distinguish between two ways of defining bibliotherapy – firstly, as an idea or principle, and secondly, as a set of historically distinct practices or forms of treatment. However, even at this level of detail, some degree of fuzziness remains. Attempts to crystallise the *idea* behind bibliotherapy have often resulted in broad and all-encompassing definitions. Liz Brewster, for instance, defines bibliotherapy as 'the premise' that 'information, guidance, and solace can be found in books'.[14] Definitions of this sort enable the maximal inclusion of as much of the perceived positive value of reading within the remit of bibliotherapy. However, as Gill Partington observes, overly inclusive definitions often do not quite articulate what it is about bibliotherapy that makes it distinctive as an approach to reading texts. To illustrate this, Partington quotes one 1981 pamphlet, which claims that 'If you have ever felt warm, weepy, excited, or renewed after reading a book, then you have experienced a form of bibliotherapy', noting drily that what it is that separates bibliotherapy as described here from 'reading in general … is not entirely clear'.[15]

Broad conceptual definitions of bibliotherapy are often accompanied by broad historical parallels and ancient origin stories. Sarah J. Jack and Kevin R. Ronan take the use of 'verbal and written materials' to 'foster emotional wellness' back to 'almost the beginning of time'.[16] In their 2016 *Lancet* article on 'the art and science of bibliotherapy', Jonathan Bate and Andrew Schuman trace what they call 'humankind's awareness of the therapeutic value of words' back to ancient Egypt and the tradition recorded in the first century BCE by the Greek historian Diodorus Siculus that 'the sacred library of Pharaoh Rameses II' had inscribed above its entrance the words 'Healing-place of the soul'.[17] Nick Canty cites the example of the Al-Mansur hospital in Cairo, founded in 1272, in which readings from the Koran formed part of the medical treatment regime.[18] Janella D. Moy likewise argues for the recognition of what she calls bibliotherapy's 'long history' by demonstrating how words and books have been ascribed medicinal powers throughout history.[19] A particular focus of Moy's brief history of bibliotherapy is ancient Greek drama. Linking Aristotle's use (in *Poetics*) of the ancient Greek medical principle of *katharsis* (or purging) for understanding how drama can move an audience with the awareness among ancient Greek writers of the power of comedy and tragedy to elicit complementary emotions, she writes that these understandings 'eventually led to the use of literature for medicinal purposes'.[20] Whole movements have been recruited to the cause as literary criticism developed along these lines. 'Some of our most familiar claims about the medical value of literature are Romantic', Brittany Pladek writes, before quoting Keats's hope that the poet might be a physician to all men and Percy Bysshe Shelley's belief that poetry 'connects, animates and sustains the life of all'.[21]

Suggestions that bibliotherapy has ancient roots and close parallels in historical literary traditions are undeniably appealing. They provide evidence for how widespread pharmacological understandings of books are, both in time and space, and show how reading, writing, and the concept of the *pharmakon* have always been interlinked. However, attempts to trace transhistorical connections can also sometimes obfuscate or mystify. Broad and all-encompassing histories and definitions can make it hard to articulate *why* bibliotherapeutic ideas arose at certain times and in certain places and *how* they intersected with particular systems and ideologies of care. When engagement with self-help manuals is equated with a bibliotherapeutic intervention, for example, as in a 2023 social science study, that difficulty is heightened.[22]

Examining how literary-therapeutic ideas functioned within particular professional and institutional settings can provide more clarity. As Laura Gray Blair shows in her contribution to this volume, asylum libraries became an integral part of the new 'moral treatment' regimes that sought to reform care of the mentally ill in early to mid-nineteenth-century Britain and America.[23] Under the moral treatment regime in place during the early 1800s at The Retreat, an asylum near York in England, its patient library was stocked with books on mathematics and natural sciences with the intention that these would 'employ the minds' of asylum residents. Patients who engaged with these books were encouraged by asylum staff to pursue single lines of study in depth. However, novels ('works of the imagination') were evidently *not* held in the library (in the belief that fictional scenarios would detrimentally encourage patients to fantasise and dissociate). Moreover, any books whose subject matter intersected with 'the peculiar notions' of individual patients were seen as especially 'objectionable' and kept out of their hands.[24]

In 1847, the American asylum superintendent John Minson Galt II provided a more extended account of how asylum libraries could assist in the treatment of the mentally ill. As at The Retreat, books in the American asylum system were viewed as a means of beneficially occupying patients' minds. However, Galt also believed that reading alleviated 'morbid thoughts and delusions' and that the general 'contentedness' that books provided would help make patients 'more manageable' for asylum staff.[25] Like literacy training in general – which was also provided in asylums – moral treatment sought to harness what Bernard Stiegler calls the 'psychotechnics' of reading, enabling asylum residents to (re)gain the power of paying attention and focus on the kinds of mental tasks that would lead to psychological recovery.[26] Like the other forms of activity prescribed in the asylum during this period – such as sewing, gardening, and farm work – reading therefore provided a positive model for behavioural reform, a template for the production of 'wellness'.[27] Rather than simply being an early stage in the evolution of a larger, transhistorical concept called 'bibliotherapy', the particularities of nineteenth-century asylum libraries show how literary-therapeutic interventions simultaneously bear the imprint of the specific institutional contexts in which they are embedded. Locating these contexts and demonstrating how they interact with bibliotherapeutic practices are key concerns across all the chapters in this collection.

Over the past hundred years, bibliotherapeutic ideas have undergone large-scale processes of development and elaboration. At the same time, the range of settings and disciplinary forms in which bibliotherapy has been practised have also multiplied. In Britain and the United States, hospital libraries were, as the African American bibliotherapist and Veterans' Administration librarian Sadie

Peterson Delaney (1889–1958) put it, the initial 'laboratory' for the development of new literary-therapeutic theories and techniques.[28] Reactive bibliotherapy was developed by hospital librarians working in American psychiatric hospitals during the 1920s. In this form of therapy, patients were provided with reading material selected to produce a 'reaction' (either positive or negative) that would assist in their ongoing treatment.[29] These hospital library systems in turn drew on the models – and sometimes the literal infrastructure – of the library services set up for soldiers during the First World War. Founded in 1919, the civilian-facing British Red Cross Society and Order of St. John Hospital Library was a direct post-war continuation of the British Red Cross Society and Order of St. John War Library established in 1914 to fulfil the reading needs of sick and wounded British soldiers. The American Library Association's War Hospital Service, meanwhile, prepared the institutional ground for the provision of comprehensive patient library services in American Veterans' Hospitals after the war.[30] More ambitious plans to extend American wartime soldiers' libraries into a post-war, nationwide 'Enlarged Program' of cultural uplift through reading targeted at adult learners and immigrant communities, however, did not ultimately pan out.[31]

Delaney took up her post as librarian at the segregated Veterans' Hospital, no. 91 in Tuskegee, Alabama, in January 1924. Her subsequent activities show how a determined library professional could adapt and expand hospital library services to support a range of bibliotherapeutic aims and practices. Writing in 1938, Delaney defined bibliotherapy as 'the treatment of a patient through selective reading'.[32] This description was to ultimately gain wide acceptance and recognition in American library circles.[33] Selective reading, as Delaney defined it, involved hospital librarians deriving as much information about individual patients' conditions as possible by consulting their attending doctors. On the basis of these prognoses, patients were then supplied with carefully chosen reading material drawn from the library's collections. This material included books, magazines, newspapers, pamphlets, book synopses, and subject-based scrapbooks compiled to facilitate patient discussion of current events. The purpose of reading in the Veterans' Hospital was, Delaney wrote, to revive 'minds long imprisoned in lethargy' by encouraging them to reconnect with old pastimes and develop their intellectual interests, a process that she believed contributed to 'the improvement and development of the whole individual'.[34]

However, bibliotherapy as Delaney conceived of it was not solely based on individual recovery, nor was it limited to equipping patients with the vocational skills they would need to obtain work after release. Selective reading at Tuskegee was also a community-based endeavour, one designed to encourage readers to identify with a collective sense of African American identity, engage with the contemporary struggle for racial recognition, and ideally become leaders in their own communities after discharge from hospital.[35] From the moment of her arrival at Tuskegee, Delaney ensured that the library contained a range of books on African history and cultural traditions, as well as African American social and political issues, and she emphasised that these books were 'used to a great extent'.[36] Describing the impact these books had on their readers, Delaney wrote that 'the hospital library' was 'aiding' them to 'lay aside all prejudice, all sense of defeat, and to take in that which is helpful and inspiring by the means of books'.[37] If, as Arthur P. Young writes, much of the initial reformist energy relating to 'social justice, economic security, and political reformation' that accompanied the end of the war soon dissipated, Delaney's activities show how bibliotherapeutic programmes within hospital libraries could be ways of applying those same ideals at the local level, forming activistic component parts within a larger political struggle.[38] A number of the chapters in this volume, particularly those by Barbara Hochman, Mary Mahoney, and Vincent Trott, expand on these themes. Each demonstrates how significant strands within American librarianship and the developing practice of bibliotherapy emerged out of – and in response to – the moral, racial, and political discourses of the 1910s and 1920s. Edmund G. C. King's chapter, meanwhile, shows how post–First World War discourses of social and cultural regeneration left their imprint on interwar British hospital librarianship.

One of the drivers behind the rising prominence of bibliotherapeutic approaches to reading – and writing, as Helen Chambers' chapter on John Galsworthy's fiction reminds us – during the early to mid-twentieth century was that, as Monique S. Dufour observes, bibliotherapy 'freshly synthesized several modern articles of faith: the value of reading, the authority of science, and the progress of medicine'.[39] Given weight by these connections, the old idea of the healing book thereby assumed a new form, as well as a new cultural and institutional authority. Bibliotherapy's expanding remit reflects another important external context: the growing profile of psychotherapy during this period, one that Freud's writing and practice in particular rendered as inextricable from a literary heritage, from Sophocles to Goethe. In the immediate aftermath of the First World War, psychotherapeutic interventions initially centred upon the figure of the nightmare-ridden, psychologically traumatised returning soldier, who needed expert help in order to reintegrate into society. However, by the middle of the twentieth century, psychotherapy had dramatically extended its range, becoming a tool for self-realisation and the treatment of emotional problems.[40] In a phenomenon that Philip Rieff dubbed 'the triumph of the therapeutic', happiness, wellbeing, and the pursuit of self-development became the new ideals of human flourishing.[41] Vast numbers of people who would not have previously considered treatment entered therapy as a way of combating unhappiness and a perceived lack of personal self-fulfilment.[42] However, the new therapy culture did not only address *individual* desires for self-development. In its most ambitious self-conceptions, the therapy movement saw itself as providing the means for 'the reconstruction of society' at large.[43]

With poetry therapy, first formulated in the 1920s by the American psychiatrists Smiley Blanton and Eli Grieffer, bibliotherapy began to be applied as a therapeutic tool in private practice. For these practitioners, the experience of reading poetry provided a unique access route to the specific 'emotional issues' of clients, which could then be worked out during the therapeutic process.[44] Clinical bibliotherapy, provided usually by a certified counsellor or therapist, evolved as a tool for use with psychiatric patients, while developmental bibliotherapy (used by educators or third-sector organisations) emerged as a text-based variant of the wellbeing-focused therapies that emerged with the positive psychology movement in the mid-twentieth century.[45] The advent of reading bibliotherapy in the 1950s provided an interactive methodology for group bibliotherapeutic practice, whereby selected reading could form the basis for group discussion, a way of generating emotional catharsis or providing insight into the experience of particular illnesses.[46] Institutional bibliotherapy, meanwhile, began to be used in an increasing range of settings beyond its initial sites of the hospital and the asylum, including schools, universities, public libraries, and prisons. A recent bibliometric analysis of the developing research literature on bibliotherapy reveals the sheer variety of conditions which bibliotherapeutic approaches in these various modes are now being used to treat. These conditions range from depression, anxiety, alcoholism, recurrent self-harm, and bulimia nervosa, to panic disorder, hoarding, compulsive buying disorder, and 'lurking' (as opposed to actively posting) on internet forums.[47]

Current practitioners draw on the legacy of previous interventions, creating new sub-divisions of practice to define their own approaches. There are divisions within 'creative bibliotherapy' for instance, if we take it that this is using (mainly) fiction or poetry in both reading and writing to promote mental wellness or to give psycho-social support. Some bibliotherapeutic work with individuals or groups relies on the 'affect' (or the emotional content) of the texts themselves, while work by other practitioners is formalised into story-based programmes. Facilitators of shared reading programmes run by Verbal, Northern Ireland, for instance, work with particular constituencies, such as at-risk youth, and aim to solicit narratives from group participants in response to selected readings. Writing, from journaling to story-telling, can also be embedded. Danni Glover's contribution to this volume, for instance, outlines the use of creative writing as a social practice and as an active ancillary to the bibliotherapeutic approach.

Bibliotherapy and the 'Transformative Powers' of Literature

There is a certain irony in the fact that, as Leah Price observes, the straightforward 'premise that books are good for you' has lately tended to be 'proclaimed with special authority by academics outside of English departments'.[48] It is a premise that sits in uneasy relation with the approaches to literature which have held sway in university Literature departments since the late-1960s revolutions in critical practice. If traditional literary criticism centred on 'upholding the canon of English literature', post-1960s trends in criticism have often tended to resist older, hierarchical systems of literary value embedded in concepts like 'the great works' and the 'timeless classic'.[49] For some practitioners within English Literature and Creative Writing, however, engaging with bibliotherapeutic approaches to reading has seemed to offer the possibility of re-establishing their disciplines on new and more secure-seeming foundations. After she set up a community outreach project entitled 'Get Into Reading' in the mid-1990s, Jane Davis (then at the University of Liverpool) was struck by how different the experience of teaching English Literature to university students was from reading poetry aloud with a more broadly representative group of readers. As the newly convened outreach group read Alfred, Lord Tennyson's poem 'Crossing the Bar' together, one of the women in the room began to cry. As Davis later reflected, 'in twenty-odd years at the university, I had never seen anyone moved to tears by a poem, but here we were, in a community centre in Birkenhead, and a woman was crying'.[50] This experience galvanised her to extend the programme into a more formal and overtly bibliotherapeutic venture – the Reader project, which aims to combat 'social isolation' and promote 'well-being' through the shared reading of 'great literature'.[51]

Reflecting on the implications of the Reader project, Robert Eaglestone observes that the shared reading approach raises some fundamental questions for the contemporary discipline of English Literature. Formal literary study has traditionally disregarded the basic emotional responses of readers. Instead, the novels and poems on university Literature degree courses are taught using various over-determining pedagogical overlays, such as literary analysis and historical context. Bypassing the intellectual distancing mechanisms of formal interpretation and providing a route back to feeling, the Reader project operates according to a different set of understandings of the role of literature. It encourages readers to work through their memories and emotions in relation to a story or text.[52] At the same time, introducing ordinary and marginalised readers to classic and canonical texts in these settings can be a way of countering charges that these works are necessarily 'elitist' or exclusionary.[53]

Davis's colleague at the University of Liverpool, Josie Billington, describes her own realisation that literary classics could be used to promote mental health in similar terms. 'The chief frustration and sadness of my own teaching life', she writes, was that the academic discipline of English Literature had 'lost a sense that literature might speak to humans' deepest needs'. In focusing narrowly on critique and historical context, any 'personal feeling a student might have for a poem or book was often deemed beside the point'. The realisation that reading could be used in the treatment of depression thereby came as 'a lifeline' for a disillusioned English Literature specialist.[54] In a group reading, poems and passages from novels can, Billington suggests, bring about their own 'realisations'. These are moments during which the text at hand and the life of the reader become synchronised by a sudden flash of recognition, so that 'life comes back … in a sort of revelation of memory' to be subsequently worked through with the aid of literature.[55]

To return to the idea of the *pharmakon*, we could say that the bibliotherapeutically informed approaches to literature outlined by Davis and Billington are notable for the emphasis they place on the internally transformative potential of books for their readers. Recent developments in literary criticism have begun to trend in the same direction. The so-called 'affective turn' and related 'postcritical' approaches to literature seek to, as Rita Felski puts it, reconcile 'academic reading and reading for pleasure'. These new critical movements focus on points of 'attachment' between text and reader, paying particular attention to affectively laden aspects of the individual reading experience such as empathy, recognition, readerly identification, and the sense of being enchanted by or swept up in a book.[56] The same sorts of ideas also circulate to much larger audiences in bibliotherapeutically themed self-help books written for the trade publishing market. In 2013's *The Novel Cure*, for instance, Ella Berthoud and Susan Elderkin write that:

> novels have the power to transport you into another existence, and see the world from a different point of view. When you're engrossed in a novel … you are seeing what a character sees, touching what a character touches, learning what a character learns. You may *think* you're sitting on the sofa in your living room, but the important parts of you – your thoughts, your senses, your spirit – are somewhere else entirely … No-one comes back from such a journey quite the same.[57]

This renewed emphasis on the emotionally transformative aspects of literature is arguably connected to another recent intersection point between literature and the languages of psychological medicine – the advent of the syllabus-level content note (or trigger warning) denoting 'distressing content'.[58] In keeping with the logic of the *pharmakon*, the flipside of the affective turn's recognition of the centrality of reader emotion is a corresponding acknowledgement that not all literary engagements are pleasant. Some, indeed, may be experienced as disturbing – or even, perhaps, as forms of emotional harm – making the mandatory listing of particularly 'challenging' books on Literature syllabi potentially problematic. Each individual reader, after all, will have a unique and perhaps far from predictable response to a text. Whether trigger warnings have any significant ability to moderate students' emotional responses to texts has not yet been demonstrated by research.[59] Preliminary evidence suggests that they can lead to student anxiety and increased anticipatory dread.[60] Literature academics, meanwhile, remain concerned that the actual effect of such warnings may be to make students less able to approach texts critically and less inclined to engage with a range of literary approaches. However, recent surveys do indicate that university students tend to approve of the use of trigger warnings.[61] Students, it seems, may appreciate their use as a sign of being taken seriously by university authorities as emotional subjects in their own right, while universities themselves have become increasingly conscious of their own therapeutic duties of care to manage and safeguard their students' emotional lives and see such warnings as one manifestation of these responsibilities.[62]

Current tendencies to talk about the power and significance of literature speak (paradoxically, perhaps) to the essential *powerlessness* many of those working in the fields of literature teaching, creative writing, and librarianship now feel about the contemporary state of literature – and reading – itself. The idea that reading literature has a profound ability to heal and transform society represents a morale-boosting rallying cry in a world where funding for the arts and humanities is being progressively withdrawn, global enrolments on Literature degree pathways are demonstrating significant decline, and teachers and academics everywhere are warning that digitally enmeshed students seem unwilling (or unable) to engage with the written word for any length of time.[63] Surveying the at-times contradictory journalistic discourse about the decline of reading in 2010s America, Leah Price remarks on the tendency of some commentators to abruptly shift registers –

sometimes in the same article – from making 'sweeping claims' about the power of books to lamenting the looming extinction of reading itself. In these frenzied responses to a perceived existential threat to the survival of literature, Price writes, commentators 'increasingly cast books at once as saviors and martyrs'.[64] Outsized fears about the obsolescence of book culture generate equally outsized claims about book culture's enduring social mission and political relevance, as well as assertions about the transformative power of reading at the level of the individual. In this climate, as Beth Driscoll argues, reading literature has arguably become a morally loaded act, if not an identity in itself, one characterised by assumptions that literary readers are empathetic, thoughtful, and purposively engaged through the act of reading with pressing ethical, social, political, and environmental issues.[65]

The understandable temptation to confront the challenges faced by literary culture (and literary education) in the twenty-first century by proclaiming the healing powers of literature, however, comes with its own risks and drawbacks. Foremost among these is the tendency to instrumentalise literature, as if to suggest that the value of books lies primarily in their real-world impact – their ability to do good in the world (or perhaps to convert their readers into *good people*).[66] For educators, an additional risk lies in the fact that they are, in effect, being asked to combine the roles of therapist, teacher, and moral manager. In the process, the classroom becomes a site in which larger, state-led and institutional politics of social and ideological transformation are carried out. In a 2022 textbook chapter, the social workers Nancy F. Cincotta and Tracy Moore define the goals of bibliotherapy as being 'to provide information about problems', 'to communicate new values and attitudes', and 'to provide solutions to problems'.[67] Their account of reading as a practice is overwhelmingly loaded with positive attributes. As they describe them, books – or at least those books assessed by the therapist as being 'developmentally and culturally appropriate' – provide 'knowledge', 'insight', 'confidence', and 'support', as well as helping 'create connections', 'foster encouragement', and 'enhance coping'.[68] Buttressed by such manifestly positive values, bibliotherapy is, Cincotta and Moore continue, 'an ideal tool for managing difficult issues' – as negatively coded in this binary moral schema as books are positively valued – including racism, bullying, and the COVID-19 pandemic.[69]

In accounts like this, we see bibliotherapeutic practice segue into something we might call bibliotherapeutic ideology. The bibliotherapist becomes a moral expert, equipped with the 'ideal tool' for effecting transformative social change (the implicitly 'good' and 'culturally appropriate' book) and accompanied by a sense of overriding moral duty to act.[70] The 'power' of books resolves in practice into the amenability of directed reading for furthering a particular sociopolitical project. This process of putting books 'to use' may involve de-emphasising certain literary features of a text in favour of others which are more amenable for addressing or 'managing' the problem at hand. In the process, reading, healing, and the inculcation of 'correct' morality ('new values and attitudes') are superimposed upon one another.[71]

'Narratives of health are', as Neil Brooks and Sarah Blanchette argue, 'intimately' and inevitably bound up with 'sociopolitical and economic contexts'.[72] However, the seriousness and moral urgency of the problems that therapeutic approaches like Cincotta's and Moore's task literature with solving raise some larger questions. What should the relationship of bibliotherapy be to literary education? How are bibliotherapeutic personnel to be trained, resourced, funded, and regulated in order to carry out these sorts of missions? What happens to bibliotherapeutic practice when medical and therapeutic norms and fashions change? Can literature ultimately bear the weight of all of these normative expectations? The tensions between the inward, unpredictable, and open-ended act of reading and therapeutic norms of progress and improvement – as well as the pressures brought to bear by institutional remits and funding limitations – are considered in various ways in the chapters that follow by Katarina Båth, Danni Glover, and Jesse Miller.

'Making literature useful can be', as Josie Billington has observed, 'its own form of forgetting its real uses'.[73] These sorts of concerns are by no means new. In 1947, the Nursing academic Norah Mackenzie expressed her own qualms about what she saw as the instrumentalism involved in some bibliotherapeutic rhetoric. 'To degrade reading to the status of being useful from a therapeutic point of view', she observed in a lecture for trainee hospital librarians, 'seems to me an abuse of one of our greatest privileges and joys'.[74] In her account of the British National Health Service's Reading Well Books on Prescription programme, Price also addresses its implicit instrumentalism. On one hand, she acknowledges the boost that this initiative provides to austerity-stricken public library services in Britain, as well as the benefits and pleasures that the prescribed titles undoubtedly confer on individual readers. However, she also mourns the way in which merely 'prescriptive' approaches subsume the essential power of literature to enrage, disrupt, or disturb under the demand that books be valued for their 'positive' and self-evidently beneficial attributes only.[75] 'In overselling' the power of books 'to calm and console', Price observes, certain palliative claims on behalf of literature 'undersell its responsibility to upset and anger us'.[76] Some of the language employed on the provider side of the Reading Well Books on Prescription programme reveals another aspect of the instrumentalism at play. Prescribing self-help books to British patient-readers is explicitly justified in terms of efficiency and value for money. A 2017 information pamphlet about the Reading Well Books on Prescription programme produced for general practitioners by the non-profit National Association of Primary Care, for instance, is subtitled 'How bibliotherapy can help your patients *and* save your practice time and money'. In a section outlining the cost-effectiveness of the scheme, the pamphlet notes that the average cost of the service amounted to only about £1 per patient.[77]

Approaches like Cincotta's and Moore's are similarly instrumental in nature. They recognise the value of reading insofar as it can be used to pursue a particular vision of progressive social change. Each of these claims on literature overlooks the fundamental ambivalence of the book as *pharmakon*, with its power to both heal and harm, without which reading's purely positive values have no real purchase. The cultural logic of the trigger warning, according to which the troubling, disturbing, or alienating aspects of literature are reframed as problems to be publicly flagged and managed (rather than intrinsic features of the work to be privately encountered and worked through in the act of reading), speaks, perhaps, to the consequences of this way of thinking. As the philosopher Boris Groys has recently noted, once a relationship is defined in terms of care, privacy concerns are often set to one side. All aspects of the body and mind under care are opened up to scrutiny (and potential intervention) according to the moral imperative of pursuing wellbeing and 'the cure'.[78] Normative associations of this sort between literary culture (assumed to be 'good'), wellbeing and happiness (assumed to be the natural outcomes of reading 'good' books), and the corresponding imperative to manage, monitor, and optimise readers' emotions are also highly visible components of the contemporary literary festival.[79] The organisers of the 2013 Cheltenham Literary Festival, for instance, engaged a technology company to monitor the smiles of attendees using a network of surveillance cameras. The supposed effectiveness of the festival's offerings in delivering wellbeing to readers was determined by the metric of observed 'smiles per hour' recorded over the course of the event.[80]

It is likely that recent events – particularly the COVID-19 pandemic and the associated global lockdowns of 2020 and 2021 – will solidify the deeply felt affective attachments between reading, wellbeing, identity, and survival that have typified book culture during the early twenty-first century. As Laura Dietz observes in her contribution to this volume, pandemic media discourses were very quick to prescribe reading as the ideal antidote to the lockdown experience. The result, she writes, was a flood of 'book recommendations, online literary events, celebrity bedtime stories, and exhortations to read through the crisis', each reflecting a practically unanimously shared faith that books would ameliorate loneliness and improve the 'health and wellbeing' of readers under pandemic conditions. Exemplifying the digitally enabled fascination with books as objects that Jessica Pressman terms 'bookishness', many thousands of readers during 2020–2021 in turn shared images of (and participated in discussions about) *their* pandemic reading choices in book-centred social media communities, such as Bookstagram, Book Twitter, BookTok, and BookTube and by commenting on literary subreddits.[81]

The significance of 'pandemic reading' as a social phenomenon and unique 'historical moment' was apparent to researchers during the COVID period itself and was accordingly subject to real-time monitoring, surveying, and research projects.[82] Data from these studies indicate that many readers responded to the pandemic by buying literary classics – either due to their reassuring familiarity or because the temporal aspects of furlough and lockdown presented opportunities to engage with aspirational 'longread' classics for the first time.[83] However, as Leah Henrickson writes, there were 'also those readers who … turned to books that reflect[ed] the uncertainty and bleakness of the times', including disease- and pandemic-related titles such as Albert Camus's *The Plague* (1947).[84] Other readers posted resonant-seeming passages from apocalyptic fiction onto their social media feeds, such as the vision in Kate Atkinson's 2002 short story, 'Charlene and Trudi Go Shopping', of a war-torn future London 'out of diesel and gin' and in which people 'burnt musty old paperbacks on bonfires and drank rum', but where there was nevertheless 'a festive atmosphere generated by communal terror'.[85] In both of these registers (the reassuring and the resonantly reflective) books arguably came to function as pandemic-period 'normality effects'.[86] They were simultaneously sources of recognition and psychologically stabilising symbols of connection with the outside world and pre-COVID life, now retrospectively recoded as 'normality' or 'the time before'. At the same time, however, books read during the pandemic were very real *physical* objects, capable of being grasped hold of by readers seeking comfort in unfamiliar and confusing times.

Towards a History of Bibliotherapies

In her recent critical survey of the developing research literature on bibliotherapy, Gill Partington suggests that thinking in terms of 'bibliotherapies' rather than 'bibliotherapy' can be one way of acknowledging the 'variety of disparate activities and ideas' now bundled within the term.[87] Taking the profusion of bibliotherapies as its starting point, this volume seeks to chart just one of the many channels through which bibliotherapeutic ideas have flowed. The word 'bibliotherapy' is itself a relatively recent coinage, but one whose time and place of origin are multiply resonant. It was coined, as we noted at the outset of this Introduction, by the American essayist and Unitarian minister Samuel McChord Crothers, initially in a series of lectures delivered from late 1914 onwards, and then in an article, 'A Literary Clinic', published in *The Atlantic Monthly* in 1916.[88] Leah Price calls Crothers's intervention 'tongue in cheek', and the story's tone is certainly playful. It concludes rather abruptly when one of the story's two speakers is called away to attend to 'a patient who had taken an overdose of war literature'.[89]

Crothers was probably not anticipating the alacrity with which librarians and psychiatrists would soon pounce on the term. He had been seeking instead, Jesse Miller suggests, to contribute to a longstanding ethical debate about the 'reading habit'.[90] However, the eagerness with which the new word was taken up, as well as the timing of its appearance (in the midst of a world war 'mediated to an unprecedented degree' through the written word), are revealing in their own ways.[91] The experiences of patient-readers and medical practitioners during the First World War provided new impetus – and new evidence – to support the idea that reading could alleviate psychological trauma, itself a concept that emerged in its modern form only towards the end of the nineteenth century.[92] What Crothers did by coining the word 'bibliotherapy' was to give shape to an idea, an ethos, and a set of practices that were already in a process of rapid development and emergence, making them tangible in ways that the library, medical, and therapeutic professions could take advantage of.

The relationship of bibliotherapy to the book relief and literary caregiving programmes carried out during the First World War provided the focus for a one-day conference held at the University of London's Institute for English Studies on 14 September 2018. 'The Book as Cure: Bibliotherapy and Literary Caregiving from the First World War to the Present' was co-organised by the editors of this volume, with plenary addresses by Jane Potter (Oxford Brookes University) and Peter Leese (University of Copenhagen). Many of the chapters included here have their origin points in papers presented at the conference. Organised under the auspices of HOBAR, the History of Books and Reading research collaboration at The Open University, the conference brought bibliotherapeutic practitioners and librarians together with academics and postgraduate students in Literature and Creative Writing and representatives from the culture and heritage industries. In doing so, it provided a forum for interdisciplinary exchange about the ways in which reading has been treated as a 'curative' force in various institutional settings both during and since the First World War.

As Partington observes, the idea that modern bibliotherapy was to a large extent 'a product of the hospital libraries of the First World War' has become 'a consensus of sorts' among scholars researching the history of bibliotherapy.[93] Fleshing out the details and contexts of this particular origin story, which are discussed in several of the chapters in the first section, is one of the main aims of this volume. Other chapters – particularly those by Hochman, Mahoney, and Trott – return to Crothers himself and the scene of his initial coinage for what they can tell us about the immediate contexts from which this version of 'bibliotherapy' emerged. However, our contributors are also conscious of the need to nuance, expand – and at times to question – some of bibliotherapy's accepted narratives of development, as well as to problematise its terminology and unpack the assumptions embedded within it. These include the extent to which bibliotherapy has operated in accordance with various ideological and political discourses of the kind flagged so far in this Introduction, both historically (in, for instance, the impact of Progressive Period social reform on early twentieth-century American practice) and in more recent ideological discourses, such as the doctrines of 'resilience' and cost-effectiveness. Bibliotherapy in practice, like reading itself, we suggest, can often be a disruptive, disturbing, and unpredictable force – something easily obscured by the normative languages of healing, progress, and utility.

The Volume

This volume is divided into three sections. Section I, 'Bibliotherapy and the First World War', is rooted in the wartime cultures that ensured bibliotherapy became part of the active treatment of soldiers' damaged minds and bodies on both sides of the Atlantic after 1914. Chapters in two further sections, 'Institutional Legacies from Libraries to Hospitals, 1919–1950' and 'Contemporary Critical Interventions', examine the expanding variety of critical contexts, both historical and more modern, in which reading and wellbeing continued to intersect. Drawing on previously unexamined archival evidence and a wide range of other source material from trench magazines to autograph books to e-novels, as well as data and information drawn from practice-based encounters, contributors describe how these discourses and practices were developed and institutionalised in various national and international contexts after the war. Finally, they examine some of the many afterlives and resonances of these ideas and practices across the twentieth and twenty-first centuries and today.

In Chapter 1, 'The Legacy of Nineteenth-Century Therapeutic Reading in the First World War Hospital', Laura Gray Blair draws attention to the legacies of the

Victorian asylum and the asylum library on the treatment of military mental health patients, showing how they influenced the treatment of shell shock after the First World War and expanding understandings of the origin of links between reading and mental states. In Chapter 2, 'Galsworthy's First World War Writing as Self-Care', Helen Chambers focuses on the wartime literary output of social reformer and author John Galsworthy (1867–1933) and outlines his inner turmoil related to aspects of the war. Chambers characterises how Galsworthy's subsequent literary works can be seen to function as a form of self-care and how this self-directed literary therapy both helped address conflicted responses to violence and released him into a new phase of writing in 1918.

Moving the interpretive lens to the United States, Vincent Trott in Chapter 3, 'The American Library Association, "Bibliotherapy" and the First World War', addresses the American Library Association's (ALA) establishment of the Library War Service, and in particular its distribution of books and scrapbooks to military hospitals. Trott posits the existence of strong links between the emergent ideas around reading as a curative practice and the ALA's wider political and moral objectives during this period. This is a theme picked up by several authors across the volume.

Remaining with materialities, the following two chapters explore little-discussed aspects of their subjects: autograph books and trench magazines. It is the filling of autograph books by convalescent soldiers, as analysed by Lindsay Davies in Chapter 4, 'Autograph Books as Alleviation in British First World War Hospitals: A Case Study', which sees them emerge as more than forms of entertainment, distraction, and community-making. Entries by soldiers narrating their experiences are assessed as a particular type of witness combined with spontaneous creativity, sometimes in visual form, which together develop a kind of expressive reflection. Véronique Duché and Amanda Laugesen in Chapter 5, in 'Print as Caregiving in Wartime: The Role of Australian First World War Trench and Hospital Magazines', provide insight into the ways in which print could act as therapy as well as entertainment. Trench and hospital journals are examined in relation to the curative power of writing for publication and crucially, in relation to how they might mediate the identities of the soldiers, adding to ways of processing experience.

Having established the historical institutional connections and developments during the war, the second section, 'Institutional Legacies from Libraries to Hospitals, 1919–1950', initially goes on to amplify the work of American librarians and institutional influence on practice in the post-war period.

Chapter 6 by Barbara Hochman, '"Return to Normalcy": American Librarians and Bibliotherapy in the Aftermath of the First World War', captures the influence of the strong social wish for a return to a former condition which had major significance for the emergent field of bibliotherapy and on ideas around book selection and control. The chapter identifies practitioners and librarians who nonetheless favoured more flexible expansive definitions, providing an essential antidote to prevailing critical contexts.

In Chapter 7, 'Can There Be a Science of Bibliotherapy? Imagining Bibliotherapy and Its Uses in a Modern Hospital', Mary Mahoney explores the attempts to create a science of bibliotherapy in the wake of the First World War. Mahoney exposes the narratives told by practitioners which eventually embraced the expressive nature of readers' own responses, paving the way for a set of empowering therapeutic possibilities.

In Edmund G. C. King's Chapter 8, 'The Curative Value of Reading: Hospital Libraries and Literary Therapeutics in Britain, 1919–1946', the institutional focus moves further into the post-war period and from the United States to Great Britain. The War Library was founded in August 1914 to provide books for the sick and wounded members of Britain's fighting forces. However, the War Library's founders were unwilling to abandon their operations with the end of hostilities in 1918. Instead, they expanded their charity into a library service for civilian hospital patients after the war as the British Red Cross Society and Order of St. John Hospital Library. Drawing on new archival research in the British Red Cross Archives, King's chapter describes how the scheme's organisers used the idea of the healing book to represent hospital libraries as essential public services. To what extent, King asks, can we regard interwar British hospital librarianship as being itself a form of bibliotherapy?

While the third section, 'Contemporary Critical Interventions', cannot provide anything like a comprehensive overview of the amount of work done in the field during this period, the chapters here focus on key challenges and debates which animate current practice.

In Chapter 9, 'The Bibliotherapy Novel: Representations of Literary Caregiving and the Crisis of Print Culture, 1919–2019', Jesse Miller examines the refunctioning of literature and literary value, focusing on representations of bibliotherapy in the novel and connecting the crisis of print culture with a move to link aesthetic experience to individual and collective health. Miller re-establishes the case for the study of literature as an important site for examining the way metaphor and narratives motivate and shape material sites and practices of reading.

Laura Dietz, in Chapter 10 '"I liked them a lot ... but I feel like I don't know them fully?": Implications of Recent Research in Immersion and Engagement for Digital Therapeutic Reading', begins with the fact that digital books are key to the widening remit and accessibility of bibliotherapy. Asking whether narrative immersion may differ when the reading is digital, this chapter presents research into the role of interactivity in bibliotherapy using digital fiction, exploring how immersion and/or the sense of authentic experience can impact readers and positing strategies to inform therapeutic reading using digital books.

Continuing the foray into contemporary practice, Katarina Båth in Chapter 11, 'Trauma and Literature: Current Bibliotherapeutic Practices and Literary Trauma Studies in Sweden', creates a dialogical narrative incorporating aspects of literary trauma studies and creative bibliotherapy. Putting pressure on the 'identification paradigm', Båth asks provocative questions about the study and use of literary depictions of traumatic experience while focusing on the relationship between trauma, memory, and literary language and positing challenges to convenors as well as those theorising around the ethics of literary testimony. Båth provides new and rich data, giving novel ways to interpret national traditions in the wider field and challenging researchers to build on her work.

Finally, Danni Glover in Chapter 12, 'Hoping Out Loud: Creative Bibliotherapy and Wellbeing Strategies', draws directly on practitioner experience in both shared reading and creative writing for therapeutic purposes. Providing insights developed in the field, in particular around the management of the therapeutic encounter, Glover also outlines some of the tensions between expected outcomes and the often more contingent, emergent, and subtly meaningful impacts such as those of generating hope for pressurised individuals.

Notes

1 Jonathan Bate and Andrew Schuman, 'Books Do Furnish a Mind: The Art and Science of Bibliotherapy', *The Lancet* 387 (20 February 2016): 742. This inscription has also been translated as 'the medicines of the soul' and is used as such by Jesse Miller to title his 2018 article, 'Medicines of the Soul: Reparative Reading and the History of Bibliotherapy', *Mosaic: An Interdisciplinary Critical Journal* 51, no. 2 (2018): 17–34.

2 We discuss Crothers in more detail later in this Introduction.

3 The effectiveness in material terms of many forms of bibliotherapy is difficult to evidence in practice, something that critics and practitioners freely acknowledge. Liz Brewster, for instance, notes that 'it has proved difficult to demonstrate an overall impact in terms of symptom reduction or decreased burden on mental health services' in her discussion of the National Institute for Health and Care Institute (NICE)'s recommendation of written resources for treatment for conditions such as depression and bulimia. See Liz Brewster, 'Bibliotherapy: A Critical History', in *Bibliotherapy*, edited by Sarah McNicol and Liz Brewster (London: Facet, 2018), 13.

4 Bernard Stiegler, 'Distrust and the Pharmacology of Transformational Technologies', in *Quantum Engagements: Social Reflections of Nanoscience and Emerging Technologies*, edited by Torben B. Zülsdorf, Christopher Coenen, Arianna Ferrari, Ulrich Fiedeler, Colin Milburn, and Matthias Wienroth (Heidelberg: AKA Verlag Heidelberg, 2011), 32.

5 Plato, *Phaedrus*, translated by Robin Waterfield (Oxford: Oxford World's Classics, 2002), 68.

6 Jacques Derrida, 'Plato's Pharmacy', in *Dissemination*, translated by Barbara Johnson (London: Athlone Press, 1981), 110.

7 Johann Wolfgang von Goethe, *The Sorrows of Young Werther*, translated by Michael Hulse (London: Penguin Classics, 1989), 43.

8 Derrida, 'Plato's Pharmacy', 99.

9 John Guillory, *Professing Criticism: Essays on the Organisation of Literary Study* (Chicago: University of Chicago Press, 2022), 47.

10 Anna Vaninskaya, 'Learning to Read Trash: Late-Victorian Schools and the Penny Dreadful', in *The History of Reading, Volume 2: Evidence from the British Isles, c.1750–1950*, edited by Katie Halsey and W. R. Owens (Basingstoke: Palgrave Macmillan, 2011), 73.

11 Martin Jarrett-Kerr, 'The Mission of English Literature', *Times Literary Supplement* (3 February 1984): 111.

12 Arleen McCarty Hynes and Mary Hynes-Berry, *Biblio/Poetry Therapy – The Interactive Process: A Handbook*, 3rd ed. (St. Cloud, MN: North Star Press, 2012), 52.

13 Hynes and Hynes-Berry, *Biblio/Poetry Therapy*, 32.

14 Brewster, 'Bibliotherapy', 3.

15 Gill Partington, *Bibliotherapy: A Survey of Literature*, Working Papers 2022/23: 03 (Exeter: Wellcome Centre for Cultures and Environments of Health, 2023), 4.
16 Sarah J. Jack and Kevin R. Ronan, 'Bibliotherapy: Practice and Research', *School Psychology International* 29, no. 2 (2008): 161.
17 Bate and Schuman, 'Books Do Furnish a Mind', 742.
18 Nick Canty, 'Bibliotherapy: Its Processes and Benefits and Application in Clinical and Developmental Settings', *Logos* 28, no. 3 (2017): 33.
19 Janella D. Moy, 'Reading and Writing One's Way to Wellness: The History of Bibliotherapy and Scriptotherapy', in *New Directions in Literature and Medicine Studies*, edited by Stephanie M. Hilger (London: Palgrave Macmillan, 2017), 16.
20 Moy, 'Reading and Writing One's Way to Wellness', 16.
21 Brittany Pladek, 'The Poetics of Palliation: Romantic Literary Therapy, 1790–1850', PhD thesis, University of Toronto, 2013, 2.
22 See, for instance, a recent article which states that 'Bibliotherapy, or reading self-help manuals, is an established treatment for sexual concerns': Hannah Warshowsky, Elizabeth A. Mahar, and Laurie B. Mintz, 'Cliteracy for Him: Effectiveness of Bibliotherapy for Heterosexual Men's Sexual Functioning', *Sexual and Relationship Therapy* 38, no. 1 (2023): 52.
23 On nineteenth-century 'moral treatment' regimes in the United States, see Len Levin and Ruthann Gildea, 'Bibliotherapy: Tracing the Roots of a Moral Therapy Movement in the United States from the Early Nineteenth Century to the Present', *Journal of the Medical Library Association* 101, no. 2 (2013): 89–90.
24 Samuel Tuke, *Description of the Retreat, an Institution Near York, for Insane Persons* (York: W. Alexander, 1813), 185.
25 Philip J. Weimerskirch, 'Benjamin Rush and John Minson Galt, II: Pioneers of Bibliotherapy in America', *Bulletin of the Medical Library Association* 53, no. 4 (1965): 517–18.
26 Cf. Bernard Stiegler, *Taking Care of Youth and the Generations*, translated by Stephen Barker (Stanford, CA: Stanford University Press, 2010), 17–18; 59.
27 Maureen Park and Robert Hamilton, 'Moral Treatment of the Insane: Provisions for Lifelong Learning, Cultural Engagement, and Creativity in Nineteenth-Century Asylums', *Journal of Adult and Continuing Education* 16, no. 2 (2010): 103.
28 Sadie Peterson Delaney, 'The Place of Bibliotherapy in a Hospital', *Opportunity* 16, no. 2 (1938): 53.
29 Debbie McCulliss, 'Bibliotherapy: Historical and Research Perspectives', *Journal of Poetry Therapy* 25, no. 1 (2012): 25.
30 Patricia A. Wolfgram, 'Hospital Libraries in the United States: Historical Antecedents', *Bulletin of the Medical Library Association* 73, no. 1 (1985): 33.
31 Arthur P. Young, 'Aftermath of a Crusade: World War I and the Enlarged Program of the American Library Association', *Library Quarterly* 50, no. 2 (1980): 191–207.
32 Delaney, 'The Place of Bibliotherapy in a Hospital', 53.
33 Betty K. Gubert, 'Sadie Peterson Delaney: Pioneer Bibliotherapist', *American Libraries* 24, no. 2 (1993): 125.
34 Delaney, 'The Place of Bibliotherapy in a Hospital', 53.
35 On discharged patients as community leaders, see the brief case history reported in Delaney, 'The Place of Bibliotherapy in a Hospital', 55.
36 Sadie M. Peterson, 'U.S.V. Hospital Library no. 91, Tuskegee, Ala.', *The Crisis* 29, no. 3 (1925): 116.

37 S. P. Delaney, 'The Negro Veteran and His Books', *Wilson Bulletin* 6, no. 10 (1932): 686.
38 Young, 'Aftermath of a Crusade', 193.
39 Monique S. Dufour, 'Reading for Health: Bibliotherapy and the Medicalized Humanities in the United States, 1930–1965', PhD, diss., Virginia Polytechnic Institute and State University, 2014, 2.
40 Jessica Grogan, *Encountering America: Humanistic Psychology, Sixties Culture and the Shaping of the Modern Self* (New York: Harper Perennial, 2013), 5–6.
41 Philip Rieff, *The Triumph of the Therapeutic* (London: Chatto & Windus, 1966); Eva Illouz, *Saving the Modern Soul: Therapy, Emotions, and the Culture of Self-Help* (Berkeley and Los Angeles: University of California Press, 2008), 12–16.
42 Illouz, *Saving the Modern Soul*, 160–1.
43 Christopher Lasch, 'Introduction', in Russell Jacoby, *Social Amnesia: A Critique of Contemporary Psychology* (1975; London: Routledge, 2017), xx.
44 Hynes and Hynes-Berry, *Biblio/Poetry Therapy*, 5.
45 Dale-Elizabeth Pehrsson and Paula McMillen, 'A Bibliotherapy Evaluation Tool: Grounding Counselors in the Therapeutic Use of Literature', *The Arts in Psychotherapy* 32, no. 1 (2005): 48.
46 McCulliss, 'Bibliotherapy', 27.
47 Zheng Xu, Ru Liu, Liping Guo, Ziyi Gao, Zicheng Gao, Xiaowei Liu, Jieyun Li, Bin Li, and Kehu Yang, 'The 100 Most-Cited Articles on Bibliotherapy: A Bibliometric Analysis', *Psychology, Health and Medicine* 28, no. 9 (2023): 2728–44.
48 Leah Price, 'Prescribed Print: Bibliotherapy after Web 2.0', *Post45* (17 September 2019).
49 Peter Widdowson, 'The Crisis in English Studies', in *Re-Reading English*, edited by Peter Widdowson (London: Methuen, 1981), 1–2.
50 Quoted in Robert Eaglestone, *Literature: Why It Matters* (Cambridge: Polity Press, 2019), 55.
51 Eaglestone, *Literature*, 56.
52 Eaglestone, *Literature*, 57–8.
53 Jonathan Rose, *Readers' Liberation* (Oxford: Oxford University Press, 2018), 192–5.
54 Josie Billington, *Is Literature Healthy?* (Oxford: Oxford University Press, 2016), 3.
55 Billington, *Is Literature Healthy?*, 82.
56 Rita Felski, 'Postcritical', in *Further Reading*, edited by Matthew Rubery and Leah Price (Oxford: Oxford University Press, 2020), 135; 138–9; 142–3.
57 Ella Berthoud and Susan Elderkin, *The Novel Cure: An A–Z of Literary Remedies* (Edinburgh: Canongate, 2013), 2.
58 For a sceptical reading, see Keith Hayward, *Infantilised: How Our Culture Killed Adulthood* (London: Constable, 2024), 234.
59 Victoria M. E. Bridgland, Payton J. Jones, and Benjamin W. Bellet, 'A Meta-Analysis of the Efficacy of Trigger Warnings, Content Warnings, and Content Notes', *Clinical Psychological Science* 12, no. 4 (2024): 751–71.
60 Helly Douglas, 'Should Teachers Be Using Trigger Warnings in Class?', *TES Magazine* (25 June 2019).
61 Richard Adams, 'Students Show "Shocking Growth in Support for Censorship", Ministers Warn', *The Guardian* (23 June 2022).
62 See Edmund G. C. King, '"Trigger Warnings", Part 1', English Political Catchwords Blog (7 November 2023). On the 'therapeutic university', see Kathryn Ecclestone and Dennis Hayes, *The Dangerous Rise of Therapeutic Education* (London: Routledge, 2019), 86–104.

63 For recent commentary along these lines, see Guillory, *Professing Criticism*, 8–9 and 239–43; Merve Emre, 'Everyone's a Critic', *The New Yorker* (23 January 2023): 62–6; Nathan Heller, 'The End of the English Major', *The New Yorker* (6 March 2023): 28–39; Tyler Austin Harper, 'The Humanities Have Sown the Seeds of Their Own Destruction', *Atlantic Monthly* (19 December 2023); Adam Kotsko, 'The Loss of Things I Took for Granted', *Slate* (11 February 2024); and Rose Horowitch, 'The Elite College Students Who Can't Read Books', *Atlantic Monthly* (November 2024): 14–16.

64 Leah Price, *What We Talk about When We Talk about Books* (New York: Basic Books, 2019), 21.

65 Beth Driscoll, *What Readers Do: Aesthetic and Moral Practices of a Post-Digital Age* (London: Bloomsbury, 2024), 94.

66 On the instrumentalisation of literature, see Derek Attridge, *The Singularity of Literature* (London: Routledge, 2004), 6–10.

67 Nancy F. Cincotta and Tracy Moore, 'Bibliotherapy', in *The Oxford Textbook of Palliative Social Work,* 2nd ed, edited by Terry Altilio, Shirley Otis-Green, and John G. Cagle (New York: Oxford University Press, 2022), 659.

68 Cincotta and Moore, 'Bibliotherapy', 659.

69 Cincotta and Moore, 'Bibliotherapy', 659–60.

70 Cf. Alvin W. Gouldner, *The Dialectic of Ideology and Technology: The Origins, Grammar and Future of Ideology* (London: Macmillan, 1976), 71.

71 Cf. Attridge, *Singularity of Literature*, 7.

72 Neil Brooks and Sarah Blanchette, 'Introduction', in *Narrative Art and the Politics of Health* (London: Anthem Press, 2021), 1.

73 Billington, *Is Literature Healthy?*, 113.

74 [Norah] Mackenzie, 'Psychology', in *Manual for Hospital Librarians*, edited by C. E. A. Bedwell (London: Library Association, 1947), 32.

75 For reflections on the current cultural tendency to resist artistic negativity, difference, and difficulty in favour of the 'likeable', see Byung-Chul Han, *The Palliative Society,* translated by Daniel Steuer (Cambridge: Polity Press, 2021), 4–6; 17.

76 Price, *What We Talk about When We Talk about Books*, 139.

77 *Reading Well Books on Prescription: How Bibliotherapy Can Help Your Patients* and *Save Your Practice Time and Money* (National Association of Primary Care, 2017), 15.

78 Boris Groys, *Philosophy of Care* (London: Verso, 2022), 87–8.

79 On the contemporary literary festival's combination of 'reverence for literature' and intense focus on the emotional responses of readers, see Beth Driscoll, 'Sentiment Analysis and the Literary Festival Audience', *Continuum* 29, no. 6 (2015): 862. See also Driscoll, *What Readers Do*, 94–5.

80 William Davies, *The Happiness Industry: How the Government and Big Business Sold Us Well-Being* (London: Verso, 2015), 36.

81 Millicent Weber, 'Online Reading during the Covid-19 Pandemic', in *Post-Digital Book Cultures: Australian Perspectives*, edited by Alexandra Dane and Millicent Weber (Melbourne: Monash University Publishing, 2021), 11–56. On 'bookishness', see Jessica Pressman, *Bookishness: Loving Books in a Digital Age* (New York: Columbia University Press, 2020).

82 Ben Davies, Christina Lupton, and Johanne Gormsen Schmidt, *Reading Novels during the Covid-19 Pandemic* (Oxford: Oxford University Press, 2022), 2. See also Abigail Boucher, Marcello Giovanelli, Chloe Harrison, Robbie Love, and Caroline Godfrey, *Reading Habits in the Covid-19 Pandemic: An Applied Linguistic Perspective* (Cham: Palgrave Macmillan, 2024).

83 Corinna Norrick-Rühl and Shafquat Towheed, 'Introduction', in *Bookshelves in the Age of the COVID-19 Pandemic*, edited by Corinna Norrick-Rühl and Shafquat Towheed (Cham: Palgrave Macmillan, 2022). 5.
84 Leah Henrickson, '"Ummmmm, guys? Don't Microwave your books": Readers, Authors, and Institutions in #PandemicReading Tweets', in *Bookshelves in the Age of the COVID-19 Pandemic*, 266.
85 Quoted in Henrickson, 'Ummmmm, guys? Don't microwave your books', 266. The story appears in Kate Atkinson, *Not the End of the World* (London: Doubleday, 2002).
86 Sally Blackburn-Daniels and Edmund G. C. King, 'Introduction: Bookshelves, Social Media and Gaming', *English Studies* 103, no. 5 (2022): 655.
87 Partington, *Bibliotherapy*, 4.
88 Samuel McChord Crothers, 'A Literary Clinic', *Atlantic Monthly* 118, no. 3 (1916): 291–301. Crothers had been using the term in public lectures since at least October 1914. See Dufour, 'Reading for Health', 2n3, and Sara Haslam and Edmund G. C. King, '"Medicinable Literature": Bibliotherapy, Literary Caregiving, and the First World War', *Literature and Medicine* 39, no. 2 (2021): 296.
89 Price, *What We Talk about When We Talk about Books*, 133; Crothers, 'A Literary Clinic', 301.
90 Miller, 'Medicines of the Soul', 21–2.
91 Cedric Van Dijck, Marysa Demoor, and Sarah Posman, 'Between the Shells: The Production of Belgian, British and French Trench Journals in the First World War', *Publishing History* 77 (2017): 77. On the First World War as a textually mediated war, see also Shafquat Towheed and Edmund G. C. King, 'Introduction', in *Reading and the First World War: Readers, Texts, Archives*, edited by Shafquat Towheed and Edmund G. C. King (Basingstoke: Palgrave Macmillan, 2015), 1.
92 On the modern genealogy of psychological trauma, see Ian Hacking, *Rewriting the Soul: Multiple Personality and the Sciences of Memory* (Princeton, NJ: Princeton University Press, 1995), 183–97.
93 Partington, *Bibliotherapy*, 9.

References

Adams, Richard. 'Students Show "Shocking Growth in Support for Censorship", Ministers Warn', *The Guardian* (23 June 2022). www.theguardian.com/education/2022/jun/23/students-shocking-growth-support-censorship-ministers-warn

Attridge, Derek. *The Singularity of Literature*. London: Routledge, 2004.

Bate, Jonathan and Andrew Schuman. 'The Art of Medicine. Books Do Furnish a Mind: the Art and Science of Bibliotherapy', *The Lancet* 387 (20 February 2016): 742–3.

Berthoud, Ella, and Susan Elderkin. *The Novel Cure: An A–Z of Literary Remedies*. Edinburgh: Canongate, 2013.

Billington, Josie. *Is Literature Healthy?* Oxford: Oxford University Press, 2016.

Blackburn-Daniels, Sally, and Edmund G. C. King, 'Introduction: Bookshelves, Social Media and Gaming', *English Studies* 103, no. 5 (2022): 653–9.

Brewster, Liz. 'Bibliotherapy: A Critical History'. In *Bibliotherapy*, edited by Sarah McNicol and Liz Brewster, 3–22. London: Facet, 2018.

Bridgland, Victoria M. E., Jones, Payton J., and Benjamin W. Bellet. 'A Meta-Analysis of the Efficacy of Trigger Warnings, Content Warnings, and Content Notes', *Clinical Psychological Science* 12, no. 4 (2024): 751–71.

Brooks, Neil, and Sarah Blanchette. 'Introduction'. In *Narrative Art and the Politics of Health*, edited by Neil Brooks and Sarah Blanchette, 1–18. London: Anthem Press, 2021.
Canty, Nick. 'Bibliotherapy: Its Processes and Benefits and Application in Clinical and Developmental Settings', *Logos* 28, no. 3 (2017): 32–40.
Cincotta, Nancy F., and Tracy Moore, 'Bibliotherapy'. In *The Oxford Textbook of Palliative Social Work*, 2nd ed, edited by Terry Altilio, Shirley Otis-Green, and John G. Cagle, 659–65. New York: Oxford University Press, 2022.
Connor, Jennifer J. 'Prescribed Reading: Patients' Libraries in North American Tuberculosis Institutions', *Libraries & Culture* 27, no. 3 (1992): 252–78.
Davies, William. *The Happiness Industry: How the Government and Big Business Sold Us Well-Being*. London: Verso, 2015.
Delaney, Sadie Peterson. 'The Negro Veteran and His Books', *Wilson Bulletin* 6, no. 10 (1932): 684–6.
Delaney, Sadie Peterson. 'The Place of Bibliotherapy in a Hospital', *Opportunity* 16, no. 2 (1938): 53–6.
Derrida, Jacques. 'Plato's Pharmacy'. In *Dissemination*, translated by Barbara Johnson, 61–171. London: Athlone Press, 1981.
Douglas, Helly. 'Should Teachers Be Using Trigger Warnings in Class?', *TES Magazine* (25 June 2019). www.tes.com/magazine/archive/should-teachers-be-using-trigger-warnings-class
Driscoll, Beth. 'Sentiment Analysis and the Literary Festival Audience', *Continuum* 29, no. 6 (2015): 861–73.
Driscoll, Beth. *What Readers Do: Aesthetic and Moral Practices of a Post-Digital Age*. London: Bloomsbury, 2024.
Dufour, Monique S. 'Reading for Health: Bibliotherapy and the Medicalized Humanities in the United States, 1930–1965', PhD, diss., Virginia Polytechnic Institute and State University, 2014.
Eaglestone, Robert. *Literature: Why It Matters*. Cambridge: Polity Press, 2019.
Ecclestone, Kathryn, and Dennis Hayes. *The Dangerous Rise of Therapeutic Education*. London: Routledge, 2019.
Emre, Merve. 'Everyone's a Critic', *The New Yorker* (23 January 2023): 62–6.
Felski, Rita. 'Postcritical'. In *Further Reading*, edited by Matthew Rubery and Leah Price, 135–44. Oxford: Oxford University Press, 2020.
Frankland, Graham. *Freud's Literary Culture*. Cambridge: Cambridge University Press, 2000.
Goethe, Johann Wolfgang von. *The Sorrows of Young Werther*, translated by Michael Hulse. London: Penguin Classics, 1989.
Gouldner, Alvin W. *The Dialectic of Ideology and Technology: The Origins, Grammar and Future of Ideology*. London: Macmillan, 1976.
Grogan, Jessica. *Encountering America: Humanistic Psychology, Sixties Culture and the Shaping of the Modern Self.* New York: Harper Perennial, 2013.
Groys, Boris. *Philosophy of Care*. London: Verso, 2022.
Gubert, Betty K. 'Sadie Peterson Delaney: Pioneer Bibliotherapist', *American Libraries* 24, no. 2 (1993): 124–5, 127, 129–30.
Guillory, John. *Professing Criticism: Essays on the Organisation of Literary Study*. Chicago: University of Chicago Press, 2022.
Hacking, Ian. *Rewriting the Soul: Multiple Personality and the Sciences of Memory*. Princeton, NJ: Princeton University Press, 1995.

Han, Byung-Chul. *The Palliative Society*, translated by Daniel Steuer. Cambridge: Polity Press, 2021.

Harper, Tyler Austin. 'The Humanities Have Sown the Seeds of Their Own Destruction', *Atlantic Monthly* (19 December 2023). www.theatlantic.com/ideas/archive/2023/12/humanities-university-conservative-critics/676890/

Haslam, Sara, and Edmund G. C. King, '"Medicinable Literature": Bibliotherapy, Literary Caregiving, and the First World War', *Literature and Medicine* 39, no. 2 (2021): 296–318.

Haslam, Sara, Miller, Jesse, and Laureen P. Cantwell Jurkovic. '"The Flow of Comfort": Bibliotherapy, the History of Literary Caregiving, and the Academic Library Today'. In *Intersections in Healing: Academic Libraries and the Health Humanities*, edited by Laureen P. Cantwell-Jurkovic, 63–83. Lanham, MD: Rowman & Littlefield, 2024.

Hayward, Keith. *Infantilised: How Our Culture Killed Adulthood*. London: Constable, 2024.

Heller, Nathan. 'The End of the English Major', *The New Yorker* (6 March 2023): 28–39.

Henrickson, Leah. '"Ummmmm, guys? Don't microwave your books": Readers, Authors, and Institutions in #PandemicReading Tweets'. In *Bookshelves in the Age of the COVID-19 Pandemic*, edited by Corinna Norrick-Rühl and Shafquat Towheed, 259–79. Cham: Palgrave Macmillan, 2022.

Horowitch, Rose. 'The Elite College Students Who Can't Read Books', *Atlantic Monthly* (November 2024): 14–16.

Hynes, Arleen McCarty, and Mary Hynes-Berry. *Biblio/Poetry Therapy—The Interactive Process: A Handbook*, 3rd ed. St. Cloud, MN: North Star Press, 2012.

Illouz, Eva. *Saving the Modern Soul: Therapy, Emotions, and the Culture of Self-Help*. Berkeley and Los Angeles: University of California Press, 2008.

Jack, Sarah J., and Kevin R. Ronan. 'Bibliotherapy: Practice and Research', *School Psychology International* 29, no. 2 (2008): 161–82.

Jarrett-Kerr, Martin. 'The Mission of English Literature', *Times Literary Supplement* (3 February 1984): 111.

King, Edmund G. C. '"Trigger Warnings", Part 1', English Political Catchwords Blog (7 November 2023). https://englishpoliticalwords.wordpress.com/2023/11/07/trigger-warnings-part-1/

Koch, Theodore Wesley. *Books in Camp, Trench and Hospital*. London: J. M. Dent, 1917.

Kotsko, Adam. 'The Loss of Things I Took for Granted', *Slate* (11 February 2024). https://slate.com/human-interest/2024/02/literacy-crisis-reading-comprehension-college.html

Lasch, Christopher. 'Introduction'. In Russell Jacoby, *Social Amnesia: A Critique of Contemporary Psychology*, xv–xxiii. 1975. London: Routledge, 2017.

Levin, Len, and Ruthann Gildea, 'Bibliotherapy: Tracing the Roots of a Moral Therapy Movement in the United States from the Early Nineteenth Century to the Present', *Journal of the Medical Library Association* 101, no. 2 (2013): 89–91.

Mackenzie, [Norah]. 'Psychology'. In *Manual for Hospital Librarians*, edited by C. E. A. Bedwell, 23–33. London: Library Association, 1947.

McCulliss, Debbie. 'Bibliotherapy: Historical and Research Perspectives', *Journal of Poetry Therapy* 25, no. 1 (2012): 23–38.

Miller, Jesse. 'Medicines of the Soul: Reparative Reading and the History of Bibliotherapy', *Mosaic: An Interdisciplinary Critical Journal* 51, no. 2 (2018): 17–34.

Moy, Janella D. 'Reading and Writing One's Way to Wellness: The History of Bibliotherapy and Scriptotherapy'. In *New Directions in Literature and Medicine Studies*, edited by Stephanie M. Hilger, 15–30. London: Palgrave Macmillan, 2017.

Norrick-Rühl, Corinna, and Shafquat Towheed, 'Introduction'. In *Bookshelves in the Age of the COVID-19 Pandemic*, edited by Corinna Norrick-Rühl and Shafquat Towheed, 1–27. Cham: Palgrave Macmillan, 2022.

Park, Maureen, and Robert Hamilton. 'Moral Treatment of the Insane: Provisions for Lifelong Learning, Cultural Engagement, and Creativity in Nineteenth-Century Asylums', *Journal of Adult and Continuing Education* 16, no. 2 (2010): 100–13.

Partington, Gill. *Bibliotherapy: A Survey of Literature*. Working Papers 2022/23: 03. Exeter: Wellcome Centre for Cultures and Environments of Health, 2023.

Pehrsson, Dale-Elizabeth, and Paula McMillen, 'A Bibliotherapy Evaluation Tool: Grounding Counselors in the Therapeutic Use of Literature', *The Arts in Psychotherapy* 32, no. 1 (2005): 47–59.

Peterson, Sadie M. 'U.S.V. Hospital Library no. 91, Tuskegee, Ala.', *The Crisis* 29, no. 3 (1925): 116–17.

Pladek, Brittany. 'The Poetics of Palliation: Romantic Literary Therapy, 1790–1850'. PhD thesis. University of Toronto, 2013.

Plato. *Phaedrus*, translated by Robin Waterfield. Oxford: Oxford World's Classics, 2002.

Price, Leah. *What We Talk About When We Talk About Books*. New York: Basic Books, 2019.

Price, Leah. 'Prescribed Print: Bibliotherapy after Web 2.0', *Post45* (17 September 2019). https://post45.org/2019/09/prescribed-print-bibliotherapy-after-web-2-0/

Reading Well Books on Prescription: How Bibliotherapy Can Help Your Patients and *Save Your Practice Time and Money*. National Association of Primary Care, 2017. https://napc.co.uk/wp-content/uploads/2017/09/Reading-well.pdf

Rieff, Philip. *The Triumph of the Therapeutic*. London: Chatto & Windus, 1966.

Rose, Jonathan. *Readers' Liberation*. Oxford: Oxford University Press, 2018.

Stiegler, Bernard. *Taking Care of Youth and the Generations*, translated by Stephen Barker. Stanford, CA: Stanford University Press, 2010.

Stiegler, Bernard. 'Distrust and the Pharmacology of Transformational Technologies'. In *Quantum Engagements: Social Reflections of Nanoscience and Emerging Technologies*, edited by Torben B. Zülsdorf, Christopher Coenen, Arianna Ferrari, Ulrich Fiedeler, Colin Milburn, and Matthias Wienroth, 27–39. Heidelberg: AKA Verlag Heidelberg, 2011.

Towheed, Shafquat, and Edmund G. C. King, 'Introduction'. In *Reading and the First World War: Readers, Texts, Archives*, edited by Shafquat Towheed and Edmund G. C. King, 1–25. Basingstoke: Palgrave Macmillan, 2015.

Tuke, Samuel. *Description of the Retreat, an Institution Near York, for Insane Persons*. York: W. Alexander, 1813.

Van Dijck, Cedric, Marysa Demoor, and Sarah Posman, 'Between the Shells: The Production of Belgian, British and French Trench Journals in the First World War', *Publishing History* 77 (2017): 67–89.

Vaninskaya, Anna. 'Learning to Read Trash: Late-Victorian Schools and the Penny Dreadful'. In *The History of Reading, Volume 2: Evidence from the British Isles, c.1750–1950*, edited by Katie Halsey and W. R. Owens, 67–83. Basingstoke: Palgrave Macmillan, 2011.

Wakefield, Donna, McEvoy, Mel, Blackburn-Daniels, Sally, and Siobhan Campbell. 'Tackling the NHS Mental Health Crisis of Working through the COVID-19 Pandemic; Pilot Creative Writing Programme in Support of Healthcare Workers', *Journal of the Royal College of Physicians of Edinburgh* 53, no. 1 (2023): 81–82.

Warshowsky, Hannah, Mahar, Elizabeth A., and Laurie B. Mintz. 'Cliteracy for Him: Effectiveness of Bibliotherapy for Heterosexual Men's Sexual Functioning', *Sexual and Relationship Therapy* 38, no. 1 (2023): 52–73.

Weber, Millicent. 'Online Reading during the Covid-19 Pandemic'. In *Post-Digital Book Cultures: Australian Perspectives*, edited by Alexandra Dane and Millicent Weber, 11–56. Melbourne: Monash University Publishing, 2021.

Weimerskirch, Philip J. 'Benjamin Rush and John Minson Galt, II: Pioneers of Bibliotherapy in America', *Bulletin of the Medical Library Association* 53, no. 4 (1965): 510–26.

Widdowson, Peter. 'The Crisis in English Studies'. In *Re-Reading English*, edited by Peter Widdowson, 1–14. London: Methuen, 1981.

Wolfgram, Patricia A. 'Hospital Libraries in the United States: Historical Antecedents', *Bulletin of the Medical Library Association* 73, no. 1 (1985): 32–8.

Xu, Zheng, Ru Liu, Liping Guo, Ziyi Gao, Zicheng Gao, Xiaowei Liu, Jieyun Li, Bin Li, and Kehu Yang, 'The 100 Most-Cited Articles on Bibliotherapy: A Bibliometric Analysis', *Psychology, Health and Medicine* 28, no. 9 (2023): 2728–44.

Young, Arthur P. 'Aftermath of a Crusade: World War I and the Enlarged Program of the American Library Association', *Library Quarterly* 50, no. 2 (1980): 191–207.

Part I

Bibliotherapy and the First World War

1 The Legacy of Nineteenth-Century Therapeutic Reading in the First World War Hospital

Laura Gray Blair

The term 'bibliotherapy' was first used during the First World War: Samuel McChord Crothers, writing in the *Atlantic Monthly*, described a fictional 'literary clinic' in which visitors' ailments would be treated with books. Rather than medical treatments or spiritual guidance, reading material would act as 'stimulants and sedatives, irritants and counter-irritants', with a library organised based on its effects on readers rather than any other cataloguing system.[1] Throughout the First World War, professional librarians ministered to soldiers on the Front as well as in hospitals in Europe and back in Britain, supplying them with books and periodicals. It is at this point in history that most surveys of the history of bibliotherapy begin, drawing lines of connection between these activities and later forms of bibliotherapeutic practice, and in the process, cementing the use of reading in therapeutic regimes as a twentieth-century phenomenon. Sara Haslam and Edmund G. C. King have traced this commonly cited genealogy: from W. B. McDaniel's categorisation of bibliotherapy as a 'war baby' in 1956 to Bate and Schuman's 2016 overview of the topic for *The Lancet* opening with a reference to Crothers' essay.[2]

However, approaches which both modern readers and practitioners today would easily categorise as 'bibliotherapeutic' were being used in lunatic asylums from the early nineteenth century and were widespread by the mid-1800s. Reading was even framed explicitly by some doctors as part of the 'cure' for insanity. By the end of the nineteenth century, most asylums for both 'pauper' and fee-paying patients held patient libraries, encouraged reading, and put in place staffing and procedures to support this activity as standard practice. Yet this era in the history of the 'healing' book has been neglected. This chapter seeks to contextualise bibliotherapeutic practices during the First World War by examining the roots of 'healing' reading in the nineteenth-century asylum, and the practical results of this background in treating soldiers at institutions requisitioned as part of the Asylum War Hospitals Scheme.

DOI: 10.4324/9781003471561-3

Healing Environments in the Institution

In the early nineteenth century, alternatives to existing systems of mental healthcare (or lack of it) began to be explored. Legislative changes supporting state intervention in the care of those deemed 'lunatics' also occurred. The 1808 County Asylums Act allowed counties in England and Wales to levy a rate to build asylums, involving the removal of the insane poor from prisons and workhouses; legislation in 1845 then *required* each county to provide an asylum for pauper lunatics.[3] Similar Acts were enacted in Ireland and Scotland, though the latter had more well-established provisions for the mentally ill. Increasing numbers of state-funded asylums were built during the nineteenth century, and by the outbreak of the First World War, England alone had over one hundred and fifteen public asylums.[4] Changes also occurred in the methods used to treat mental illness. Contrasting with earlier conceptions of the mind, Roy Porter has described the growing sense that insanity was not an 'overthrow' of Reason, but an error of it.[5] 'False principles' shaped by associations such as sight, smell, and sound could be developed, but these problems of reasoning could also be corrected. The 'madman' could be influenced by his surroundings and experiences and return to sanity.

The space of the institution changed in significant ways in order to facilitate the correction of Reason. *Traitement moral* was popularised by Philippe Pinel (1745–1826), the superintendent of the Bicêtre Hospital in Paris, and gained traction across Britain, Europe, and the United States. Rather than physical punishment and mechanical restraints, 'non-restraint' became considered best practice, promoted by British asylum doctors such as Robert Gardiner Hill and John Conolly.[6] Under 'moral treatment', staff were expected by their superintendents and state inspectors to provide moral authority, discipline, and order, and patients were expected to engage in a regime including 'useful' work, attending religious services, and appropriate leisure activity (dependent on their condition and good behaviour).[7] The asylum itself was seen as a material aspect of care, providing a healing environment for the patients to experience at all times. 'Neatness' and 'cheerfulness' were highly important, and 'objects of interest' were deemed essential.[8] Images of Victorian asylums, even for pauper patients, demonstrate the array of potted plants, ornaments, and birdcages lining rooms filled with typically Victorian furniture, wallpaper, and soft furnishings. The asylum space was to be homely, with what Andrew Scull described as a 'tireless insistence' upon making the institution mimic the ideal Victorian home.[9]

The architecture and landscape of the asylums were also carefully planned. The York Retreat – one of the most influential asylums for the nineteenth century – was designed to allow for what Barry Edginton describes as a 'type of sociability' linked to the family unit.[10] Asylum design became a particular topic of discussion in medical journals.[11] Asylum windows were to be large and unbarred; there should be spaces for recreation and shared meals; corridors should be wide; galleries and wards to have appropriate ventilation but adequate warmth and light.[12] Various plans of asylum design were experimented with to allow an ideal and practical combination of supervision, communication, recreation, and segregation. These ranged from radial plans, with a central tower and radiating wings based on Jeremy Bentham's famous 'panopticon' (as at the 1818 Cornwall County Asylum), to corridor-based plans with central administration blocks and flanking wards (as at the 1831 Middlesex County Asylum at Hanwell), to the later colony plan featuring groups smaller detached buildings emphasising an even more 'domestic' surrounding (as used in 1890s additions to the Royal Edinburgh Asylum).[13]

Asylums were set where possible away from larger metropolitan areas, in spacious grounds which often resembled the aristocrat's landscape park and garden, frequently featuring ornamental planting and lawns, and sometimes greenhouses or more elaborate gardens.[14] Sports were facilitated with bowling greens, cricket pitches, and even curling (as was the case at the Royal Edinburgh Asylum, which utilised its frozen pond for this purpose).[15] Many asylums ran their own bakeries, farms, kitchen gardens, and even breweries – fulfilling a double purpose in making the asylum cost-effectively self-sufficient and providing patients with 'useful work' as part of their rehabilitation. Workshops further allowed patients to take part in crafts and trades such as basketweaving, tailoring, shoemaking, bookbinding, and printing.[16] Recreation also became an essential aspect of the treatment regime. Patients had access to musical instruments, were entertained by musical and theatre troupes or formed their own, wrote and published their own literary work, and produced artwork.[17]

Institutions were additionally expected to give patients access to books and periodicals, with many developing significant library holdings for the use of their patients, carefully considering the choice of books, and assigning reading with a variety of 'medical' purposes.[18] Even as the optimism surrounding the efficacy of 'moral treatment' waned and asylum populations grew, these aspects of nineteenth-century asylum endured, with a patient library becoming a standard inclusion in institutions treating mental illness. The term 'bibliotherapy' had not yet been conceived of, but asylum doctors such as W. A. F. Browne, working at the Crichton Royal Institution, clearly viewed books as healing agents. He described reading as 'moral medicine'.[19] (During the First World War, Crichton would house soldiers with psychological injury as well as civilian patients displaced by the Asylum War Hospitals Scheme, with which this chapter is concerned.)

The Healing Book

Throughout the First World War, newspapers across Britain appealed for the public to send books and magazines to soldiers: Sara Haslam provides an example in *The Times* recommending 'small, cheap books of good literature and fiction' in 1915.[20] This sort of reading was administered via camp libraries run by organisations such as the YMCA. It is evident that great emphasis was placed on books at the Front. Edmund King's discussion of author E. W. Hornung's involvement with the Arras library hut during the war contains considerable evidence of the efforts put into the provision of reading material and a comfortable environment for soldiers to engage with it.[21] Marcella Sutcliffe asserts that the provision of reading material to soldiers was underpinned by two motivations: firstly, the need to maintain morale and provide comfort; and secondly, an aim to 'capitalise on the potential of assembled men' to shape provision according to 'good taste'.[22] The domestic environment of the huts and moral instruction provided by books were utilised as an attempt at social control and disease prevention in addition to enjoyment.[23] The American librarian Theodore W. Koch, on staff at the Library of Congress, visited Britain before America's entry into the war and saw Helen Mary Gaskell's work with the War Library first-hand. In his account of 1918, Koch noted that some officers believed the provision of books could aid in the reduction of venereal disease.[24] Reading was a means of encouraging soldiers to spend time on 'appropriate' activities which would contribute to military health and order, very much like asylum patients were encouraged to develop their 'moral' (reasoning) powers through the consumption of proper literature.

However, soldiers fighting at the Front and those recovering from physical and psychological injury at home were different groups, and for the latter, the function of the 'healing book' took an alternative form. For less able-bodied soldiers admitted into hospitals back in Britain, moral concerns about military conduct and disease prevention through social control were not as relevant. Instead, I believe that Sara Haslam's conceptualisation of the provision of books as representative primarily of caregiving is most applicable.[25] These approaches, focused on maintaining soldiers' morale and creating a sense of comfort and caregiving, perhaps more closely fit with Crothers' satirised 'literary clinic' than his true hope for reading practice. Jesse Miller has argued that Crothers portrayed the fictional clinic as having an ultimately negative impact on its patients, with the neurasthenic middle-classes guided to use literature as an escape from the problems of modernity.[26] Miller posits that instead, Crothers seeks to promote a reading practice functioning as a 'means of engaging the world in an active and vigorously creative manner'.[27] Crothers' ideal reader would not use books as a coping mechanism but as an impetus to act. However, while Crothers' essay criticised the early twentieth-century conceptions of the relationship between reading and health (ethical, psychological, and/or physiological), those who were invested in the notion of reading's ability to heal seem in many ways to have taken the idea of the 'literary clinic' to heart. American librarians wholeheartedly embraced the term 'bibliotherapy' and throughout the twentieth century professionalised the practice.[28] British librarians, whilst largely eschewing 'bibliotherapy' as a descriptor, leaned into what Haslam and King have characterised distinctly as 'literary caregiving'.[29]

Marcella P. Sutcliffe has argued that the reading of soldiers during the First World War should be framed in relation to wider pre-war debates about the 'value' of books in society.[30] She notes D. H. Lawrence's assertion in 1913 that one could 'shed' sickness through books, but the perceived relationship between books and health was a complex one. During the nineteenth century, the publishing landscape had become increasingly characterised as a looming threat to the public. Ten thousand books a year 'flooded' the world of the English-speaking reader, threatening to overwhelm them altogether.[31] The press began to be characterised as a flood, a plague, or a torrent.[32] Books were also compared more directly to drugs, whether medicinal or illicit. Michael Shoenfeldt writes that Milton saw books as 'salutary drugs necessary to achieve moral and physiological health'.[33] Conversely, physician John Reid described how circulating libraries could 'for the most part be compared to a chest of liqueurs', and John Harvey Kellogg likened excessive reading to the use of alcohol or opium.[34] But this pathologisation of reading as 'dangerous' naturally suggested that there was 'safe' and beneficial reading.[35] Despite arguments about how and what people should read, by the start of the First World War, reading had long been conceived of as a suitable activity for those suffering from illness and was considered a cornerstone in the life of a soldier. Koch, in his discussion of hospital libraries, could even draw on the book-drug metaphor in a more positive, and explicitly medical, way: he wrote that 'from the standpoint of the neurologists, books, like drugs, are classified into stimulants and depressants'.[36]

Examination of medical and social discourses around reading and health can shed light on why, for injured soldiers, reading could be considered medicine. The ideas which underpinned the clinic Crothers depicted, and the subsequent approaches taken by hospital librarians, developed from a nineteenth-century conception of 'healthy' and 'unhealthy' reading fleshed out in Victorian institutions, and discussion of hospitalised soldiers' reading closely mirrors discussion of that of asylum patients. I argue that the perception of reading as a beneficial practice for those recovering from traumatic psychological and physiological injury is a result of medical and social discourse developed during the nineteenth century, particularly in the context of treating 'lunatics'. This discourse developed in both Britain and the United States, with doctors travelling across these areas to learn from, collaborate with, and sometimes compete with their medical peers in implementing new aspects of moral treatment. Asylum doctors contributed to the idea of 'restorative reading' significantly, and their mid-nineteenth-century philosophies are mirrored in discussions of soldiers' reading.

Koch wrote that the work of librarians during the war showed 'the truth of the maxim that reading is to the mind what medicine is to the body'.[37] American ambassador Henry Van Dyke responded to Koch's 1917 paper 'Books in camp, trench and hospital', writing that good books counted alongside human fellowship and music as 'three of the best medicines and tonics in the world'.[38] These were not new sentiments – W. A. F. Browne, as mentioned earlier, was writing in the 1840s of his view that the library might 'directly' act as 'part of the remedy' for mental illness and that the library should receive as much care as a laboratory.[39] Where American war hospital librarians began recommending courses of reading specific to their patients, and librarians and physicians later even created specific forms for these prescriptions, the medicalisation of reading practice had already begun in earnest in British asylums. Browne discussed 'prescribing' patient activities including reading; his son James Crichton Browne later recommended courses of study which were 'foreign to feeling' in order to heal the mind 'snapped asunder' by stress, preventing the formation of a 'mental false joint'.[40]

The ways in which books could act as medicine, however, were perceived slightly differently by Koch or Van Dyke than by Browne or his son. Elsewhere I have argued that reading in the asylum was framed as beneficial in several different (but interconnected) ways: as 'useful' work, as a means of building therapeutic relationships and reinforcing desirable behaviour, as a distraction or challenge, as a form of comfort and connection, and finally as acceptable entertainment to improve wellbeing.[41] As moral treatment fell from favour, it was the three latter approaches which became most influential for those using books in therapeutic environments.

Overlapping Approaches

At the Endell Street Military Hospital, the environment was often described as one of 'gentleness', with a 'wonderful atmosphere of sympathy and home'. The domesticity of the hospital, in contrast with others of the period, set it apart as one where care for the psychological welfare of patients was especially important.[42] Literary caregiving was an important aspect of this domestic environment: nurses would read to patients, and volunteer librarians handled their literary needs. Standard lamps were donated by St. Leonard's School for soldiers to read by.[43] Sara Haslam has argued that for the sick soldier, books provided an experience of care by 'activating the memory of familial affection and familiar routine, distracting and entertaining, demonstrating the gratitude and the comparatively small but significant sacrifices of the donating public or by helping men to cope in other ways'.[44] At the Middlesex Asylum in Colney Hatch, books – and the care demonstrated by those involved in their provision – represented something similar to patients. Superintendent W. G. Marshall wrote in 1858 that books 'tend[ed] to render the Patients more contented with their temporary home' and 'engender[ed] feelings of kindness and gratitude, that someone is endeavouring to ameliorate their condition'.[45] The Commissioners in Lunacy (and at the point of the war, the Board of Control) had encouraged the engagement of asylum patients with literature regardless of their physical condition or abilities. They demanded that attendants should read out loud for those too unwell to read or who lacked the skill.[46] The view was that for the 'insane' patient, books could represent a connection to the world which they were removed from, and it was important for all patients to be able to access that connection regardless of their own capacity to read.

In asylums, staff recognised that books – increasingly available to their nineteenth-century patients – were a key means of keeping patients entertained where their normal routines and habits were unavailable to them. J. Burchell Spring, chaplain at the Bristol Asylum, offered up the following reminder to readers of his report in 1874:

> When it is remembered how much consolation well chosen books bring with them to the healthy and the sane, we need not be surprised if they should be valued by those who are shattered in mind and body, and who, in a measure, are shut out from those thousand distractions which meet us in the busy world.[47]

D. C. Campbell, Superintendent at Essex, emphasised the need to keep a patient from 'brooding over his own morbid thoughts', and Dr. M'Culloch at the Joint Counties Asylum in Wales suggested that the library worked to 'soothe, divert and strengthen the diseased mind'.[48] Haslam notes Helen Mary Gaskell's similar belief that books were a 'necessity' for sick and wounded soldiers, characterising her approach as one 'calculated to make connections' and to 'fill an emotional vacuum'.[49] Distraction from their illness, trauma, and grief was ideally served through reading. Books and magazines offered comfort even for those who weren't able to fully partake. At the Dundee Asylum in 1855, the directors noted that the presence of books was important therapeutically even for those unable to read. They still could gain pleasure from the act of turning pages, or looking at illustrations.[50] Similarly, the volunteer librarian Beatrice Harraden wrote that some soldiers liked to have copies of the magazine *John Bull* near them, 'ready for the moment when returning strength gives them the incentive to take even a glance of some of its pages'.[51] The *presence* of books contributed to their sense of wellbeing, representing a return to 'normal' activities.

Social and medical discourse had proliferated in the nineteenth century as to the *types* of books most suitable for readers. Items such as adult education advocate John Lubbock's *One Hundred Books* list had been published, debated, and adapted by those invested in guiding readers in 'suitable' and 'healthy' reading.[52] In asylums, doctors had moved from suggesting that imaginative works were 'to be avoided' (Samuel Tuke) to encouraging patients to read rollicking military stories to distract and cheer them (W. A. F. Browne).[53] A key early practice in asylum-based therapeutic reading was the individualised approach taken by those such as Browne (and more frequently the asylum chaplain-cum-librarian), emblematic of ideal moral treatment practices. By the beginning of the twentieth century, detailed individual approaches to reading access had fallen away as patient numbers increased and optimism faltered. But the librarian – in selecting or releasing books – remained an interface between the patient and their reading material. Twentieth-century librarians resurrected individualised practice. In the 1920s, G. O. Ireland even created a specific prescription form for recommending and restricting literature for psychiatric patients.[54]

The Asylum War Hospitals Scheme

Reading in the asylum and reading in the First World War hospital have further connections – as well as utilising therapeutic ideologies surrounding reading which were developed in asylums, more practically many soldiers were treated using asylum buildings and associated resources. Before the First World War, the army had a single unit for soldiers experiencing mental illness at the Royal Victoria Military Hospital near Southampton, but this admitted only around 120 patients per year.[55] More often, soldiers with mental illnesses were discharged from service and admitted to the large system of public asylums. Military hospitals for physically wounded patients were more well organised. However, soon after the beginning of the war, it became clear to authorities that many more beds than existed in military hospitals in England and Wales were going to be required for soldiers returning from fighting. As greater numbers of soldiers returned from the Front, physically and mentally wounded – or both – authorities struggled to appropriately house them during rehabilitation.

Suitable places for receiving the sick and wounded needed to be found. As discussed earlier in this chapter, philosophies emphasising community, occupation, and leisure had governed the architecture and organisation of asylums, rendering them readymade environments for the treatment and rehabilitation of war wounded. In a 1920 report to the Secretary of State for the Home Department, Commissioners of the Board of Control Marriott Cooke and C. Hubert Bond identified that lunatic asylums' 'extensive grounds, good workshops, and large recreation halls' were influential in the choice of asylums as sites for War Hospitals. These features offered 'opportunities for exercise, occupation and amusement which enhanced the rapidity and completeness of their recovery, and tended to relieve the monotony of hospital life'.[56] Asylums taken for physiologically wounded patients required some adaptation, but those for military 'mental cases' required little intervention.[57]

In October 1914, the Board of Control contacted all public asylums informing them of this need, initiating discussions about making beds available for service patients.[58] Moss Side Hospital at Maghull, Liverpool, was the first asylum to be handed over to the military authorities for rehabilitating soldiers, in December 1914.[59] In January 1915, it was made clear to the Board of Control that 50,000 beds would be needed, and arrangements were made to provide 15,000 in asylums by clearing some asylums of their patients and transferring them elsewhere. Initially, nine asylums were chosen for the scheme: Newcastle City, West Riding, Lancashire County, Birmingham City, Norfolk County, Cardiff City, West Sussex County at Chichester, Bristol City, and London County at Horton. Six of these nine asylums were established in nineteenth century, with the earliest opening in 1814. However, it soon became clear that even clearing these hospitals entirely of their patient populations would not provide sufficient accommodation for wounded soldiers, and other asylums were soon involved in the war effort. Twenty-four were eventually in use.[60] By 1918, beds for 'mental cases' accounted for around one-seventh of all beds in the war hospitals.[61] The impact was keenly felt by the civilian patient population, who were moved to other institutions, losing their familiar wards and staff, access to their families, and sometimes fellow patients.[62] J. L. Crammer has additionally argued that administration during this period caused a significantly elevated death rate for civilian patients.[63]

Little scholarly work has been produced on the Asylum War Hospitals Scheme. Ian Beech has surveyed the impact on the Cardiff Mental Hospital; Brendan Kelly has explored the treatment of shell shock at the Richmond War Hospital in Dublin; and Steven Cherry has provided an account of the Norfolk Lunatic Asylum (known during the scheme as the Norfolk War Hospital).[64] No wider exploration of the scheme exists, barring contemporary reports of the scheme, such as that by Cooke and Bond. Academic studies of asylums included in the scheme deal most significantly with the administration and staffing of the War Hospitals, and often treat the War Hospital period as a separate era in an asylum's history. The potential for continuity in approaches to patient care – seemingly an obvious aspect, given staff, buildings, and facilities remained much the same – has not been thoroughly explored. Much work has also been produced on the treatment of mental and nervous cases during the First World War, particularly relating to shell shock.[65] These studies focus primarily on the medical conceptualisation of the disorder, its diagnosis, and medical treatment. Far less attention has been paid to the wider curative 'atmosphere' of hospitals. Jeffrey Reznick has argued that the 'chief features' of the military hospital – the pavilion ward and the curative regime of 'fresh air' – demonstrate the endurance of 'central features of nineteenth-century institutional architecture'. Reznick identifies, as I have discussed earlier, that for Victorian medical authorities, the institution itself could be seen as an 'instrument of cure'.[66] If this endurance might be said to apply to ward design and the fresh air regime, could it not also apply to other aspects of nineteenth-century medical and asylum practice? Alongside access to spacious grounds and provision for occupation and leisure activities such as sports, soldiers would also have gained access to the libraries developed for the civilian asylum population.

Napsbury and Springfield War Hospitals

Napsbury, opened in 1905, is a modern combination of villas and a main echelon-style complex. Prior to its construction, architect Roland Plumbe and asylum doctor Hugh Gardiner Hill had embarked on a survey in the north of England and Scotland.[67] They sought to find the most successful examples of asylum architecture and practices and combine these to produce the 'ideal' asylum in Napsbury. They visited asylums famous for pioneering moral treatment, such as the Royal Edinburgh Asylum. Gardiner Hill himself had a pedigree in the topic, as his father was Robert Gardiner Hill, who was mentioned earlier as instrumental in introducing non-restraint to the British asylum system via his work at the Lincoln Asylum.[68] They also spoke with Dr Sibbald, a Scottish Commissioner in Lunacy, Deputy Commissioner at the time of Dr David Skae's tenure at the Royal Edinburgh.[69] Under Skae's guidance, the patient library was continually replenished, with patients being encouraged to read widely, and he provided detailed reports on the Library's success year after year.[70] Especially emphasised in the report they produced for the County Council was the benefits of asylums being designed to feel 'homelike', from their architecture, to decorations, to recreation available to the patients.[71]

A few months into the war, Napsbury was requisitioned by the War Office to help provide beds for wounded soldiers. Dr Lancelot Rolleston, Medical Superintendent at Napsbury, quickly offered the use of part of the asylum as a War Hospital, and by the 14th of May 1915, the Napsbury War Hospital was officially receiving soldiers who were suffering from shell shock and other mental conditions.[72] Only a couple of months later, the War Office notified the Board of Control that yet more beds were needed for soldiers, and soon the entire asylum was turned over for use as a War Hospital. About 1,332 patients were moved to other asylums, leaving only 81 'harmless cases' to work on the farm and in the grounds. The original 300-350 beds remained reserved for soldiers suffering with 'severe nervous disorder', whilst the rest were for the 'ordinary sick and wounded'.[73] The Board of Control emphasised that the soldiers would enjoy their 'full share of the amenities of the institution', presumably including the library contained within its walls.[74]

At Napsbury, the chaplain R. A. Squires had acted as librarian. He wrote each year about the state of the Library and the ways in which reading was facilitated in the wards – a central library kept in the Chaplain's room was distributed amongst open shelving in each ward. In 1907, the Library consisted of around 2,000 volumes, arranged alphabetically and fully catalogued (unfortunately no catalogues appear to have survived).[75] By 1909, the number of works in the Library had increased to around five or six thousand volumes.[76] Expenditure on books, newspapers, periodicals, and stationery was noted in annual reports from 1906, where £35, 13 shillings, and 2 pence was spent. The year 1907 saw an increase to £44, 2 shillings, and 11 pence, the year 1909 saw another increase to £90, 17 shillings, and 7 pence – at least £20 of this was spent directly on Library books, as the Chaplain wrote that this grant was spent on 'books of popular instruction', 'so as to satisfy actual demands'. He wrote that he hoped to make the existing selection of fiction last a little while longer.[77]

By the time the war started in 1914, the Library at Napsbury was fairly substantial. In late 1914, another 1050 books were added to the Library, and expenditure on library books, periodicals and newspapers for 1913-14 totalled over £100.[78] The assistant chaplain, A. Treeve Stephens, noted that the books were in 'great demand' after the War Hospital opened in May 1915.[79] The quarterly maintenance accounts during the life of the War Hospital show that significantly less was spent on newspapers and periodicals during this period than in the years before, which given the state of the war is not surprising. Library books were not bought at regular intervals at Napsbury, but there was a significant purchase midway through the war between November 1916 and February 1917, where yet another 1050 library books were purchased for the soldiers from W. H. Smiths.[80] The Board of Control, in overseeing a military mental hospital, continued library administration as they had done for their civilian population – adding to reading provision, maintaining library stock, and retaining the chaplain as librarian.

Asylum libraries were developed over the course of decades, and despite the fact that many – like the libraries ministering to soldiers during the First World War – were dependent on donations to develop their holdings, care was taken to ensure that titles were suitable for asylum patients. They would therefore have contained plenty of material deemed appropriate for recuperating soldiers. While records of the books available at Springfield and Napsbury do not survive, catalogues from other nineteenth-century asylums do. In the mid-nineteenth century, the libraries at Crichton Royal Institution, the Royal Edinburgh Asylum, and the Murray Royal Asylum (the former two which took military psychiatric patients during the First World War) are recorded.[81] These libraries contained a wide range of materials including fiction, history, biography, educational materials, and more. A register of issues from the library at the Parkside Asylum in Chester also demonstrates that a large proportion (around 77%) were fiction.[82] The library at Napsbury was almost certainly similar, shaped by the same public discourse, doctors' publications, financial constraints, and governmental oversight. The inherited asylum librarian would provide an additional level of security when it came to mediating soldiers' interaction with reading material.

However, some books were more appropriate than others. As with Gaskell's War Library, work done by librarians at Endell Street was personalised, and requests by individual patients were taken seriously. The rule of the library was 'to provide every book asked for, on whatever subject and in whatever language', from detective novels to handbooks dealing with the subject of machinery.[83] The men at Endell Street were not without guidance, however. Haslam has noted that newspaper coverage of the library approvingly reported that men were encouraged to widen their reading to 'classic' works such as Tennyson's.[84] As the Tukes had facilitated at the Retreat in York one hundred years earlier, soldiers' reading was conceived of as a kind of diversion – a form of escape from their immediate situation – but it was still important that gatekeepers of the libraries could shape their reading. Appeals for literature published in newspapers can give some sense of the types of reading authorities wanted to encourage. Mr Walter Ashley, in charge of a camp library, was quoted in the *Newcastle Journal* in November 1915. He appealed for books but specified that they should be 'suitable for a library of this kind' – 'good modern novels' like the works of Wilkie Collins, Charles Dickens, Charles Reade, Charlotte Brontë, George Eliot, Nathaniel Hawthorne, and Charles Kingsley.[85] Dickens' work in particular was favoured by asylums, being used for group readings at Hanwell in London and appearing as the sixth most popular author at the Parkside Asylum library. There, Reade appeared as the seventh most popular, and Collins eighth.[86]

At Springfield War Hospital (formerly the Wandsworth Asylum), there is further evidence of the links between therapeutic practice in the asylum and in the twentieth-century war hospital. Springfield opened to patients in 1841, and Hugh Gardiner Hill worked as superintendent before his involvement with Napsbury. The separate 'Annexe for Idiot Children' at Springfield was utilised from 1915 until after the end of the war as a specialist centre for soldiers suffering from mental trauma. The concerns of the authorities and the public about the stigmatisation of soldiers being treated in asylums led to a clear separation from the rest of the 'pauper lunatic' patients – they even built a large fence separating the main hospital from the annex.[87]

Like other hospitals during the First World War, the Springfield War Hospital produced its own publication, the *Gazette*.[88] This magazine demonstrates that soldiers weren't just left with the offerings of the asylums where they were residing. In a March 1918 issue of the *Gazette*, now with a circulation of around 11,000 issues per month, a small note appears.[89] This appeal reveals that the Springfield War Hospital has its own Librarian (very possibly the Chaplain) and that the Hospital is soliciting donations for itself, separate from the main asylum. This method, and the material which is requested – fiction, travel, history, geography, natural history, and illustrated books and periodicals – is particularly interesting. Throughout the nineteenth century, asylums had produced their own periodicals written by patients in what is another example of nineteenth-century asylum practices establishing forms of therapeutic activity later applied in the war hospital.[90] There, librarians and patients themselves would make requests of their readers for books and periodicals as a humanitarian cause, and the type of material requested was virtually identical. The Springfield *Gazette*, produced at an asylum-turned-hospital, utilised the same traditions forged by the asylum sector to appeal for the same resources.

Conclusion

For patients in the nineteenth and twentieth centuries, reading was an essential activity sought out by and recommended to them. Reports of how both groups interacted with their books demonstrate how they valued reading material. Reports from Crichton evidence the lengths that patients would go to in the mid-nineteenth century: one man would steal books given to others, whereas another would mutilate books unless he was given new ones.[91] Koch's descriptions of soldiers' interactions with their books are similar: men would hide them to prevent them from being removed, read them until the paper covers disintegrated, or 'carry [them] in their pockets like a treasure trove'.[92] The view of reading as a practice which could provide therapeutic benefit to the reader was one which developed significantly over the course of the nineteenth century, and this philosophy was already embedded in medical practice by the beginning of the First World War. I contend that the promotion of reading in medical settings such as asylums contributed to a growing perception that reading could be a beneficial practice.

The therapeutic environment of the War Hospitals of the early twentieth century – both in terms of architecture and organisation – was shaped by a century of development in British asylum practice regarding occupational therapy and therapeutic recreation. Soldiers were encouraged to engage in recreational activities much in the same way that asylum patients had been throughout the nineteenth century and at the War Hospitals were able to make use of patient libraries developed over the course of the previous decades. Therefore, the history of proto-bibliotherapeutic practice in the nineteenth-century British asylum is inextricably linked to the experiences of soldier patients in War Hospitals. Asylum doctors laid down the foundations for reading to be considered a powerful aid in keeping soldiers' minds healthy or returning them to health. Histories of First World War reading would benefit from further examination of reading conducted within the Asylum War Hospitals Scheme as a distinct practice from other hospital library schemes due to its historical context.

Acknowledgement

This work was supported by the Wellcome Trust, Grant number 212863/Z/18/Z.

Notes

1 Jesse Miller, 'Medicines of the Soul: Reparative Reading and the History of Bibliotherapy', *Mosaic: An Interdisciplinary Critical Journal* 51, no. 2 (2018): 21.

2 W. B. McDaniel, 'Bibliotherapy – Some Historical and Contemporary Aspects', *American Library Association Bulletin* (October 1956): 584–589; Jonathan Bate and Andrew Schuman, 'The Art of Medicine. Books Do Furnish a Mind: the Art and Science of Bibliotherapy', *Lancet* 387 (February 2016): 742–743, both cited by Sara Haslam and Edmund G. C. King, ' "Medicinable Literature": Bibliotherapy, Literary Caregiving, and the First World War', *Literature and Medicine* 39, no. 2 (2021): 296.

3 For an overview of the law surrounding insanity until 1845, see Kathleen Jones, *Law and Conscience, 1744–1845: The Social History of the Care of the Insane*, Abingdon: Routledge, 1998.

4 Sarah Rutherford, 'Landscapers for the Mind: English Asylum Designers, 1845–1914', *Garden History* 33, no. 1 (2005): 61.

5 Roy Porter, *Mind Forg'd Manacles: A History of Madness in England from the Restoration to the Regency*, London: Athlone Press, 1987, 191.

6 For a useful overview of non-restraint, see Leslie Topp, 'Single Rooms, Seclusion and the Non-Restraint Movement in British Asylums, 1838–1844', *Social History of Medicine* 31, no. 4 (2018): 754–773.

7 Leonard D. Smith, *Cure, Comfort and Safe Custody: Public Lunatic Asylums in Early Nineteenth-Century England*, London: Leicester University Press, 1999, 191.

8 Jane Hamlett, *At Home in the Institution: Material Life in Asylums, Lodging Houses and Schools in Victorian and Edwardian England*, Basingstoke: Palgrave Macmillan, 2015, 19–20.

9 Andrew Scull, 'The Domestication of Madness', *Medical History* 27 (1983): 245.

10 Barry Edginton, 'Moral Architecture: The Influence of the York Retreat on Asylum Design', *Health & Place* 3, no. 2 (1997): 92.

11 See for example John Bucknill, 'Asylum Architecture and Arrangements', *Asylum Journal of Mental Science* 3, no. 21 (April 1857): 385–396.

12 Edginton, 'Moral Architecture', 94.

13 See Jeremy Taylor, *Hospital and Asylum Architecture in England, 1840–1914: Building for Health Care*, London: Mansell, 1991; the work of Peter Cracknell and the team at 'County Asylums', www.countyasylums.co.uk/about/ [accessed 25 May 2024]; and the work of Harriet Richardson, 'Historic Hospitals: An Architectural Gazetteer' https://historic-hospitals.com [accessed 25 May 2024].

14 Rutherford, 'Landscapers for the Mind', 62–63.

15 See Steven Cherry and Roger Munting, ' "Exercise Is the Thing"? Sport and the Asylum c.1850–1950', *International Journal of the History of Sport* 22, no. 1 (2005): 42–45; Rob Ellis, 'Asylums and Sport: Participation, Isolation and the Role of Cricket in the Treatment of the Insane', *International Journal of the History of Sport* 30, no. 1 (2013): 83–101.

16 For an overview of some aspects of therapeutic work, see Jennifer Laws, 'Crackpots and Basket-cases: A History of Therapeutic Work and Occupation', *History of the Human Sciences* 24 (2011): 65–81; the use of printing and writing as a therapeutic activity is explored by Mila Daskalova, 'Printing as Poison, Printing as Cure: Work and Health in the Nineteenth-Century Printing Office and Asylum', *Book History* 24, no. 1 (2021): 58–84 and in her thesis, 'Printing and Periodical Culture in the Nineteenth-Century Asylum', PhD diss., University of Strathclyde, 2022.

17 See, for example, Emily Jessica Turner, 'Patients' Creative Work and "Expressive Possibilities" ' in *New Moon*, *Under the Dome*, and *The Hydra*, 1844–1918', PhD diss., University of Sussex, 2019; Daskalova, 'Printing and Periodical Culture' (2022); Benjamin Reiss, *Theatres of Madness: Insane Asylums and Nineteenth-Century*

American Culture, Chicago: University of Chicago Press, 2008; Jessica Campbell, 'The Healing Arts? An Examination of Madness, Creativity and Experience in British Asylum Culture c.1840–1914', PhD diss., University of Edinburgh, forthcoming; Maureen Park, *Art in Madness: Dr W. A. F. Browne's Collection of Patient Art at Crichton Royal Institution, Dumfries*, Dumfries: Dumfries and Galloway Health Board, 2010; Ute Oswald, '"Distraction from Hurtful Thoughts" – "Von trüben Gedanken ablenken": Recreational Activities as Agents of Healing in Nineteenth-Century British Asylums', *Medizinhistorisches Journal* 56 (2021): 30–57; and Rosemary Golding, *Music and Moral Management in the Nineteenth-Century English Lunatic Asylum*, London: Palgrave Macmillan, 2021.

18 Several scholars have explored medical libraries for patient use, notably Antonia J. Bunch, *Hospital and Medical Libraries in Scotland: An Historical and Sociological Study*, Glasgow: Scottish Library Association, 1975; and Jennifer Connor, 'Medical Library History: A Survey of the Literature in Great Britain and North America', *Libraries & Culture* 24 (1989): 459–474. Studies of asylum bibliotherapy are few and often US-focused, such as Lisa M. Dunkel, 'Moral and Humane: Patients' Libraries in Early Nineteenth-Century American Mental Hospitals', *Bulletin of the Medical Library Association* 71, no. 3 (1983): 274–281; and Len Levin, 'Bibliotherapy: Tracing the Roots of a Moral Therapy Movement in the United States from the Early Nineteenth Century to the Present', *Journal of the Medical Library Association* 101, no. 2 (2013): 89–91. My own PhD thesis discusses asylum bibliotherapy in the British Isles: see Laura Gray Blair, '"Library as Laboratory": Moral Treatment, Patient Libraries and Reading in Nineteenth-Century British Asylums', PhD diss., Queen Mary University of London, 2024.

19 Dumfries and Galloway Archives and Local Studies, DGH1/2/2/2/1, Annual Reports 1st–18th, Crichton Royal Institution, W. A. F. Browne, Medical Superintendent, Crichton Royal Institution, Annual Report, 1844, 20.

20 'The Queen and the War Library', *Times* [London, England] 4 December 1915: 11, quoted in Sara Haslam, 'Reading, Trauma and Literary Caregiving 1914–1918: Helen Mary Gaskell and the War Library', *Journal of Medical Humanities* 41 (2020): 312.

21 Edmund G. C. King, 'E. W. Hornung's Unpublished "Diary," the YMCA, and the Reading Soldier in the First World War', *English Literature in Transition, 1880–1920* 57, no. 3 (2014): 369–70.

22 Marcella P Sutcliffe, 'Reading at the Front: Books and Soldiers in the First World War', *Pedagogica Historica* 52, no. 1–2 (2016): 105.

23 Sutcliffe, 'Reading at the Front', 108.

24 Theodore Wesley Koch, *War Libraries and Allied Studies*, New York: G. E. Stechert & Co, 1918, 69; Koch's visit to the War Library service is dealt with by Sara Haslam, 'Reading, Trauma and Literary Caregiving', 307, 310–313.

25 Haslam, 'Reading, Trauma and Literary Caregiving', 313–314.

26 Miller, 'Medicines of the Soul', 26.

27 Miller, 'Medicines of the Soul', 21.

28 Mary Mahoney explores this topic in her thesis, 'Books as Medicine: A History of the Use of Reading to Treat the Self and Its Diseases in the Anglophone World, 1800-1940', PhD diss., University of Connecticut, 2018, and in her online exhibit, 'From Library War Service to Science: Bibliotherapy in World War I', https://booksasmedicine.com/libraryw arservice/. [accessed 08 January 2024].

29 Haslam and King, 'Medicinable Literature', 299.

30 Sutcliffe, 'Reading at the Front', 104.

31 [John Murray] 'Books and Reading', *The Quarterly Review* 162 (April 1886), 504.

32 Kelly J. Mays, 'The Disease of Reading and Victorian periodicals', in *Literature in the Marketplace: Nineteenth-Century British Publishing and Reading Practices*, edited by John O. Jordan and Robert L. Patten, Cambridge: Cambridge University Press, 1995, 169.
33 Michael Shoenfeldt, 'Reading Bodies', in *Reading, Society and Politics in Early Modern England*, edited by Kevin Sharpe and Steven N. Zwicker, Cambridge: Cambridge University Press, 2003, 220.
34 John Reid, *Essays on Hypochondriasis and Other Nervous Affections*, 3rd edn, London: Longman, Hurst, Rees, Orme and Brown, 1823, 103; John Harvey Kellogg, *Ladies' Guide in Health and Disease: Girlhood, Maidenhood, Wifehood, Motherhood*, New York: Modern Medicine Publishing, 1893, 207.
35 Ashleigh Blackwood, 'Toxic Texts and Reading Remedies: Literary Medicine in Eighteenth-Century Print Cultures', *Literature and Medicine* 34 (2016): 279.
36 Koch, *War Libraries*, 145.
37 Koch, *War Libraries*, 116.
38 Koch, *War Libraries*, ix.
39 Dumfries and Galloway Archives and Local Studies, DGH1/2/2/2/1, Annual Reports 1st–18th, Crichton Royal Institution, W. A. F. Browne, Medical Superintendent, Crichton Royal Institution, Annual Report, 1841, 19–20; and Annual Report, 1844, 20.
40 James Crichton Browne, Medical Superintendent, Newcastle Asylum, Annual Report, 1866, 19.
41 Laura Blair, 'Library as Laboratory'.
42 Jennian F. Geddes, 'Deeds *and* Words in the Suffrage Military Hospital in Endell Street', *Medical History* 51 (2007): 87.
43 Geddes, 'The Women's Hospital Corps', 114.
44 Haslam, 'Reading, Trauma and Literary Caregiving', 314.
45 W. G. Marshall, Physician (Female Side), Colney Hatch Asylum, Annual Report, 1858, 31.
46 This occurred at multiple asylums, but is notable at the very large Hanwell (Middlesex) Asylum in 1873. Visiting Commissioners, Hanwell Asylum, Annual Report, 1873, 19.
47 J. Burchell Spring, Chaplain, Bristol Asylum, Annual Report, 1874, 34.
48 D. C. Campbell, Medical Superintendent, Essex Asylum, Annual Report, 1854, 19–20; Dr. M'Cullough, Medical Superintendent, Joint Counties Asylum, Annual Report, 1859, 24.
49 Haslam, 'Reading, Trauma and Literary Caregiving', 309–310.
50 Directors, Dundee Royal Asylum, Annual Report, 1855, 9–10.
51 *John Bull*, Saturday 11 November 1916, 3. This article quotes Harraden's 'What our soldiers read', published in *Cornhill Magazine* in November 1916.
52 'Sir John Lubbock's Liberal Education', *Pall Mall Gazette*, Monday 11 January 1886, 4.
53 Samuel Tuke, *Description of the Retreat, an Institution Near York, for Insane Persons of the Society of Friends: Containing an Account of Its Origin and Progress, the Modes of Treatment, and a Statement of Cases*, Philadelphia: Isaac Pierce, 1813, 114–115; DGH1/2/2/2/1, W. A. F. Browne, Annual Report, Crichton, 1839–1840, 19–20.
54 G. O. Ireland, 'Bibliotherapy – The Use of Books as a Form of Treatment in a Neuropsychiatric Hospital', *Medical Bulletin* 5 (1929): 443.
55 Peter Barham, *Forgotten Lunatics of the Great War*, New Haven: Yale University Press, 41.
56 Marriott Cooke, and C. Hubert Bond, *History of the Asylum War Hospitals in England and* Wales, London: His Majesty's Stationery Office, 1920, 1–2.

57 Jennifer Farquharson, '"Passing the Border": the Civilian and Soldier Patient in the Scottish Asylum, 1914–1934', PhD diss., Glasgow Caledonian University, 2019, 49–50.
58 Judith Devine and Philip Barton Wright, 'The Impact of World War I on Asylums in the UK', *British Journal of Mental Health Nursing* 3, no. 6 (2014): 264.
59 Edgar Jones, 'Shell Shock at Maghull and the Maudsley: Models of Psychological Medicine in the UK', *Journal of the History of Medicine and Allied Sciences* 65 (2010): 369.
60 Cooke and Bond, *History of the Asylum War Hospitals*, 1–2.
61 Peter Barham, *Forgotten Lunatics*, 45.
62 Claire Hilton, *Civilian Lunatic Asylums during the First World War: A Study of Austerity on London's Fringe*, Cham, Switzerland: Palgrave Macmillan, 2021, 54.
63 J. L. Crammer, 'The Extraordinary Deaths of Asylum Inmates during the 1914–1918 War', *Medical History* 36, no. 4 (1992): 430–441.
64 Ian Beech, 'The Universal Khaki: The Impact of the Asylum War Hospital Scheme on Cardiff City Mental Hospital, 1915–1920', *Llafur: Journal of the Welsh People's History Society* 9, no. 2 (2005): 4–26; Brendan D. Kelly, 'Shell Shock in Ireland: The Richmond War Hospital, Dublin (1916–19)', *History of Psychiatry* 26, no. 1 (2014): 50–63; Steven Cherry, *Mental Health Care in Modern England: The Norfolk Lunatic Asylum/St. Andrew's Hospital c.1810–1998*, Woodbridge: Boydell Press, 2003.
65 For example, see Fiona Reid, *Broken Men: Shell Shock, Treatment and Recovery in Britain 1914-30*, London: Bloomsbury, 2012.
66 Jeffrey S. Reznick, *Healing the Nation: Soldiers and the Culture of Caregiving in Britain During the Great War*, Manchester: Manchester University Press, 2004, 43.
67 This survey is mentioned in the minutes of the Standing Sub-Committee of Visitors for Napsbury at several points in 1898. See London Metropolitan Archives (LMA), H50/A/01/001 Napsbury Standing Sub-Committee of Visitors, Minutes Vol. 1.
68 Camilla Haw and Graeme Yorston, 'Thomas Prichard and the Non-Restraint Movement at the Northampton Asylum', *Psychiatric Bulletin* 28 (2004): 140–142.
69 H50/A/01/001, 4 July 1898, 55–56.
70 See for example David Skae, Physician, Royal Edinburgh Asylum, Annual Report, 1861, 33.
71 In particular, the Alt-Sherbitz asylum near Leipzig was praised by the Committee at Napsbury, emphasising non-restraint, homeliness, liberty, and recreation. H50/A/01/001, 4 July 1898, 74–75.
72 LMA, H50/A/01/024 Napsbury Standing Sub-Committee of Visitors, Minutes Vol. 24 (1915), 3.
73 LMA, H50/A/01/026 Napsbury Standing Sub-Committee of Visitors, Minutes Vol. 26 (1916–17), 26–29.
74 LMA, H50/A/01/023 Napsbury Standing Sub-Committee of Visitors, Minutes Vol. 23, cited by Barham, *Forgotten Lunatics*, 57.
75 LMA, MCC/MIN/05/070, R. A. Squires, Chaplain's Report, *The Third Annual Report of the Visiting Committee of the Middlesex County Lunatic Asylum at Napsbury, 1907-1908*, London: Harrison & Sons, 1908, 15.
76 LMA, MCC/MIN/05/070, Report of the Commissioners in Lunacy, 12 June 1909, *The Fifth Annual Report Relating to the Middlesex County Lunatic Asylum at Napsbury, 1909-1910*, London: Harrison & Sons, 1910, 74–75.
77 Squires, *Fifth Annual Report*, 73.
78 Financial statement for Napsbury Hospital for the year ending 31 March 1914, H50/A/01/023, 3 (tucked into volume).

79 LMA, H50/A/01/024, A. Treeve Stephens, 'Annual Report of the Assistant Chaplain', Napsbury Standing Sub-Committee of Visitors, Minutes Vol. 24, 15.
80 Napsbury Sub-Committee Minutes 1916–17, H50/A/01/026, 158.
81 Dumfries and Galloway Archives and Local Studies, DGH1/6/17/1, C.R.I. Scrapbook, *Catalogue of the Library of the Crichton Royal Institution*, Dumfries: Crichton Press, 1853; Lothian Health Services Archive, GD16/52, *Catalogue of the Library of the Royal Edinburgh Asylum*, Morningside, Edinburgh: Royal Asylum Press, 1861; University of Dundee Archive Services, THB29/11/2/1, *Catalogue of the Library of Murray's Royal Institution*, Perth, compiled by M. W. J., Perth: Robert Whittet, 1863.
82 Cheshire Archives NHM/8/30, Library Issue Register for the New Cheshire Asylum, 1877–1899.
83 Flora Murray, *Women as Army Surgeons: Being the History of the Women's Hospital Corps in Paris, Wimereux and Endell Street; September 1914–October 1919*, London: Hodder and Stoughton, 1920, 195.
84 Haslam and King, 'Medicinable Literature', 306.
85 'Books Read by Soldiers: the Kind of Library Required', *Newcastle Journal*, 26 November 1915, 4.
86 Catherine M. E. Macfie, Matron, Hanwell Asylum, Annual Report, 1856, 51–52; Cheshire Archives NHM/8/30, Library Issue Register for the New Cheshire Asylum, 1877–1899, analysed in Blair, 'Library as Laboratory'.
87 Barham, *Forgotten Lunatics*, 55–56.
88 Many periodicals were produced by soldiers in the trenches and in military hospitals. Perhaps the most well-known is the *Hydra*, produced at Craiglockhart War Hospital and contributed to by Wilfred Owen. See for example Meredith Martin, '"Therapeutic Measures": The Hydra and Wilfred Owen at Craiglockhart War Hospital', *Modernism/Modernity* 14 (2007): 35–54.
89 LMA, H46/SP/Y/01/001, *Springfield War Hospital Gazette*, 15 March 1918.
90 The asylum periodical, especially in Britain, has only recently received proper scholarly attention. See in particular: Turner, PhD diss. (2019) Daskalova, PhD diss. (2022).
91 DGH1/2/2/2/1, W. A. F. Browne, Medical Superintendent, Crichton Royal Institution, Annual Report, 1840, 19–20.
92 Koch, *War Libraries*, 82.

Bibliography

Primary and archive sources

[Murray, John]. 'Books and Reading', *The Quarterly Review* 162 (April 1886): 504.

'Books Read by Soldiers: the Kind of Library Required', *Newcastle Journal* 139.21992 (26 November 1915): 4.

'Sir John Lubbock's Liberal Education', *Pall Mall Gazette* 43.6497 (Monday 11 January 1886): 4.

'The Queen and the War Library', *Times* [London, England] 41029 (4 December 1915): 11.

Bucknill, John. 'Asylum Architecture and Arrangements', *Asylum Journal of Mental Science* 3.21 (April 1857): 385–396.

Campbell, D. C. 'Report of the Medical Superintendent', *Report of the Committee of Visitors, Report of the Medical Superintendent, and Other Papers Relating to the Asylum: Printed by Order of the Court of Quarter Session, January 1854 [for 1853].*

Chelmsford: Meggy and Chalk, 1854. https://wellcomecollection.org/works/k4kuhmqm. [accessed 08 January 2024].

Cheshire Archives, NHM/8/30, Library Issue Register for the New Cheshire Asylum, 1877–1899.

Cooke, Marriott, and C. Hubert Bond. *History of the Asylum War Hospitals in England and Wales*. London: His Majesty's Stationery Office, 1920.

Crichton Browne, James. 'To the Chairman and Committee of Visitors', *First Annual Report for 1865/Newcastle-upon-Tyne Borough Pauper Lunatic Asylum*. Newcastle-Upon-Tyne: Daily Journal Office, 1866. https://wellcomecollection.org/works/kujympt3. [accessed 08 January 2024].

Dumfries and Galloway Archives and Local Studies

DGH1/2/2/2/1, Annual Reports 1st–18th, Crichton Royal Institution.

DGH1/6/17/1, C.R.I. Scrapbook, *Catalogue of the Library of the Crichton Royal Institution*, Dumfries: Crichton Press, 1853.

Ireland, G. O. 'Bibliotherapy – The Use of Books as a Form of Treatment in a Neuropsychiatric Hospital', *Medical Bulletin* 5 (1929): 443.

John Bull, 20.545 (Saturday 11 November 1916): 3.

Kellogg, John Harvey. *Ladies' Guide in Health and Disease: Girlhood, Maidenhood, Wifehood, Motherhood*. New York: Modern Medicine Publishing, 1893.

Koch, Theodore Wesley. *War Libraries and Allied Studies*. New York: G. E. Stechert & Co, 1918.

London Metropolitan Archives (LMA)

H46/SP/Y/01/001, *Springfield War Hospital Gazette*, March 1918.

H50/A/01/001 Napsbury Standing Sub-Committee of Visitors, Minutes Vol. 1.

H50/A/01/023 Napsbury Standing Sub-Committee of Visitors, Minutes Vol. 23.

H50/A/01/024 Napsbury Standing Sub-Committee of Visitors, Minutes Vol. 24.

H50/A/01/026 Napsbury Standing Sub-Committee of Visitors, Minutes Vol. 26.

Lothian Health Services Archive, GD16/52, *Catalogue of the Library of the Royal Edinburgh Asylum*. Morningside, Edinburgh: Royal Asylum Press, 1861.

Macfie, Catherine M. E. 'Matron's Report', *The Eleventh Report of the Committee of Visitors of the County Lunatic Asylum at Hanwell: January Quarter Session, 1856*. London: John Thomas Norris, 1856. https://wellcomecollection.org/works/wtb5fhst. [accessed 08 January 2024].

Marshall, W. G. 'Letter to the Committee of Visitors', *The Seventh Annual Report of the Committee of Visitors of the County Lunatic Asylum at Colney Hatch: January Quarter Session, 1858*. London: John Thomas Norris, 1858. https://wellcomecollection.org/works/yq46jq96. [accessed 08 January 2024].

M'Cullough, David M. 'Report of the Medical Superintendent', *The Sixth Annual Report of the Committee of Visitors of the Joint Lunatic Asylum for the Counties of Monmouth, Hereford, Brecon, Radnor, and City of Hereford, for the Year 1858*. Abergavenny: Catharine Wilson, 1859. https://wellcomecollection.org/works/bam2v89n. [accessed 08 January 2024].

MCC/MIN/05/070, R. A. Squires, Chaplain's Report, *The Third Annual Report of the Visiting Committee of the Middlesex County Lunatic Asylum at Napsbury, 1907–1908*. London: Harrison & Sons, 1908.

MCC/MIN/05/070, Report of the Commissioners in Lunacy, 12 June 1909, *The Fifth Annual Report Relating to the Middlesex County Lunatic Asylum at Napsbury, 1909–1910*. London: Harrison & Sons, 1910.

Reid, John. *Essays on Hypochondriasis and Other Nervous Affections*, 3rd edn. London: Longman, Hurst, Rees, Orme and Brown, 1823.

Skae, David. 'Physician's Report', *Annual Report of the Royal Edinburgh Asylum for the Insane: For the Year 1860*. Edinburgh: Royal Asylum Press, 1861. https://wellcomecollection.org/works/ehd6z7gg. [accessed 08 January 2024].

Spring, J. Burchell. 'Chaplain's Report', *Report of the Committee of Visitors of the Lunatic Asylum for the City and County of Bristol for the Year 1873, Together with the Reports of the Medical Superintendent & Chaplain*. Bristol: Leech and Taylor, 1874. https://wellcomecollection.org/works/dujcanj7 [accessed 08 January 2024].

Thirty-fifth Annual Report of the Directors of the Dundee Royal Asylum for Lunatics: Submitted, in Terms of Their Charter, to a General Meeting of the Directors, 18 June 1855, with the Report of the Medical Officers. Dundee: Northern Warder Office, 1855. https://wellcomecollection.org/works/vj49j4bb. [accessed 08 January 2024].

Tuke, Samuel. *Description of the Retreat, an Institution Near York, for Insane Persons of the Society of Friends: Containing an Account of Its Origin and Progress, the Modes of Treatment, and a Statement of Cases*. Philadelphia: Isaac Pierce, 1813.

University of Dundee Archive Services, THB29/11/2/1, *Catalogue of the Library of Murray's Royal Institution, Perth, compiled by M. W. J.* Perth: Robert Whittet, 1863.

Visiting Commissioners, *The Twenty-Eighth Report of the Committee of Visitors of the County Lunatic Asylum at Hanwell: January Quarter Session, 1873*. London: Harrison and Sons, 1873. https://wellcomecollection.org/works/ntf6sek2. [accessed 08 January 2024].

Secondary sources

Barham, Peter. *Forgotten Lunatics of the Great War*. New Haven: Yale University, 2004.

Bate, Jonathan and Andrew Schuman. 'The Art of Medicine. Books Do Furnish a Mind: the Art and Science of Bibliotherapy', *Lancet* 387 (February 2016): 742–743.

Beech, Ian. 'The Universal Khaki: The Impact of the Asylum War Hospital Scheme on Cardiff City Mental Hospital, 1915–1920', *Llafur: Journal of the Welsh People's History Society* 9, no. 2 (2005): 4–26.

Blackwood, Ashleigh. 'Toxic Texts and Reading Remedies: Literary Medicine in Eighteenth-Century Print Cultures', *Literature and Medicine* 34 (2016): 278–298.

Blair, Laura Gray. '"Library as Laboratory": Moral Treatment, Patient Libraries and Reading in Nineteenth-Century British Asylums', PhD diss. Queen Mary University of London, 2024.

Bunch, Antonia J. *Hospital and Medical Libraries in Scotland: An Historical and Sociological Study*. Glasgow: Scottish Library Association, 1975.

Campbell, Jessica. 'The Healing Arts? An Examination of Madness, Creativity and Experience in British Asylum Culture c.1840–1914', PhD diss. University of Edinburgh, forthcoming.

Cherry, Steven. *Mental Health Care in Modern England: The Norfolk Lunatic Asylum/St. Andrew's Hospital c.1810–1998*. Woodbridge: Boydell Press, 2003.

Cherry, Steven and Roger Munting. '"Exercise Is the Thing"? Sport and the Asylum c.1850–1950', *International Journal of the History of Sport* 22, no. 1 (2005): 42–58.

Connor, Jennifer. 'Medical Library History: A Survey of the Literature in Great Britain and North America', *Libraries & Culture* 24 (1989): 459–474.

Cracknell, Peter, et al. 'County Asylums', www.countyasylums.co.uk [accessed 25 May 2024].

Crammer, J. L. 'The Extraordinary Deaths of Asylum Inmates during the 1914–1918 War', *Medical History* 36, no. 4 (1992): 430–441.

Daskalova, Mila. 'Printing and Periodical Culture in the Nineteenth-Century Asylum', PhD diss. University of Strathclyde, 2022.

Daskalova, Mila. 'Printing as Poison, Printing as Cure: Work and Health in the Nineteenth-Century Printing Office and Asylum', *Book History* 24, no. 1 (2021): 58–84.

Devine, Judith, and Philip Barton Wright. 'The Impact of World War I on Asylums in the UK', *British Journal of Mental Health Nursing* 3, no. 6 (2014): 264–267.

Dunkel, Lisa M. 'Moral and Humane: Patients' Libraries in Early Nineteenth-Century American Mental Hospitals', *Bulletin of the Medical Library Association* 71, no. 3 (1983): 274–281.

Edginton, Barry. 'Moral Architecture: The Influence of the York Retreat on Asylum Design', *Health & Place* 3, no. 2 (1997): 91–99.

Ellis, Rob. 'Asylums and Sport: Participation, Isolation and the Role of Cricket in the Treatment of the Insane', *International Journal of the History of Sport* 30, no. 1 (2013): 83–101.

Farquharson, Jennifer. '"Passing the Border": The Civilian and Soldier Patient in the Scottish Asylum, 1914–1934', PhD diss. Glasgow Caledonian University, 2019.

Geddes, Jennian F. 'Deeds *and* Words in the Suffrage Military Hospital in Endell Street', *Medical History* 51 (2007): 79–98.

Golding, Rosemary. *Music and Moral Management in the Nineteenth-Century English Lunatic Asylum*. London: Palgrave Macmillan, 2021.

Hamlett, Jane. *At Home in the Institution: Material Life in Asylums, Lodging Houses and Schools in Victorian and Edwardian England*. Basingstoke: Palgrave Macmillan, 2015.

Haslam, Sara. 'Reading, Trauma and Literary Caregiving 1914–1918: Helen Mary Gaskell and the War Library', *Journal of Medical Humanities* 41 (2020): 305–321.

Haslam, Sara, and Edmund G. C. King. '"Medicinable Literature": Bibliotherapy, Literary Caregiving, and the First World War', *Literature and Medicine* 39, no. 2 (2021): 296–318.

Haw, Camilla, and Graeme Yorston. 'Thomas Prichard and the Non-Restraint Movement at the Northampton Asylum', *Psychiatric Bulletin* 28 (2004): 140–142.

Hilton, Claire. *Civilian Lunatic Asylums during the First World War: A Study of Austerity on London's Fringe*. Cham, Switzerland: Palgrave Macmillan, 2021.

Jones, Edgar. 'Shell Shock at Maghull and the Maudsley: Models of Psychological Medicine in the UK', *Journal of the History of Medicine and Allied Sciences* 65 (2010): 368–395.

Jones, Kathleen. *Law and Conscience, 1744-1845: The Social History of the Care of the Insane*. Abingdon: Routledge, 1998.

Kelly, Brendan D. 'Shell Shock in Ireland: The Richmond War Hospital, Dublin (1916–19)', *History of Psychiatry* 26, no. 1 (2014): 50–63.

King, Edmund G. C. 'E. W. Hornung's Unpublished "Diary", the YMCA, and the Reading Soldier in the First World War', *English Literature in Transition, 1880–1920* 57, no. 3 (2014): 361–387.

Laws, Jennifer. 'Crackpots and Basket-cases: A History of Therapeutic Work and Occupation', *History of the Human Sciences* 24 (2011): 65–81.

Levin, Len. 'Bibliotherapy: Tracing the Roots of a Moral Therapy Movement in the United States from the Early Nineteenth Century to the Present', *Journal of the Medical Library Association* 101, no. 2 (2013): 89–91.

Mahoney, Mary. 'Books as Medicine: A History of the Use of Reading to Treat the Self and Its Diseases in the Anglophone World, 1800-1940'. PhD diss. University of Connecticut, 2018.

Mahoney, Mary. 'From Library War Service to Science: Bibliotherapy in World War I', https://booksasmedicine.com/librarywarservice/. [accessed 08 January 2024].

Martin, Meredith. '"Therapeutic Measures": The Hydra and Wilfred Owen at Craiglockhart War Hospital', *Modernism/Modernity* 14 (2007): 35–54.

Mays, Kelly J. 'The Disease of Reading and Victorian Periodicals'. In *Literature in the Marketplace: Nineteenth-century British Publishing and Reading Practices*, edited by John O. Jordan and Robert L. Patten, 165–194. Cambridge: Cambridge University Press, 1995.

McDaniel, W. B. 'Bibliotherapy – Some Historical and Contemporary Aspects', *American Library Association Bulletin* 50.9 (October 1956): 584–589.

Miller, Jesse. 'Medicines of the Soul: Reparative Reading and the History of Bibliotherapy', *Mosaic: An Interdisciplinary Critical Journal* 51, no. 2 (2018): 17–34.

Murray, Flora. *Women as Army Surgeons: Being the History of the Women's Hospital Corps in Paris, Wimereux and Endell Street; September 1914–October 1919*. London: Hodder and Stoughton, 1920.

Oswald, Ute. '"Distraction from Hurtful Thoughts" – "Von trüben Gedanken ablenken": Recreational Activities as Agents of Healing in Nineteenth-century British Asylums', *Medizinhistorisches Journal* 56 (2021): 30–57.

Park, Maureen. *Art in Madness: Dr W. A. F. Browne's Collection of Patient Art at Crichton Royal Institution, Dumfries*. Dumfries: Dumfries and Galloway Health Board, 2010.

Porter, Roy. *Mind Forg'd Manacles: A History of Madness in England from the Restoration to the Regency*. London: Athlone Press, 1987.

Reid, Fiona. *Broken Men: Shell Shock, Treatment and Recovery in Britain 1914-30*. London: Bloomsbury, 2012.

Reiss, Benjamin. *Theatres of Madness: Insane Asylums and Nineteenth-Century American Culture*. Chicago: University of Chicago Press, 2008.

Reznick, Jeffrey S., *Healing the Nation: Soldiers and the Culture of Caregiving in Britain during the Great War*. Manchester: Manchester University Press, 2004.

Richardson, Harriet. 'Historic Hospitals: An Architectural Gazetteer', https://historic-hospitals.com [accessed 25 May 2024].

Rutherford, Sarah. 'Landscapers for the Mind: English Asylum Designers, 1845-1914', *Garden History* 33, no. 1 (2005): 61–86.

Scull, Andrew. 'The Domestication of Madness', *Medical History* 27 (1983): 233–248.

Shoenfeldt, Michael. 'Reading Bodies', In *Reading, Society and Politics in Early Modern England*, edited by Kevin Sharpe and Steven N. Zwicker, 215–243. Cambridge: Cambridge University Press, 2003.

Smith, Leonard D. *Cure, Comfort and Safe Custody: Public Lunatic Asylums in Early Nineteenth-Century England*. London: Leicester University Press, 1999.

Sutcliffe, Marcella P. 'Reading at the Front: Books and Soldiers in the First World War', *Pedagogica Historica* 52, no. 1–2 (2016): 104–120.

Taylor, Jeremy. *Hospital and Asylum Architecture in England, 1840-1914: Building for Health Care*. London: Mansell, 1991.

Topp, Leslie. 'Single Rooms, Seclusion and the Non-Restraint Movement in British Asylums, 1838–1844', *Social History of Medicine* 31, no. 4 (2018): 754–773.

Turner, Emily Jessica. 'Patients' creative work and "expressive possibilities" in *New Moon*, *Under the Dome*, and *The Hydra*, 1844-1918'. PhD diss. University of Sussex, 2019.

2 Galsworthy's First World War Writing as Self-Care

Helen Chambers

On 3 August 1914, at Wingstone Farm, his house on the edge of Dartmoor, John Galsworthy (1867–1933) wrote in his diary, anticipating not only the social but the very personal trauma to come:

> A miserably anxious day, ourselves hovering on the edge of this war [...]. I hate and abhor war of all kinds; I despise and loathe it. And the thought of the million daily acts of its violence and hateful brutishness keeps riving my soul. I try not to think of all the poor creatures who are suffering and will suffer so terribly.[1]

An altruistic and immensely compassionate man, Galsworthy remained throughout the war morally and emotionally opposed to it.[2] Hypersensitive to the suffering on all sides, he responded with an outpouring of literary activity in various forms and for various reasons. In addition to the public ways in which he contributed directly to the war effort by his very substantial fundraising through his writing and later magazine editing, he also used writing to overcome his own often deeply conflicted feelings. During the early days of the war, these feelings had left him emotionally sickened and creatively paralysed – a kind of 'war sickness' – but as this chapter will show, he was also able to heal through his writing. A further outcome of his writing was the raising of very substantial funds for the war effort through the sale of manuscripts.[3] My focus in this chapter, however, is how Galsworthy used his writing to address a range of subjects about which he had strong and often complex feelings. These included not only his opposition to the increasing levels of xenophobic patriotism (this despite his own deep and abiding love for the English countryside and its inhabitants) but also his almost unbounded compassion for the sick and wounded of any nationality, his empathy with ordinary Germans whose lives were caught up in the war (and which he could not publicly express), and his support for conscientious objectors and other forms of passive resistance. At a very personal level he also confronted, as he wrote, the death of his mother about whom he had long held ambivalent feelings, his own externally subdued emotional and sexual attitudes, and the final loss of his Christian faith.

This chapter, therefore, examines and charts the trajectory of Galsworthy's wartime literary activity, showing how, from his early rapid and prolific writing to raise

DOI: 10.4324/9781003471561-4

general funds for the war effort in order to partially appease his guilt about not joining up, through his various cathartic outpourings addressing complex issues close to his heart, to his targeted work for disabled servicemen and other causes, it can usefully be placed under the rubric of what Sara Haslam has called 'responsive literary caregiving' (rather than 'top-down' literary provision).[4] This model, which encompasses any form of non-institutionalised non-politically driven textually related therapeutic activity, whether reading to one's self or others, writing for various reasons, or facilitating the charitable provision of reading or writing materials to others, is a concept which can be located within the broad framework of bibliotherapy but directed toward emotional and psychological well-being. Literary self-care, as I use it in this chapter, is related to this concept, offering a development of it: referring to a self-directed intervention in which a person addresses and attempts to relieve, through their own actions, the psychological distress and pain of personal trauma or moral anguish and thus improving their own physical and/or psychological well-being. The established literature on bibliotherapy rarely highlights creative writing, the nearest perhaps being Debbie McCullis when she wrote about 'client-directed bibliotherapy', part of which involves creative writing in which the writer and their fictional character both address an area of concern.[5] The use of poetry writing as therapy, discussed by Lengelle and Meijers, does touch on this aspect of bibliotherapy in the broadest sense, though generally as a directed or group activity.[6] However, Lengelle and Meijer's theoretical 'black box' framework is very relevant to my discussion in this chapter. Galsworthy's reaction to the outbreak of war and associated atrocities could be considered his 'boundary experience', and his early rapid writing responses were, I suggest, his 'first story'. Later I will discuss how Galsworthy constructed what this framework refers to as a 'second story', illustrating therefore an example of how 'the aim of therapeutic writing is to work toward a more life-giving perspective or (be helped to) develop [...] a "second story" [with] a shift in perspective, acceptance, or meaning found/constructed'.[7] I propose that all of Galsworthy's vast output of wartime writing fits not only within the broader framework of bibliotherapy (at least of 'creative bibliotherapy') but more specifically as a form of responsive literary caregiving. It can be seen as a prototype case study in literary self-care specifically through entirely self-directed writing, and many decades before creative writing became an established therapeutic modality.

Biographical Context

Born near London into a conservative upper middle-class family, Galsworthy, despite a conventional mid-Victorian education, including considerable sporting achievements, always considered himself something of an outsider. After Harrow, he read law at New College, Oxford, was called to the bar in 1890, and though he never practiced, his legal knowledge informed much of his writing. In 1892, while taking a 'gap year' voyage to Sydney and the South Pacific with a university friend, and failing to find a passage to Samoa to meet Robert Louis Stevenson, he went on to Adelaide where in March 1893 he boarded the fast passenger clipper *Torrens* for

Cape Town. It was at Port Adelaide that he first encountered Joseph Conrad, then serving as the *Torrens*'s First Officer, and thus began 31 years of close friendship.

Back in London, Galsworthy had, by 1895, begun a discrete but passionate affair with the unhappily married wife of his cousin Arthur. Beautiful, elegant, and highly intelligent, Ada Nemesis Cooper *née* Pearson (1864–1956) was a talented near-professional grade pianist, a translator, and a composer of songs.[8] The couple only married after John Galsworthy Senior's death in 1904. Galsworthy's writing career began in 1897 and, with family money, no children, and later well provided for in his father's will, he was not, unlike his friends Joseph Conrad and Ford Madox Ford, obliged to write in order to earn a living and support a family. Instead, he saw writing as his lifelong vocation, conscientiously working at it almost daily even while travelling. Outwardly calm, mild-mannered, emotionally stable, and with strong support from Ada he had, by the outbreak of war, published eight novels, two short story collections, and nine plays including the very successful *The Silver Box* (1906) and *Strife* (1909), both plays with themes of social injustice. His best-known pre-war novel was *The Man of Property* (1906), a detached, lightly satirical, and at times scathing portrait of his own class, particularly those whose wealth derived from property development and stock market speculation. Although never formally affiliated with a political party, Galsworthy was essentially Liberal. He had a very strong social conscience and, increasingly facilitated by his influential social and political connections, was an active campaigner, pamphleteer, and petitioner for a range of causes including (among others and at various levels of intensity) workers' rights, minimum wages, tenants' rights, prison reform, animal rights (particularly causes related to horses, dogs, and wild birds), censorship reform, women's suffrage, divorce law reform, maternal and child health during the war, disabled servicemen, internment of 'enemy aliens', and, after the war, housing reforms and food security. Jill Felicity Durey has examined in detail Galsworthy's empathy and compassion as an integral part of his engagement, through his writing, with many of these reforms, pre- and post-war as well as wartime, about which he personally felt very strongly, and usefully links social and historical context with Galsworthy's emotional life and literary output.[9] In the broadest bibliotherapeutic context, his writing at times directly led to social reforms – a shared benefit. Durey devotes a chapter to his controversial but successful play *Justice* (1910), for example, which specifically addressed the evils of prolonged solitary confinement in prisons and led to a change in the law in 1910.[10]

Galsworthy's literary responses to the war were wide-ranging, and his output can be summarised as follows: rapid early revision of current work in progress with the very substantial USA proceeds dedicated entirely to war relief funds; targeted government-initiated propaganda and explanatory writing aimed at the American periodical-reading public in order to encourage American intervention; two emotionally charged rapidly written long romantic novels; a series of rather more tightly crafted short stories and sketches in which, directly or indirectly, he overtly expressed his ambiguous and painful feelings about the war; what he called 'humanist' essays on social reforms and post-war reconstruction written not only to raise funds but also as powerful therapeutic expressions of his own attitudes;

soothing nostalgic reflections on nature and the English countryside; and lastly, throughout 1918 until early 1919, by his professional editorial activity in reactivating a disabled soldiers' magazine originally entitled *Recalled to Life* then *Reveille*. Galsworthy's significant involvement with *Reveille* and what he called 'the sacred work' of rehabilitating disabled servicemen for a meaningful post-war life, using physical, psychological, and occupational therapy, has been discussed in detail by Jeffrey Reznick, who has examined this aspect of Galsworthy's activity, not only as literary history but also from the perspective of disability studies and of material culture studies.[11] Reznick writes that 'Galsworthy's very act of writing about, and his very actions connected with, disabled soldiers were as much about his self-empowerment in the face of perceived disability as they were about propaganda', an argument that is crucial to focus on Galsworthy's literary self-care.[12] Reznick, moreover, lightly anticipates a definition of literary self-care, though limiting his reflections to Galsworthy's writings on disability: 'Galsworthy sought to overcome his sense of paralysis [...] through engagement in the occupation he knew best, namely writing'.[13] Durey, on the other hand, focuses on Galsworthy's compassionate output towards a range of causes, without addressing the internalised and empowering self-care aspects of his writing. This chapter therefore extends both Reznick's and Durey's work in its consideration of a wider range of Galsworthy's (mostly fictional) war writing in order to establish the trajectory of his literary self-care in the light of a bibliotherapeutic critical framework. I place his substantial compassionate output aimed ostensibly at garnering funds for the war effort and at raising public awareness of specific social issues resulting from war, into the context of bibliotherapy in its broadest sense. This chapter demonstrates that all of Galsworthy's wartime writing constituted self-therapy from the most obvious (doing something for the war effort without enlisting) to the compassionate and at times cathartic 'writing out' of his own deep-seated torment.

Soon after the outbreak of war, on 15 November 1914, Galsworthy made one of his most significant diary entries. It declares his acute moral turmoil and offers a revelation which he then sought to mediate by purposeful writing:

> The heart searchings of this War are terrible; the illumination of oneself rather horrible. I think and think what is my duty, and all the time I know that if I arrived at certain conclusions I shouldn't do that duty. This is what comes of giving oneself to a woman body and soul. A[da] paralyses me and has always paralysed me. I have never been able to face the idea of being cut off from her.[14]

Letters and diaries are essential to establishing the timeline and the trajectory of Galsworthy's war writing – from the immediate shock, horror, diffuse anxiety guilt, internal conflict, and temporary creative paralysis, as expressed above, through therapeutic writing in which he sought to absolve his guilt and as emotional catharsis, to a flourishing creative output arguably starting in 1916 but most obviously just before the end of the war. My focus will be on the short stories and sketches with wartime themes, mostly published in newspapers and periodicals, and collected immediately post-war in *Tatterdemalion* (1920)[15] and on his rather curious wartime novels. It is also worth noting here that his diaries and letters contain very little comment about the critical reception of any of his wartime writings, and show how, apart from acknowledging praise from his friends, he remained unconcerned by its reception, as long as it sold well enough in England and in America to raise money for the war effort.

'Making Money for the Country': Galsworthy's Early Responses to War

Galsworthy's diary entries from Dartmoor during the last days of July and the first few days of August 1914, in addition to noting his daily activities of writing, reading, walking, and riding, include a concentration of ominous phrases, such as 'these war-clouds are monstrous', 'war clouds still black', 'this awful catastrophe [...] the suddenness of this horror is appalling', 'Too ghastly for words [...] the nightmare of it'.[16] Agonising about what he could actively do to justify why he did not enlist he wrote on 15 November:

> In cool blood I suppose what I am doing – that is writing on – novels and stories – and devoting all I can make, especially from America – no mean sum [about £1200 already by November] to Relief – is being of more use than attempting to mismanage Relief Funds, or stretcher-bearing at some hospital, or even training my elderly unfit body in some elderly corps.[17]

The context is critical here. Earlier, on 5 September 1914, he had rather exaggerated, in a letter to his friend the writer Ralph Mottram, his own perceived disability: 'If I weren't married and old [he was 47] and blind and bald and game in the shoulder I believe these atrocities would make me go and forswear all my convictions [...]'. In a conscious process of self-justification, therefore, Galsworthy had already constructed an image of himself as physically disabled and therefore inevitably to be judged unfit for service (he did indeed suffer from poor eyesight and a relatively minor unresolved shoulder injury), thus rationalising his fear of being separated from Ada. In reality, he remained an active equestrian and regular energetic hill walker throughout the war years and afterwards. Perhaps he was also displacing his own feelings when he expressed his great relief that Peggy, his favourite mare, was after the army's first local mustering on 5 August 'rejected as unsound'? It is worth noting here that as late as 22 July 1918, after being obliged by the new Manpower Bill to present himself for army service, Galsworthy received his definitive rejection (on the grounds only of weak eyesight) and his discharge certificate. This he copied out and kept among his papers, perhaps because it served to retrospectively vindicate his tormented decision in 1914.

At a public level, Galsworthy had very quickly sprung into action. By 1 August he had enquired about ambulance classes and attended a local meeting to establish a Nursing Fund, and on 5 August wrote to *The Times* proposing an urgent War Relief Fund. By 9 August he had already donated a substantial amount to relief organisations and was writing his first fund-raising piece for *Scribner's Magazine*, called 'First Thoughts on this War', in which he expressed in an outburst of anger and bitterness some of his core values, such as his antipathy to jingoistic patriotism and to dogmatic Christianity.[18]

Late in 1914, Galsworthy wrote his first wartime short story, 'The Mother Stone', in which 'five elderly gentlemen discuss after dinner the causes of war', with an anecdote by the narrator on how the first diamond discovery in Southern Africa in 1860 eventually led to the Boer War and thence to global German ascendency.[19] After writing on 5 August that he was 'in despair of doing any new work',[20] Galsworthy's first and most substantial literary activity during that first week or so of the war was however to rapidly finish and revise *The Freelands* (1915), a rather academic sociological novel he had started in 1913, dealing with pre-war landowning families and the rights of tenant farmers in England. By mid-August 1914, he had 'settled down to finish *The Freelands* and make money (for the country)' and by 25 August he wrote: 'started my spurt to finish *The Freelands*. A big price is promised by Scribner's for the serial. So much American money will come in handy for relief funds'.[21] Taking advantage of his literary reputation Galsworthy was thus able to assuage in part at least his painful and ambivalent feelings of powerlessness; finishing this novel, which sold badly but raised money through serialisation, amounted to his first steps in literary self-care. He also contributed to the fund-raising charity books starting to appear, writing the foreword for *The Queen's Gift Book* in aid of disabled servicemen, and pieces for several other charity books all of which also amounted to early steps in the identification and 'treatment' of his own mental paralysis and perceived physical disability described above.[22]

'Chief Literary Men at Wellington House': Writing Information and Propaganda

Galsworthy's official war writing needs to be placed in its politico-literary context. While many young men, including Robert Graves, Siegfried Sassoon, Edward Thomas, Edmund Blunden, Wilfred Owen, Ivor Gurney, and Isaac Rosenberg, were serving (and some dying) at the Front, older writers took on more political roles. We know from Galsworthy's diary that he was summoned from Devon by telegram on 2 September 1914 and 'went up to a meeting (in London) of chief literary men at Wellington House to concert measures of putting forward principles for which England is fighting'.[23] This was the event convened by Liberal politician Charles Masterman, recently appointed as head of a secret new government department, the War Propaganda Bureau, generally referred to as 'Wellington House'.[24] Masterman had invited a group of 25 well-known writers including, as well as Galsworthy, Arnold Bennett, H. G. Wells, G. K. Chesterton, J. M. Barrie, John Buchan, Hall Caine, Conan Doyle, and John Masefield. Several of those invited agreed to write pamphlets and magazine articles, all aimed at countering German propaganda in the United States by promoting the official British position on the war. The government approached and funded commercial and university presses to publish, as seemingly independent works, the output of this bureau, which amounted to about 1,400 pamphlets and other publications during the war years.[25]

Though not invited to Masterman's Wellington House meeting, the Anglo-German Ford Madox Ford (until 1919 still using his birth name Hueffer), who had endured xenophobic insults at the outbreak of war, later joined Masterman's initiative and rapidly wrote a large number of propaganda pieces for *Outlook* before he was enlisted as a second lieutenant in 1915 in the Welch Regiment and which were published in 1915 as *When Blood is Their Argument* and *Between St Dennis and St George*. Lucinda Borkett-Jones argues convincingly in a finely nuanced essay that Ford, in his propaganda pieces, was not so much rejecting his German heritage but re-framing it to create a legitimate enemy Other.[26] This activity might also be construed as a form of literary self-care as defined earlier, since it served to highlight, analyse, and resolve his own ambivalence about his German roots and cultural identity.[27]

Ford's erstwhile friend and collaborator Joseph Conrad, trapped temporarily in Poland with his family at the outbreak of war, and at 56 too old to enlist, became ill and depressed after returning to England and wrote very little during the war apart from charity book pieces and *The Shadow-Line* (1917). This semi-autobiographical tale of a young merchant service officer's first command of a sailing ship, set in South East Asian waters in the late 1880s and dedicated to his son Borys serving in France, 'and all others who like himself have crossed in early youth the shadow-line of their generation', can also be read as a war metaphor. H. G. Wells satirised his own wartime activities in his best-selling novel *Mr Britling Sees It Through* (1916) and then withdrew from propaganda work.[28] D. H. Lawrence, vehemently opposed to the war, wrote a great deal of poetry, notably the collection *Look! We Have Come Through!* (1917) as his own literary self-care, struggled with the suppression of *The Rainbow* and drafted *Women in Love*. He and his German-born wife Frieda were expelled from Zennor near Land's End in Cornwall, suspected of spying. Overall, Galsworthy's literary responses to the war were more varied both in type and in quality, and far more prolific, than those penned by these key examples of his fellow writers.

Very conscious of the dangers of propaganda, Galsworthy wrote his American pieces to explain, level-headedly, the British position, as well as to help himself to find a measured distance from the horrors of the war and, of course, to raise money. Many of his journalistic pieces, including his 'humanist' essays, were first published in American periodicals and subsequently collected into two volumes. *A Sheaf*, which one critic rather extravagantly called 'a prose of pure gold that issues from a burning heart' – another found it 'ethically significant' – was published in 1916.[29] The second, *Another Sheaf* (1919), was also well-received, with its emphasis on post-war social reconstruction, including national food security. Reznick summarises this output: 'These companion volumes represent the largest concentration of Galsworthy's humanitarian writings before, during and immediately after the Great War'.[30]

The Wartime Novels: Fiction as Emotional Catharsis

After his intensive early fund-raising activity, Galsworthy, during some of the darkest days of the war, launched into a phase of what can be described as therapeutic creative writing, eventually producing, as well as numerous short stories discussed later, two interesting though by now almost forgotten romantic novels and a short satirical one. The two romantic works, *Beyond* (1917) and *Saint's Progress* (1919), include passages that were fairly sexually explicit for their time, and both have interesting and appealing central female characters, Gyp Winton and Noel Pierson. They were genre successors to his only romantic pre-war novel *The Dark Flower* (1912), a prose poem describing three episodes in the life of a sculptor, Mark Lennan. The third part of this novel, in which the married middle-aged sculptor becomes involved with a very young woman, is a therapeutic working out of Galsworthy's guilty feelings immediately after breaking off his short-lived (and almost certainly non-consummated) affair with the 19-year-old Margaret Morris, a talented and innovative London dancer and choreographer, and perhaps finally put to rest in *Beyond* in the character of the young dancer, Daphne Wing.

So what aspects of literary self-care was Galsworthy working through in these wartime novels? The first novel, *Beyond*, though set just before the war, which is only hinted at, was originally very long, written rapidly, and revised even more rapidly. He began it at Christmas 1914 and wrote throughout 1915 finishing on 2 January 1916. 'One year and seven days work; length 120,000 – the longest book I have written. It is very different to any of my others, but most like *The Dark Flower*'.[31] It is as though he was now writing out his otherwise repressed emotions which he had kept under control since *The Dark Flower* and during the early part of the war. There are faint echoes of Ada's childhood, unhappy first marriage, and her rescue by Galsworthy. But apart from these rather tenuous autobiographical gestures, the main themes of the novel, viewed retrospectively in relation to literary self-care, are its great outpouring of romantic and sexual feeling and presentation of a sympathetic disabled minor character. The novel centres on Gyp, a beautiful and illegitimate young woman who is something of an outsider, with a rebellious and unconventional personality and who certainly is one of Galsworthy's most appealing female characters. Gyp's beloved father Charles Winton is disabled 'after six years' service in India and Egypt, having lost his right hand in a charge against dervishes' (14) which, from the dating of the narrative, would have been during Kitchener's war in the Sudan in 1896. Significantly, given Galsworthy's ongoing involvement with disabled servicemen many of whom had limb prostheses, Winton has an impressive prosthetic leather hand. Gyp is attracted to and marries a strange, almost diabolical, Swedish violinist called Fiorsen, but after becoming pregnant leaves him to bring up their daughter alone. She then falls in love and lives in a rural idyll with a respectable young lawyer Brian Summerhays (a Galsworthy-like figure), who is killed in a spectacular riding accident. It was more popular than *The Freelands,* also not about war but, unlike *The Freelands* was a 'full blooded love story'.[32] It tends towards melodrama at times and suffers from sections which are over-written, including elaborate botanical metaphors for sexual activity. Marketed by Scribner's for its 'sensitivity and intimacy',[33] it sold quite well, despite or because of hostile reviews which emphasised Galsworthy's obsession with sex and 'a blinding mist of the erotic', though American reviewers were more flattering than British ones.[34] A number of his friends and literary peers wrote praising the novel including Edward Garnett and Thomas Hardy.[35] It seems that Galsworthy, who had quite intensely emotional though discretely expressed attitudes toward sex, was using this novel as a catharsis for these unexpressed feelings.

The second of these 'therapeutic' novels, *Saint's Progress* (1919), is more tightly written and firmly situated in the wartime present. Galsworthy began it in mid-1917, wrote hard between July and the end of that year, and finished it on 10 April 1918. Set in London in 1916–1917, it concerns a liberated young woman Noel Pierson and her father Edward, the eponymous 'saint', an idealistic but moralistic clergyman. Noel at 18 has become pregnant after spending a last night with her lover, a young officer, before he goes off to war and is killed. She rejects the idea of an abortion and is financially and emotionally supported by her father, despite the disapproval of his London parish. Galsworthy expresses unequivocally in this novel his sympathy for all victims of war regardless of nationality. At one point while Noel excitedly watches a burning Zeppelin above London, her father imagines with horror the German victims inside.[36] Noel then becomes sexually attracted to a much older, disabled soldier, Jimmy Fort, a liaison of which her father disapproves, and only after Edward is driven out of his parish to become an army chaplain in Egypt does Noel find some peace and happiness with Jimmy. Noel, in conversation with her father, also expresses support for conscientious objectors. As well as these familiar themes reflecting his compassion for all victims of war, the novel reflects Galsworthy's increasingly strong anticlerical stance and the loss of his Christian faith, further accelerated by the war, and his deep scepticism about all established religion, even though in this novel the clergyman is a sympathetic character. The book got mixed, at times lukewarm, reviews on both sides of the Atlantic though friends including J. M. Barrie and Thomas Hardy both enjoyed it, as did the critic and novelist W. L. George.[37] In terms of its cathartic function, as well as the issues mentioned above, the novel can be seen retrospectively as Galsworthy's most extensive fictional working out to date of his hostile attitude to dogmatic religion; there is however nothing in his diary or letters to indicate this intention, he merely called it, on 10 April 1918 while revising it, 'a curious book'.[38]

In 1918 Galsworthy also wrote, in short intense bursts of activity, a brief, abortive, mildly satiric novel *The Burning Spear: Being the Experiences of Mr John Lavender in Time of War*. This was first published in 1919 under the pseudonym 'A. R. P.-M'. Galsworthy later called it 'a revenge of nerves'. In a superficial almost trivial way, he mocks and satirises patriotic prose, including some of his own earnest humanistic proposals, and also his own work with disabled soldiers, hiding behind his anonymity.[39] As one critic puts it 'John Lavender is John Galsworthy made clownish, aging and wretched'.[40]

'A Mere Masseur': Hands-on Work in France and Its Literary Aftermath

On 3 October 1916, Galsworthy wrote to his friend the French critic André Chevrillon that he 'badly wanted a rest from the head and pen, and one can only rest from that by working with the hands'.[41] The amount of writing in 1916, which included producing and revising *Beyond*, writing 'A Stoic' and his fine story 'The Apple Tree' (see below), and revising his futuristic play *The Foundations,* was indeed intense. Galsworthy and Ada had recently accepted an invitation from their friend Dorothy Allhusen to spend the winter of 1916–1917 as volunteers at the *Hôpital Bénévole* which she had established as a convalescent home for French soldiers with rheumatic disorders and with shell-shock or other 'neurasthenic' problems. In a large house called Le Martouret, just outside the small provincial town of Die, in the mountainous south-eastern French *département* of the Drôme, Allhusen had rented part of what was already, since the 1860s, a well-equipped hydrotherapy centre specialising in rheumatic disorders.[42] Galsworthy took intensive lessons in 'Swedish massage' in London, to enable him to work as a masseur with the physically and mentally damaged *poilus*. Ada, with her nimble pianist's fingers, was to mend and maintain the hospital linen. It was Galsworthy's experience in France which generated, on his return, an intense period of writing about disability. This began during the 11 days the couple spent in March in Cassis near Marseilles, immediately after leaving Le Martouret, when Galsworthy wrote 'Flotsam and Jetsam', the first of the stories about disabled soldiers drawn from his experience there. This was followed in June 1917 by 'Cafard' and at some stage the following year 'Poirot and Bidan: A Recollection', and these three stories of disabled soldiers were later included in the *Tatterdemalion* collection. These three tales, all written as a direct result of his 'working with his hands' in France, suggest that this period of hands-on learning and physical care-giving experience at Le Martouret, which was intensely physically active, while ostensibly a break from writing, can be considered as an indirect aspect of his own ongoing literary self-care, not an explicit moving away from it but rather a means of displaying how he had overcome his own perceived physical disability.

Of these sensitive sketches inspired by the few months at Le Martouret, two – 'Flotsam and Jetsam' and 'Cafard' – concern psychologically damaged soldiers, while 'Poitou and Bidan' portray individuals with physical mobility problems. 'Flotsam and Jetsam' is a vivid and sympathetic portrayal of two severely shell-shocked French (but not entirely French) soldiers, who find themselves lost and adrift.[43] 'Flotsam' is a Breton fisherman longing for the sea, who consoles himself drinking, and climbing tall pine trees like masts, and gains satisfaction from making nets out of string, while 'Jetsam' (part-English) is a glassblower whose shell-shock makes him speechless and almost catatonic and who wanders vaguely around trying to escape. This sketch also includes an immediately recognisable vignette of the historic centre of the old town of Die's 'most quaint – all yellowish-grey, with rosy-tiled roofs. It had once been Roman, once a walled city of the Middle Ages', after which follows another page and a half of evocative description.[44] 'Poirot and Bidan'[45] first appeared in August 1918 in *Reveille* and is more of a portrait than a story of two patients, both with severe arthritis caused by long periods in the trenches and with contrasting attitudes to illness and rehabilitation.

The pleasantly sentimental 'feel-good' story 'Cafard' gains its title from the French word that not only means 'cockroach' but also refers to the black beetle of despair gnawing at the brain, symbolising depression or the 'black dog'.[46] It may well have originated from Galsworthy's own observations at Le Martouret or an incident relayed to him by a patient. Jean Liotard, a young soldier suffering shell shock, walks out one summer day and lies down on the sandy bank of the river Drôme. Terrified of being returned to the Front, he experiences deep fear and anguish and reflects on the Germans he had killed: 'something wrenched at his ribs. They were only Boches, but their wives and children, their mothers – faces questioning, faces pleading for them …'.[47] A small, scruffy but very real black dog approaches him, he gains its confidence by feeding it biscuits and feels cured of his own '*cafard*'.[48] Liotard's anguish about the collateral victims of war clearly mirrors Galsworthy's own, as also expressed in other works.

The longer story 'Spindleberries' has topographical reflections of Le Martouret and was also written in 1918, after the Galsworthys had returned to England. The narrator Richard Scudamore, a well-known painter, recalls in vivid visual detail in several vignettes and with each memory stimulated by the sight of a spray of pink spindleberries, a series of encounters with a woman called Alicia, an increasingly eccentric painter whom he had once loved. Their final encounter is in winter in France in 1904, when

> He had hired a little *château* in front of the Glandaz mountain – himself, his wife, their eldest girl, and Alicia […] with an absorbing view over the pantiled old town of Die […] and a ruined monastery high in the amphitheatre of the Glandaz mountain

here describing the beautiful landscape in which the Galsworthys hiked when not working.[49] This pleasant story, an impressionist tale about regeneration of artistic talent, can also be considered part of the rehabilitation phase of Galsworthy's literary self-care; Scudamore's Christmas visit to this specifically identified sub-Alpine region reflects not only Galsworthy's happy winter memories there 18 months earlier but also how, like the painter, he rediscovers his talent and begins afresh in a new style.

More Literary Fragments of War Experiences

In addition to the Martouret tales a number of other stories and sketches, also eventually collected in *Tatterdemalion*, clearly reveal the extent to which Galsworthy used his writing to further work out his feelings about a war which had highlighted his own self-doubts, thrown him into a personal moral dilemma and had raised new personal and social issues about which he was ambivalent or at times deeply troubled. It is this writing, alongside his emotional outpourings in the war novels discussed above which were both personal catharsis and further targeted fundraising to justify his non-combatant role, which constitute the main elements of his literary self-care, that is identifying an issue and working through it in a fictional or quasi-fictional manner. He explores in this way a number of important themes, some of which mirrored his own war experiences. It is therefore in this little-known volume, rather than in the novels, that we see the full range of Galsworthy's responses to war. The collection is divided unequally into two parts, 'Of Wartime' and 'Of Peacetime'. The 'peacetime' stories, apart from 'Spindleberries', are slight; several were in fact actually written during wartime not peacetime and two of those, 'A Strange Thing' (1916) and 'The Nightmare Child' (1917), have faint echoes of war, while one, 'Manna' (1916) is overtly and deliberately anti-clerical.[50]

Galsworthy's empathy with ordinary Germans is first revealed in the slightly sentimental story 'Defeat' (1916), a tale of a sympathetic but ultimately bitter encounter in London between a young officer and a prostitute.[51] The young German woman, calling herself 'May Belinski' and pretending to be Russian, has spent half her earnings on a Promenade concert at the Queens Hall, indulging in one of her regular 'music baths' to listen to Beethoven and Mozart.[52] Outside she meets a recently invalided young officer, also leaving the concert, attracts him back to her sordid room in Bloomsbury, and reveals her true nationality. They have a long conversation about the war, including mentioning a burning Zeppelin and its occupants. He cannot bring himself to have sex with her but nevertheless gives her money. As they stand by the window together, seduced by the moonlight, he muses 'Poor girl! […] and after all, fellow-feeling was bigger than principalities and powers! Fellow feeling was all pervading as this moonlight which she had said would be the same in Germany'. The moment and the feeling end abruptly with triumphant cries as newspaper vendors and crowds, celebrating a major German defeat, invade the street and, reflexively, the officer leans out and enthusiastically joins in the cheering. May, totally disillusioned and anticipating the imminent defeat of Germany, rips up his banknotes in despair and when he has left, collapses.

> She, who had just one shilling in this great town of enemies, who wrung her stealthy living out of the embraces of her foes! And suddenly in the moonlight she sat up and began to sing with all her might – '*Die Wacht am Rhein*'.[53]

Two contrasting stories describe the prevailing xenophobic nationalism and the treatment of ordinary Germans as enemy aliens.[54] In both 'The Bright Side' and 'The Dog It Was That Died', Galsworthy expresses his anger and despair about the internment of enemy aliens. His German brother-in-law, the painter Georg Sauter (1866–1937), the husband of Galsworthy's sister Lilian, and father of Galsworthy's much-loved nephew Rudolf ('Rudo') were interned, and these events affected Galsworthy deeply. Detained for 13 months in Wakefield, South Yorkshire, in December 1915, Georg Sauter was virtually deprived of visitors, the only one he had being Galsworthy, who was permitted only a single 30-minute visit, travelling from south Devon to Yorkshire and back within 24 hours. Galsworthy petitioned the government about this internment but was unsuccessful, possibly because of the interference of the militantly jingoist Northcliffe popular press. In

'The Bright Side', Max Gerhardt – a German leather craftsman from the Black Forest region – has been settled in London for 18 years and is married to Dora (Dolly), the daughter of a Putney carpenter and with whom he has three children. He is suddenly and brutally interned, which Galsworthy, for narrative convenience, locates not in Yorkshire but at the Alexandra Palace, London (where Rudo was interned), thus allowing Dolly her weekly visits. Dolly endures increasingly xenophobic comments from her neighbours and stops reading the newspapers, an action which reflects Galsworthy's hatred of the popular press. Like Galsworthy, who petitioned for the release of his brother-in-law, Dolly goes to Whitehall and pleads unsuccessfully for Max's release. We get a glimpse of the squalid conditions of the internees 'an encampment of brown blankets, slung and looped up anyhow, dividing from each other countless sordid beds, which were almost touching, and a whiff of huddled humanity'.[55] Eventually, in 1919, Max, like Georg Sauter, is released, an ill and broken man. 'The Dog It Was That Died' is a contrasting tale about a long-established half-British half-German family called Holsteig, middle-class this time, so more like the Sauters. Like them, the husband is interned and, like Sauter, is eventually repatriated to Germany. The story overall is more subtle and less sentimental than 'The Bright Side'. The xenophobic middle-class British view is expressed here through a neighbour called Harburn, and the whole tale is recounted by a Galsworthy-like frame narrator Cumbermere.

Several short sketches seem to be based directly on Galsworthy's wartime observations, and all reveal his compassionate nature. In 'Recorded' (1915), the narrator encounters a poor family in a train compartment, the wife and children travelling to farewell the soldier husband, all described in realistic and sympathetic detail. 'The Recruit' (1917), in which a very young and illiterate farm boy tries unsuccessfully to sign up for the Royal Marines, suggests an encounter or an anecdote from rural Devonshire.[56] 'The Peace Meeting', written in the late summer of 1917, at the same time as Galsworthy sent a plea for '800 extreme conscientious objectors', also reads as though based on personal observation.[57]

In contrast to 'Cafard', Galsworthy offers a different conjunction of dogs and war in 'In Heaven and Earth' (1917). This sharp very short Maupassant-like story, told by a painter to a group of friends during an after-dinner storytelling competition (theme: 'the queerest thing seen during the war'), is about a man who feels morally obliged to ask the vet to shoot a local dog for stealing eggs and thus eating food destined for others at a time when food was scarce, but who then breaks down inconsolably over the dog's body while digging its grave. The narrator then marvels at how

> the same creatures who are blowing each other to little bits all the time, bombing babies, roasting fellow creatures in the air and cheering while they roast [...] are capable of feeling like that about shooting a wretched ill cur of a dog, no good to anybody.[58]

Very soon after returning from Le Martouret, Galsworthy wrote a delicate story 'The Grey Angel' (1917), his most detailed and sensitive working out of his complex feelings towards his mother. It tells of an elderly English woman living alone in southern France. The town is not named, but there are several references to Arles, which the Galsworthys visited for the first time in 1917[59] including its antiquity, inhabited by 'ancient peoples, the Romans, Gauls, Saracens and all, and still looked out toward the flat Camargue';[60] it also possesses some small hill town features, perhaps of Die itself. The unnamed 'Grey Angel' lives alone with a maid and a parrot, separated by the war from her son and daughter. 'Her predilection for things French came from childish recollections of school-days in Paris and a hasty removal thence by her father during the revolution of '48. […] Unto her seventy-eighth year, her French accent had remained unruffled […] and her face had the pale, unwrinkled, slightly aquiline perfection of the French marquise type' a description which matches perfectly Georg Sauter's portrait in oils of Blanche Galsworthy, who spent her last years alone, though in Torquay, not France.[61] The fictional 'Grey Angel' fills her days knitting socks and scarves and visiting French soldiers in the local hospital, carrying various carefully budgeted, thoughtful but not always appropriate gifts, cigarettes, games, books, and magazines. Eventually, she fatally neglects her own health for fear of causing trouble to others; her son and daughter (as did Galsworthy and his sister Lilian) rush to her bedside, and she dies content.

Mothers and fathers and their relationships with their adult children feature throughout Galsworthy's writing and echo his own life story. Frances Freeland in *The Freelanders* and the unnamed 'Grey Angel' are the final working out of Galsworthy's ambivalent relationship with his mother, who was quietly self-sacrificing, engendering guilt in others.[62] Furthermore, it was around the same time, just after returning from France in spring 1917 that Galsworthy, in 'The Indian Summer of a Forsyte' wrote his last ambiguously sympathetic portrayal of his own father, as Old Jolyon. This type of autobiographical writing could be considered a distinct subgenre of literary self-care.[63]

Nature and Landscape Writing as Literary Self-Care

As well as incorporating detailed description of landscape and vegetation into his wartime novels, notably as overdone metaphors in *Beyond*, Galsworthy wrote a number of reflective shorter pieces during the war which might count as nature writing, with sketches and stories based on his rural experiences in the Sussex and Devonshire landscapes in which he always found calm and relief. In some pieces, the landscape and vegetation are part of the fabric of the story or novel, not only 'The Apple Tree' (see below) but also 'A Strange Thing' (1916) in which the unique atmosphere of the Devonshire countryside and the effects of unintended pregnancy during war time are the main themes.[64] Here the narrator, on a solitary rural walk, stumbles into the village wedding of the prettiest girl around; a little later he encounters a worn-out-looking woman of 35 who had come incognito to watch the wedding, which is in fact that of her illegitimate daughter, given up at birth having been conceived during a one-night stand with a local lad later killed during the Boer War.

The greatest influence on this kind of nature writing was almost certainly the Argentinian-born writer W. H. Hudson (1841–1922) whom Galsworthy had known for many years in London and greatly admired, as did Conrad and Ford. In February 1916, the Galsworthys visited Hudson at his nursing home in Cornwall, and again the following month. It was immediately after this second visit that Galsworthy began 'The Apple Tree' (1916), one of his finest long stories which not only celebrates the beautiful Devon landscape but explores the notion of 'chivalry'. A happily married man revisits, with his wife, the site of a brief love affair 26 years earlier and recalls his rather callous abandonment of this pretty and naïve rural girl for a more sophisticated urban wife, with the tragic outcome of the affair only revealed at the end. It appeared in *Five Tales* (1918) and was among the first significant works to signal Galsworthy's creative regeneration. He had, after the cathartic outpourings of the two novels and the tighter generally better structured but often quite sentimental shorter pieces begun again to write works of better overall literary quality.

'A Second Flowering': Writing Regenerated

While all of the *Five Tales* invoke subjects about which Galsworthy felt strongly and had already been trying to work through, these stories are more robust, more tightly controlled, and less self-indulgent than the earlier pieces rapidly written to highlight particular social or personal emotional issues. They were, I suggest therefore, part of Galsworthy's 'second story', to use the framework of Lengelle and Meijers. The writing of several of the *Five Tales* coincided with the period when he was also finishing *Saint's Progress*, which suggests that this novel marked the end of his need for intense emotional relief through writing. In the first of the *Five Tales,* 'The First and the Last' (actually started late in 1913), a respectable lawyer protects his dissolute brother allowing him to escape a murder charge and is one of Galsworthy's many explorations of guilt *versus* responsibility. He had begun the second, 'A Stoic', on 5 February 1916, a few days after finishing *Beyond*, and no two works could be more different in style, tone, and content. He wrote 'Wingstone. Lovely day. Began a new story *A Stoic* writing out of doors in the sun'.[65] The story features Sylvanus Heythorp, a sympathetically portrayed elderly man, who is arranging his inheritance, and it is almost a precursor to *In Chancery*, the next volume of the *Forsyte Saga*. 'The Apple Tree' is discussed above. 'The Juryman', in which a young mentally fragile 'neurasthenic' soldier is being tried for 'desertion' (here attempted suicide) because he cannot envisage separation from his deeply loved wife, again expresses Galsworthy's sympathy for anti-war protesters, as well as transiently unveiling again his own great fear in August 1914 of being separated from Ada. The last tale, one of Galsworthy's best pieces of short fiction, 'The Indian Summer of a Forsyte' (1917), mentioned above, heralded his return to consistently higher quality impressionistic but tightly compressed and psychologically well-tuned writing, without the slightly overblown melodrama of the wartime romantic novels. This tale was eventually incorporated as one of the 'Interludes' in the single volume *Forsyte Saga* in 1922. Like a number of other pieces dating from his return from France ('Spindleberries', 'The Grey Angel', and 'Cafard'), 'Indian Summer' has a peaceful and elegiac quality. The critical reception of *Five Tales* was generally favourable.[66]

Galsworthy's diary entries not only allow insight into the motives for his writing during the war but also chart his recovery and mark the point when therapeutic writing had, he thought, finally cured him of the 'war sickness' that negatively affected his creative output. On 28 July 1918, he noted:

> We stayed on at Wingstone till the end of August and, during which I began the Second Part of *The Forsyte Saga*, to be called *The Second Flowering* [subsequently *In Chancery*]. The idea of making *The Man of Property* the first volume of a trilogy cemented by *Indian Summer of a Forsyte* and another short episode came to me on Sunday and I started the same day.[67]

In retrospect the original title was appropriate, and the dates are very significant in charting Galsworthy's own psychological/creative healing as well as his physical recovery from his perceived sense of overall disabilities, effectively dealt with by his activities at Le Martouret in 1916–17.

In Chancery (1920) is set 20 years earlier, against a background of the end of Queen Victoria's reign; here Galsworthy displaced his residual internal conflicts about the recent war back towards the Boer War. He depicts the opposing attitudes of the British population to that war, and he not only has Young Jolyon Forsyte's son Jolly volunteering (though not for patriotic reasons) and then die pointlessly of typhoid fever in South Africa but also allows two women, Jolly's sister Holly and her much older half-sister June, to travel out as volunteer nurses. *In Chancery* is tightly constructed, full of finely drawn psychological portraits, a polished and finished work, and Galsworthy's testimony to his own full recovery. After finishing it, he almost immediately embarked on the third volume *To Let* (1921) set contemporaneously, 20 years after *In Chancery*, and which also includes numerous echoes of Galsworthy's war time preoccupations.

There is thus abundant evidence that Galsworthy cured his own 'war sickness' in part by writing vast amounts of fiction, some undeniably second rate. Yet it is clear from careful reading of these texts and Galsworthy's diaries – which also detail significantly his own systematic revision and careful re-reading of the novels – that this process (which corresponds to Lengelle and Meijers 'transformational space'[68]), from initial rapid drafting to re-reading and revision, was overall a cathartic cleansing. None of this, despite its importance to a full understanding of Galsworthy's wartime literary output, was apparent to his critics or his friends nor recorded by himself.[69] Other writing, notably the nature writing and the considerable amounts of poetry Galsworthy wrote during the war, also provided more gentle forms of (self) therapy. Fiction has been my focus here, but, little republished, his poetry was at the time also a means to air his intense and conflicted feelings. He finished only one (unsuccessful) wartime play, *A Bit o' Love*, started in 1913. Galsworthy's immediate post-war activity included not only *In Chancery* and *To Let* but an important new play 'The Skin Game' (1919), about two families in conflict, and which can be read as a war metaphor. He went on to write the less impressive second Forsyte trilogy *A Modern Comedy,* much of which explores father–daughter relationships, by following through the 1920s the lives of Soames Forsyte, his daughter Fleur, and her earnestly idealistic Galsworthy-like husband Michael Mont.[70] As well as a third trilogy *The End of the Chapter*, the second volume of which *Flowering Wilderness* (1932) centred around his final working out of his hostility to dogmatic religion of any shade, he wrote several now forgotten plays and an excellent long story called 'Soames and the Flag'.[71] Galsworthy's chief concern was now his long-standing campaign for internationalism in literature, which led to him becoming the founding president of PEN in 1921.

Thus we see that in the majority of the stories and sketches in the *Tatterdemalion* collection and in other works discussed above, including three almost-forgotten novels, Galsworthy, as well as writing information pieces for 'Wellington House', and fund-raising through his wartime novels and stories, used creative writing as his wartime literary self-care. In works of romantic and satirical fiction and in quasi-autobiographical sketches and stories, he expressed his own fears, ambivalence, guilt, frustration, anger, and hatred of war, as well as recalling ephemeral but happy times in France, Devon, and Sussex, either in wartime or pre-war peacetime. The outbreak of war had created a (for him unprecedented) state of cognitive dissonance leading to emotional turmoil and intense anxiety. His writing progressively helped him to rationalise his feelings, overcome his mental distress, and allow him to progress with further substantial and successful writing, beginning with *Five Tales* and thence to the second and third volumes of *The Forsyte Saga*, overall his most enduring success.

Notes

1 H.V. Marrot, *The Life and Letters of John Galsworthy* (London: William Heinemann, 1935), 395–6.

2 James Gindin, *John Galsworthy's Life and Art: An Alien's Fortress* (Ann Arbor: University of Michigan Press, 1987), 348; for details, see for example 'First Thoughts on this War' (1914) and 'Second Thoughts on this War' (1915) both in John Galsworthy, *A Sheaf* (London: William Heinemann; New York: Scribner's, 1916), 224–41; 288–312.

3 Gindin, *John Galsworthy's Life and Art*, 347.

4 Sara Haslam, 'Reading, Trauma and Literary Caregiving, 1914–1918: Helen Mary Gaskell and the War Library', *The Journal of Medical Humanities* 41 (2018): 305–21.

5 Debbie McCulliss, 'Bibliotherapy: Historical and Research Perspectives', *Journal of Poetry Therapy* 25, no. 1 (2012): 23–38.

6 R. Lengelle and F. Meijers, 'Mystery to Mastery: An Exploration of What Happens in the Black Box of Writing and Healing', *Journal of Poetry Therapy* 22, no. 2 (2009): 57–75.

7 Lengelle and Meijers, 'Mystery to Mastery', 59.

8 Ada, born illegitimate with her biological father uncertain, was adopted by Dr Emanuel Cooper of Norwich and travelled extensively in Europe with her mother Anna Pearson during her teens.

9 Jill Felicity Durey, *John Galsworthy's Compassion: All Beings Great and Small* (Cham: Palgrave Macmillan, 2021).

10 Gindin, *John Galsworthy's Life and Art*, 206–7; Durey, *John Galsworthy's Compassion*, 63.

11 Jeffrey S. Reznick, *John Galsworthy and Disabled Soldiers of the Great War* (Manchester: Manchester University Press, 2009).

12 Reznick, *John Galsworthy and Disabled Soldiers of the Great War*, 11.

13 Reznick, *John Galsworthy and Disabled Soldiers of the Great War*, 13.

14 Marrot, *The Life and Letters of John Galsworthy*, 411.

15 John Galsworthy, *Tatterdemalion* (London: William Heinemann, 1920).

16 Marrot, *The Life and Letters of John Galsworthy*, 395.

17 Marrot, *The Life and Letters of John Galsworthy*, 412.

18 Later collected with a number of other magazine pieces reflecting his early responses to war, such as 'France' and 'Reveille' in *A Sheaf*.

19 Galsworthy, *Tatterdemalion*, 173–8. An anecdote possibly heard during his South African travels in 1893. Biographers all state that Galsworthy went only to 'High Constantia', a winegrowing area very close to Cape Town. However, in one of his very early stories, 'The Spirit of the Karroo' in *From the Four Winds* (1897), he also describes the landscape of the hinterland in detail, and these two stories suggest that he went much farther inland within the Western Cape. On the *Torrens* homebound in 1893 he re-read Olive Schreiner's *The Story of an African Farm* (see Marrot, 87), partly set in the Karroo, and may also have acquired his sense of place from that novel.

20 Marrot, *The Life and Letters of John Galsworthy*, 408.

21 Marrot, *The Life and Letters of John Galsworthy*, 409. Published on 18 August 1915, *Freelands*, unconnected with the war, did not appeal to the public in the tense emotional atmosphere of wartime and sold badly with its main value being fundraising. Galsworthy, by then a very well-known author, was able to command substantial amounts for serialisation – here £1500 from Scribner's for serial rights. Galsworthy does not in his diaries or letters mention any disappointment about its poor sales and thus it seems to have fulfilled what had become its main purpose: therapeutic writing specifically for war relief fundraising.

22 His diary indicated many such contributions which continued throughout the war. See also Reznick, *John Galsworthy and Disabled Soldiers of the Great War*, 17–19.

23 Marrot, *The Life and Letters of John Galsworthy*, 409.

24 See for example Peter Buitenhuis, *The Great War of Words: Literature as Propaganda, 1914-18 and After* (London: Batsford, 1989) for an authoritative account of this initiative.

25 Gary Messinger, *British Propaganda and the State in the First World War* (Manchester: Manchester University Press, 1992), 40–44. By June 1915, 2.5 million publications of various sorts had been circulated, and by August 1916 300 books and pamphlets in 21 languages had been published (40–41). Popular writers commissioned, in addition to Galsworthy, included Anthony Hope Hawkins, Arthur Conan Doyle and G. K. Chesterton, among others.

26 Lucinda Borkett-Jones, '"My Friend the Enemy": Ford's Construction of the German Other in Wartime' in *Homo Duplex: Ford Madox Ford's Experience and Aesthetics of Alterity*, edited by Isabelle Brasme (Montpellier: Presses Universitaires de la Méditerranée, 2020), 87–104.

27 The literary expression of Ford's wartime experiences was only revealed much later, in his *Parade's End* tetralogy (1924–1928) and his fictionalised autobiography *No Enemy* (1929).

28 See Haslam for a detailed analysis of Wells's novel within the context of literary caregiving.

29 Earle E. Stevens and H. Ray Stevens, *John Galsworthy: An Annotated Bibliography of Writings about Him* (De Kalb, IL: Northern Illinois University Press, 1980), 99, 112.
30 Reznick, *John Galsworthy and Disabled Soldiers of the Great War*, 7.
31 Marrot, *The Life and Letters of John Galsworthy*, 416–17.
32 Marrot, *The Life and Letters of John Galsworthy*, 457.
33 Gindin, *John Galsworthy's Life and Art*, 385.
34 Stevens, *John Galsworthy*, 102, 104.
35 Marrot, *The Life and Letters of John Galsworthy*, 458–9.
36 This fictional event can be dated to 23 September 1915 and recalls Galsworthy and Ada watching a Zeppelin raid during the night of their wedding anniversary (Marrot, 423).
37 Stevens, *John Galsworthy*, 112–17; Marrot, *The Life and Letters of John Galsworthy*, 462–6.
38 Marrot, *The Life and Letters of John Galsworthy*, 441.
39 See also Reznick (180) who, reprinting a significant chapter, situates the novel within the context of Galsworthy's disability work.
40 Alec Fréchet, *John Galsworthy: A Reassessment* (Basingstoke: Macmillan, 1982), 85.
41 Marrot, *The Life and Letters of John Galsworthy*, 759.
42 I am grateful to Christian Rey (Valence, France) for generously sharing with me his notes and images of Le Martouret.
43 Galsworthy, *Tatterdemalion*, 51–74.
44 Galsworthy, *Tatterdemalion*, 62–4.
45 Galsworthy, *Tatterdemalion*, 179–87.
46 Galsworthy, *Tatterdemalion*, 106–17.
47 Galsworthy, *Tatterdemalion*, 109–10.
48 The Galsworthys were famously great dog lovers and Ada mentioned in a letter from Cassis the day after leaving Le Martouret (Marrot 426–7) how they would miss 'the dearest little dog that had adopted us weeks ago'.
49 Galsworthy, *Tatterdemalion*, 221.
50 Three stories in the collection, 'Two Looks' (1904), 'Fairyland' (1912), and 'Buttercup Night'(1913) were written before the war and are therefore not relevant.
51 Galsworthy, *Tatterdemalion*, 27–50.
52 Galsworthy and Ada had been to a Promenade concert (Beethoven's 7th symphony) on 16 September 1916, and on 28 September he began 'Defeat' (Marrot, 423–4).
53 Galsworthy, *Tatterdemalion*, 48–50. A 19th-century patriotic anthem, popular in Germany during the Franco-Prussian and First World wars.
54 Both dated 1919 so probably written then, as both refer to the end of war.
55 Galsworthy, *Tatterdemalion*, 92.
56 Galsworthy, *Tatterdemalion*, 126–36.
57 Galsworthy, *Tatterdemalion*, 137–46; Marrot, 430.
58 Galsworthy, *Tatterdemalion*, 169–72.
59 See also 'France, 1916–1917: An Impression' in *Another Sheaf* (1919), 73–5. This essay also includes detailed descriptions of Le Martouret and the landscape around Die as well as Arles.
60 Galsworthy, *Tatterdemalion*, 5.
61 Galsworthy, *Tatterdemalion*, 3; see File:Georg Sauter – Blanche Bailey Galsworthy.jpg – Wikimedia Commons.
62 See for example Marrot, *The Life and Letters of John Galsworthy*, 55–8; Galsworthy's piece 'A Portrait of My Mother'.
63 Lengelle and Meijers, 'Mystery to Mastery', 63.

64 Galsworthy, *Tatterdemalion*, 255–70.
65 Marrot, *The Life and Letters of John Galsworthy*, 417.
66 Stevens, *John Galsworthy*, 110–11.
67 Marrot, *The Life and Letters of John Galsworthy*, 443.
68 Lengelle and Meijers, 'Mystery to Mastery', 59–60.
69 Galsworthy read his work in progress to his wife Ada, who also typed for him, so it is extremely unlikely that she was unaware of this cathartic process, even though I can find no written evidence of her awareness.
70 *The White Monkey* (1924), *The Silver Spoon* (1926), and *Swan Song* (1928).
71 In *On Forsyte Change* (1930), a collection of interesting short stories forming a Forsyte family back story.

References

Borkett-Jones, Lucinda. '"My Friend the Enemy": Ford's Construction of the German Other in Wartime'. In *Homo Duplex: Ford Madox Ford's Experience and Aesthetics of Alterity*, edited by Isabelle Brasme, 87–104. Montpellier: Presses Universitaires de la Méditerranée, 2020.

Buitenhuis, Peter. *The Great War of Words: Literature as Propaganda, 1914-18 and After*. London: Batsford, 1989.

Durey, Jill Felicity. *John Galsworthy's Compassion: All Beings Great and Small*. Cham: Palgrave, 2021.

Fréchet, Alec. *John Galsworthy: A Reassessment*. Basingstoke: Macmillan, 1982.

Galsworthy, John. *The Dark Flower*. London: William Heinemann, 1913.

Galsworthy, John. *A Sheaf*. London: William Heinemann; New York: Charles Scribner's Sons, 1916.

Galsworthy, John. *Beyond*. New York: Charles Scribner's Sons, 1917.

Galsworthy, John. *Five Tales*. London: William Heinemann, 1918.

Galsworthy, John. *Saint's Progress*. New York: Charles Scribner's Sons, 1919.

Galsworthy, John. *Another Sheaf*. London: William Heinemann, 1919.

Galsworthy, John. *Tatterdemalion*. London: William Heinemann, 1920.

Galsworthy, John. *In Chancery*. London: William Heinemann, 1920.

Galsworthy, John. *The Burning Spear*. New York: Charles Scribner's Sons, 1923.

Gindin, James. *John Galsworthy's Life and Art: An Alien's Fortress*. Ann Arbor: University of Michigan Press, 1987.

Haslam, Sara. 'Reading, Trauma and Literary Caregiving, 1914–1918: Helen Mary Gaskell and the War Library', *Journal of Medical Humanities* 41 (2018): 305–321.

Lengelle, R. and Meijers, F. 'Mystery to Mastery: An Exploration of What Happens in the Black Box of Writing and Healing', *Journal of Poetry Therapy* 22, no. 2 (2009): 57–75.

Marrot, H.V. *The Life and Letters of John Galsworthy*. London: William Heinemann, 1935.

McCulliss, Debbie. 'Bibliotherapy: Historical and Research Perspectives', *Journal of Poetry Therapy* 25, no. 1 (2012): 23–38.

Partington, G. 'Bibliotherapy: A Survey of Literature. Working Papers 2022/23:03'. Exeter: Wellcome Centre for Cultures and Environments of Health, 2023.

Reznick, Jeffrey S. *John Galsworthy and Disabled Soldiers of the Great War*. Manchester: Manchester University Press, 2009.

Stevens, Earle E. and H. Ray Stevens. *John Galsworthy: An Annotated Bibliography of Writings about Him*. De Kalb, IL: Northern Illinois University Press, 1980.

3 The American Library Association, 'Bibliotherapy' and the First World War

Vincent Trott

In 1956 the librarian W. B. McDaniel wrote that 'bibliotherapy' is 'unquestionably a war baby. It is a hospital library baby of World War I'.[1] McDaniel was referring to the work of the American Library Association (ALA) and its Library War Service which provided books to servicemen in camps and military hospitals between 1917 and 1921.[2] As the historian Arthur P. Young has argued, librarians working in these military hospitals developed 'an almost evangelical faith in the curative power of controlled reading'.[3] This belief was central to the practice of what would become known as 'bibliotherapy', an approach widely publicized and theorized by hospital librarians in the United States during the 1920s and 1930s.[4] The ALA's role in military hospitals during and shortly after the First World War, however, has received little attention. Studies of the ALA during the conflict, including Young's, have focused primarily on the provision of books to soldiers in training camps and overseas. These works have revealed much about soldiers' reading habits and the ALA's organizational history, but less about the provision of books in military hospital libraries.[5]

This chapter illuminates the development of bibliotherapy by examining how notions of curative reading informed the work of hospital librarians during and shortly after the First World War. Drawing on reports and promotional materials from the ALA archives, it pays particular attention to the emergence of what Jesse Miller has described as 'the trope of the literary clinic – the system of metaphors describing books as medicine, readers as patients, and reading as a form of therapy'.[6] In doing so, this chapter complicates the idea that bibliotherapy was 'born' during the First World War. It demonstrates not only that a belief in curative reading predated the conflict but also that this notion did not gain serious traction with ALA librarians until 1919. This chapter also provides a more complete account of the emergence of bibliotherapy in American military hospitals by examining the ideological context in which it developed. Crucially, it argues that bibliotherapy was never central to the agenda of the Library War Service. Rather, the ALA's work during the First World War, in both camps and hospital libraries, was shaped primarily by political, moral and educational imperatives. Bibliotherapeutic approaches emerged within this context and were frequently intertwined with it.

DOI: 10.4324/9781003471561-5

This chapter takes a chronological approach. It begins by discussing the development of the Library War Service in 1917 and the various ideological drivers which underpinned its work. It then examines the expansion of the ALA's role in hospital libraries in 1918 and the factors which informed its provision of books in this setting. Finally, by focusing on the ALA's work shortly after the Armistice, this chapter demonstrates how hospital librarians increasingly extolled the value of therapeutic reading when promoting the Library War Service.

The Library War Service

Soon after the USA intervened in the First World War in April 1917, librarians, politicians and military officials recognized the value of supplying reading material to the troops. Three months earlier, Librarian of Congress Herbert Putnam had sent his colleague Theodore Wesley Koch to England to report back on the provision of reading material to British soldiers.[7] The ALA shared Koch's findings at its annual conference in Louisville, Kentucky in June 1917, highlighting the work of the various British agencies which supplied books and magazines in camps and military hospitals.[8] At the end of the conference, the ALA formed a War Service Committee to oversee similar initiatives in the United States. The US Commission on Training Camp Activities (CTCA) – which managed troop morale, recreation and entertainment – assigned the ALA, under the direction of Putnam, responsibility for managing libraries in the 32 training camps across the United States. What became known as Library War Service would eventually extend its provision overseas, supplying reading material to soldiers near the Western Front.[9] By 1920, it had collected and distributed approximately 10 million books and magazines, employing over a thousand library workers across its facilities.[10]

Initially, librarians did not foreground therapeutic reading when promoting the Library War Service. This was hardly surprising, for the ALA's primary purpose was to provide books to fit and healthy recruits. When advertising its work, the ALA stressed the educational and recreational benefits of books, highlighting the importance of technical and military literature and the value of reading for pleasure.[11] In its early promotional materials, the Library War Service urged the public to donate reading material, stressing that soldiers needed books for 'study, recreation and diversion in lonely moments'.[12] The ALA's booklists, which catalogued the books provided by the camp libraries, reflected these priorities. They included technical works, such as *Descriptions and Instructions for the Use of Rifle and Hand Grenades*, as well as a wide range of fiction, informed by soldiers' reading habits and public library borrowing trends. Soldiers were offered escapist works, such as the adventure stories of Rider Haggard, as well as more cerebral novels by the likes of Tolstoy and Turgenev.[13] By ensuring that soldiers' various reading preferences were catered to, ALA librarians closely followed the approach – outlined by Theodore Koch – which British charities employed when providing books for soldiers during the conflict.[14]

Nevertheless, ALA promotional materials did sometimes draw a direct connection between reading and health. In September 1917, the Library War

Service newsletter, the *War Library Bulletin*, quoted the author Henry Van Dyke, who had stressed the importance of books for 'the hospital wounded … trying to gain strength of body and mind to go back to the battle … Human fellowship, good books, and music are three of the best medicines and tonics in the world'.[15] In the following issue of the *War Library Bulletin*, the ALA echoed Van Dyke's sentiments, arguing that 'Health in Mind means health in body. Libraries will increase the strength of our armies. Libraries for our soldiers will help win the war. They are more than a recreation'.[16] The ALA thus presented its work as integral to the military effort as a whole, promoting reading as essential for the maintenance of physical strength and martial masculinity.

Anecdotal evidence fuelled these beliefs, and soldiers themselves praised the work of the ALA for similar reasons. The *War Library Bulletin* printed the words of a soldier at Washington's Camp Lewis in April 1918, who had said that the library service 'has enabled me to keep up my spirits and health more than anything else, to have a couple of hours free occasionally to sit in a comfortable library and read'.[17] The ALA's belief that reading might help to sustain an individual's psychological and physical wellbeing, evident in all of these promotional materials, would underpin later efforts to promote and systematize bibliotherapy. At this stage, however, librarians did not explicitly refer to reading in therapeutic terms. While the language of bibliotherapy arose in an embryonic form in these pronouncements, articles and anecdotes tended to portray reading as beneficial for the maintenance of soldiers' morale and mental health, rather than as a curative process.

Distinct moral and ideological motivations also shaped the work of the Library War Service. The CTCA, led by the social reformer Raymond Fosdick, sought to regulate soldiers' behaviour with the intention of ensuring they conformed to codes of masculine respectability. Prior to the war, the regular army in the United States had been plagued by heavy drinking and high rates of venereal disease. Following American intervention, many military leaders and social reformers alike were determined to ensure the mass influx of new recruits upheld conventional standards of morality.[18] In accordance with the goals of the CTCA, the ALA, at its June 1917 conference, had promoted reading as a wholesome pastime which would deter soldiers from pursuing less salubrious sources of entertainment. They were concerned not only with relieving the 'depressing tedium' of military life but also with 'dangerous temptation'.[19] In this sense, reading was connected to a soldier's health, insofar as it might discourage him from frequenting bars or brothels. ALA librarians – many of whom shared Fosdick's reforming zeal and a desire to uphold middle-class morality – thus implicitly linked the act of reading to the maintenance, perhaps even the reform, of a soldier's mental wellbeing and moral fibre, even if they did not explicitly espouse a therapeutic agenda. The CTCA and the Library War Service, then, were products of the Progressive Era's widespread preoccupation with social reform.[20]

Entrenched racism also informed the CTCA's ethos. The army was segregated, and so too were its training camps and recreational facilities. As the historian Chad Williams has demonstrated, the commission took a 'paternalistic' view of Black soldiers, stigmatizing them as distinctly susceptible to immoral temptations.[21]

White officers shared these concerns, especially after the American Expeditionary Force had crossed the Atlantic. Lieutenant John Melvin's letter to an ALA librarian at Boston Public Library, for example, asked for donations of books to his base in France with the hope this might 'cut down venereal disease' within the ranks. Despite the prevalence of this problem among white soldiers, Melvin was concerned that nearly 3,000 African American soldiers at the base were 'made far too much of by the French women'. As the Regimental Censor, Melvin believed 'books will keep them in camp'.[22] The significance attached to reading, then, was also shaped by pre-existing moral prejudices, in this case, concerns regarding unrestricted Black sexuality and interracial mixing.

A desire to reform men – and the moral and political assumptions at its core – also informed the educational activities of the CTCA. The US army, after testing new recruits, soon realized illiteracy was a far greater problem than many had predicted, with results demonstrating that 50.6 per cent of Black soldiers and 21.5 per cent of white soldiers were unable to read or write.[23] In certain units, the problem may have been more severe than this. When relaying his concerns regarding venereal disease, Lieutenant Melvin had also noted that two-thirds of his regiment were illiterate.[24] The CTCA, in conjunction with the YMCA and the ALA, therefore provided basic classes in literacy for soldiers. In addition to supplying the books which facilitated this learning, ALA librarians themselves also helped soldiers to read. A librarian at Fort Sam Houston in Houston, Texas, for example, noted that she was teaching three pupils, one of whom 'knew only one letter' and 'was still struggling with the alphabet'.[25]

Despite its prevalence among those born in the United States, politicians and educationalists often viewed illiteracy as primarily a problem within the nation's immigrant communities.[26] Shortly before the war, classes in literacy became part of 'Americanization' programmes in the United States, which aimed to teach immigrants civic values and citizenship. These initiatives were often driven by a desire to improve the lives of immigrants and did not necessarily require those who had recently settled in the United States to renounce their old-world heritage. Nevertheless, the Americanization movement gained momentum after the outbreak of the conflict in Europe inflamed anti-immigrant sentiment within the United States, especially as rumours of German espionage and industrial sabotage on American soil began to circulate.[27] A fear that 'hyphenated' Americans (those who claimed a dual national heritage) posed a threat to American security intensified efforts to 'Americanize' immigrants. Increasingly, immigrants were expected to abandon their 'hyphenated' identity amid clamours for '100% Americanism'.[28] These impulses were given credence by President Woodrow Wilson, who in December 1915 denounced citizens of foreign birth who 'had poured the poison of disloyalty into the very arteries of our national life'.[29]

Many librarians had also participated enthusiastically in Americanization initiatives before US intervention. A 1916 article in the *Bulletin of the American Library Association*, for example, stressed the importance of 'Americanizing Books and Periodicals for Immigrants'.[30] The same periodical also published an article that year by H. H. Wheaton, who oversaw Americanization programmes coordinated by the Bureau of Education. Wheaton urged ALA librarians to establish Americanization initiatives, such as night schools, which would help to remedy the fact that five million recent immigrants to the United States, many of them illiterate, were unable to speak the English language.[31] Even if they were not illiterate, some soldiers, especially those who had emigrated from Eastern Europe, may not have been able to read or write in the Roman alphabet.

The ALA's growing support for 'Americanization' would also inform its work during the war. Public libraries in the United States disseminated propaganda, which included campaigns to encourage immigrant communities to assimilate.[32] A similar approach shaped the work of the Library War Service in camp libraries. In October 1918, *Outlook* magazine celebrated the ALA's work in this area, explaining that 'Camp Librarians are co-operating with military officials in a Nation-wide endeavor to Americanize men of all nationalities in the ranks before they are sent abroad'. Its author, George F. Worts, highlighted the task that lay before them at Camp Devens in Massachusetts, where 40 different languages were spoken among the troops. Worts also observed that 'In the light of New England's reputation for erudition, camp officials at Devens have viewed with some alarm the large number of illiterates among the incoming soldiers. Many of these can scarcely write their own names'.[33]

To assist with Americanization, the librarians at Camp Devens had a number of tools at their disposal, including Edward Everett Hale's novel *The Man Without a Country* (1863), which extolled the value of patriotism and national belonging. ALA librarians placed the book on every table in the camp library. Perhaps of more direct benefit to soldiers were textbooks, such as the 'fifty-seven easy readers in English' that were available at the library in Camp Wadsworth, South Carolina.[34] The ALA took pride in this work, and readers no doubt appreciated its efforts, not least because many immigrants wanted to assimilate and avail themselves of the educational opportunities on offer. A librarian at Camp Wadsworth proudly noted that an Italian immigrant, when asked whether he was Italian, had replied, 'No, Sir, I am American, but I speak Italian'.[35] At this stage, then, the efforts of the ALA were corrective rather than curative, centred as much on making men literate in 'Americanness' as they were on helping them to read and write. As the war progressed, political imperatives like these continued to shape the activities of the Library War Service even as it began to promote the therapeutic benefits of reading in hospitals. As the following sections argue, these curative and ideological motivations were frequently intertwined. The emergence of bibliotherapy in the United States was influenced not only by medical or literary concerns but also by broader political priorities.

Hospital Libraries

Since the autumn of 1917, many librarians had provided reading material for patients in hospitals attached to training camps, but a more systematic hospital library service did not begin until the spring of 1918, when the ALA assumed responsibility for running military hospital libraries, working closely with the

American Red Cross. In June 1918, 22 librarians were serving in military hospital libraries.[36] In charge of the hospital library service was Caroline F. Webster of New York State Library, who oversaw the rapid expansion of the scheme. By April 1919, ALA librarians were working in 66 different hospitals.[37]

Within this setting, the relationship between reading and health gradually became more central to the ALA's promotional efforts. This was not an entirely novel concept. Volunteers working in Britain for the War Library – a charity formed by Helen Mary Gaskell at the start of the conflict – had already stressed the palliative value of reading when supplying literature to convalescent servicemen in British military hospital libraries. The War Library, which became affiliated with the British Red Cross in 1915, was one of the key agencies Theodore Koch had discussed in his report for the ALA in early 1917.[38] The ALA's work in military hospitals also drew on pre-war precedents. Although McDaniel suggested that bibliotherapy was a 'war baby', Arthur P. Young's assertion that it 'came of age during World War I' is perhaps more apt.[39] McDaniel himself had acknowledged that hospital libraries were nothing new by the time of the First World War. Some hospitals had provided patients with books since at least the early nineteenth century in the United States, and a more systematized hospital library service also predated the First World War.[40] A major pioneer in this area was the librarian E. Kathleen Jones, who would go on to play an important role in managing the ALA's work in hospital libraries during and shortly after the war.[41] Jones reflected on the development of hospital libraries in an article for the journal *Modern Hospital* in 1922. According to Jones, the library she had helped to establish in 1904 at McLean, a psychiatric hospital in Waverley, Massachusetts, was one of the first in the United States. Here, trained librarians provided carefully selected books to patients. A few other hospitals then followed suit, establishing organized libraries run by professional librarians. By the time of the First World War, some of these libraries had begun to recognize the 'value of recreational reading as a therapeutic agent', though these libraries were rare and 'might have been counted on the fingers of one hand'.[42]

For these reasons, bibliotherapy was not central to the ALA's mission when it began working in military hospitals. Though librarians sometimes alluded to the curative power of reading, the language of bibliotherapy would only begin to gain serious traction following the Armistice, after ALA librarians had been working in military hospitals for some time. When they began their work, these librarians did not typically draw explicit links between reading and health and instead focused on the recreational and educational benefits of books. In this sense, they built upon the practices the ALA had developed in the training camps, where ideological concerns often shaped its work. This was especially the case when the ALA began to manage library services in the new 'reconstruction hospitals'. These were dedicated treatment centres for discharged soldiers, which aimed to equip men with skills that would allow them to become productive citizens once they were released from hospital. In these hospitals, teachers and medical practitioners ran vocational workshops, often employing emerging ideas of occupational therapy.

This focus on rehabilitation, as the historian Beth Linker had demonstrated, was driven by a distinct political agenda. The huge cost of paying pensions to disabled veterans of the Civil War motivated many Progressive Era reformers to seek less costly methods of caring for men who had been severely injured in conflict. These reformers came from a variety of backgrounds and included prominent social workers, lawyers, medical experts and politicians. Spurred on by medical advancements and imbued with an unerring faith in scientific expertise, many reformers believed that disabled ex-servicemen could be rehabilitated through various forms of physical and vocational therapy, which in turn would restore their ability to work. This belief was fuelled by the notion of the Protestant work ethic and a belief in the 'redemptive value of work'.[43] A widespread faith in these ideals encouraged President Woodrow Wilson to appoint two prominent reformers – Julian Mack (a circuit judge) and Julia Mathrop (director of the United States Children's Bureau) – to draft the legislation which became the War Risk Insurance Act. Passed by Congress in October 1917, the Act replaced military pensions with a system of life insurance and the expanded provision of rehabilitation for disabled veterans.[44] It also led to the establishment of the Division of Special Hospitals and Physical Reconstruction and the creation of new rehabilitation centres at military hospitals in the United States. Two hospitals – Walter Reed General Hospital in Washington DC and Letterman Hospital in San Francisco – were transformed into dedicated reconstruction hospitals, and 14 new facilities were built to handle the influx of disabled soldiers returning from base hospitals in France following the Armistice.[45] These hospitals practised vocational therapy and contained 'curative workshops' in which patients could develop various practical skills, including woodworking, telegraphy, sign-painting and carpentry.[46]

These initiatives were the product of a therapeutic mindset that infused American culture during the late nineteenth and early twentieth centuries. The historian Jackson Lears has argued that this ethos was a secular response to the peculiar dislocations of modernity, which drove people to seek a renewed sense of selfhood. Growing fears that cases of 'neurasthenia' were on the rise led to a greater concern for emotional wellbeing, driving this therapeutic impulse.[47] Champions of the Arts and Crafts movement also emphasized the therapeutic value of traditional craftsmanship as an antidote to the increasingly mechanized nature of industrial work.[48] A similar belief in the efficacy of shop work would inform the therapeutic philosophy espoused at the reconstruction hospitals.

The Division of Special Hospitals and Physical Reconstruction also oversaw an extensive programme of recreational activities which was administered by the American Red Cross. According to a bulletin from the Surgeon General's Office, recreation induced a 'general spirit that facilitates recovery', while sport and other games had a physical benefit, providing 'beneficial therapeutic exercise for all patients'. Recreation also had a vocational justification, in that it would allow men to provide a 'better service to the army, navy and society'. Reading was one of a number of recreational activities – including amateur theatricals, singing, music and indoor games – overseen by the American Red Cross, with the ALA maintaining 'a library of technical works, approved fiction, current magazines, periodicals and newspapers'.[49] The ALA's primary purpose, in the eyes of the Surgeon General's Office, was twofold: to facilitate vocational training by providing the requisite technical literature and to provide reading materials that might enable recreation and distraction. This bulletin did not present reading itself as a therapeutic activity.

The ALA did not initially promote its work in these terms either. Its annual report published in June 1918 outlined the two key elements of its role in the reconstruction hospitals. First, it aimed to 'support the efforts of agencies and workers in occupational therapy and vocational rehabilitation by supplying to them books and special librarians'. Second, it intended to offer 'technical and clerical' training to patients that could be undertaken in the libraries.[50] The ALA's goal was to *facilitate* the therapeutic work taking place in the hospital, while also providing an educational service that would help to equip patients with new skills. A report from New Haven General Hospital in September 1918, likewise, emphasized the vocational value of books. Its librarian noted that 'I have here books which will make better soldiers of the men who go back into the army, and better citizens of all of them after the war is over'.[51] An advert for the ALA in the magazine *Carry On*, published specifically for disabled soldiers and sailors in the reconstruction hospitals, also highlighted its 'fine library of the most modern books on technical vocational subjects'.[52] Books had a crucial educational function, inculcating vocational skills and ideals of citizenship, but they were not necessarily presented as therapeutic in their own right. All these pronouncements reflected the ALA's political motivations. Books were part of a broader reconstructive mission centred on transforming men into productive citizens. Before the Armistice, this included preparing men for a potential return to the army. After the war, the focus shifted to equipping men with the skills needed for post-war civilian work.

ALA booklists reflected these underlying imperatives. Works such as *Elements of Modern Field Artillery* and *Field Book for Machine Gunners* served a clear technical purpose when it seemed likely that soldiers might have to return to the battlefields.[53] Other recommended booklists centred on skills that soldiers might need in civilian life. One bibliography, issued when the ALA commenced its work in the reconstruction hospitals, included books on politics and government, economics, vocational guidance, engineering, chemistry and botany, among others.[54] There was also an appetite for these books among the soldiers. Shortly after the armistice, one hospital librarian noted there was a demand for works on 'wood-carving, metal work, civil service preparation, electricity, mechanical drawing'.[55] Convalescents also read for pleasure, with fiction in high demand. A report from the hospital library at Camp Wadsworth in South Carolina observed that the soldiers 'crave stories of adventure, especially exciting western stories'. Librarians recognized this, despite their political imperatives, and happily supplied convalescents with books for escapist purposes. Around two-thirds of the books circulating in one month were works of fiction.[56]

Hospital librarians certainly took the individual reading needs of patients into account. As they did in camps, many encountered men who were illiterate or at least unable to read the Roman alphabet. Other servicemen, meanwhile, were not physically or mentally able to read books. The ALA therefore began to create and distribute scrapbooks for soldiers, a scheme which had been recommended by Theodore Koch in 1917. When Koch had reported on the British provision of books to soldiers during the war, he credited Rudyard Kipling with the idea of supplying scrapbooks to convalescent soldiers, a practice adopted by Helen Mary Gaskell's War Library in military hospitals.[57] These scrapbooks contained clippings from popular newspapers and magazines, prioritizing humour, short articles and colourful illustrations. In April 1918, the American Red Cross began to assist the ALA with a similar scheme to distribute scrapbooks to soldiers in military hospitals.[58] The Red Cross also instructed volunteers, including high school students, to make scrapbooks for American soldiers in France.[59] The ALA's decision to create and distribute scrapbooks aptly reflects the intertwined educational, recreational, political and nascent curative motives that shaped its work in the hospital libraries.

Scrapbook making itself was nothing new and had emerged as a popular pastime in the United States during the late nineteenth century, often as a way for individuals to collate content that interested them from a disparate range of printed media.[60] There was also a tradition of charitable scrapbook-making, in which children and church groups provided these reading materials to those who were poor or sick.[61] The ALA's initiative built on these precedents and served a vital purpose in military hospitals. One librarian, reporting in 1918 from Walter Reed General Hospital, noted that 'picture scrapbooks are of value for the entertainment of the illiterate, and likewise for the men not long removed from the operating table and still a bit dulled by the ether'.[62] Another ALA report explained that scrapbooks were ideal for 'weak men who could not hold or pay attention to books'.[63] Many patients appreciated the scrapbooks, too. In one hospital ward, according to an ALA librarian, 'the men literally flocked around the table' when shown a collection of scrapbooks.[64] Though librarians did not explicitly articulate the therapeutic value of reading at this stage, they increasingly recognized the restorative potential of scrapbooks.

Scrapbooks were not solely a way of making reading accessible. Ellen Garvey has argued that 'scrapbook makers imposed their will on what they read'.[65] But it is equally true that scrapbook makers imposed their will on what *others* read. The provision of scrapbooks, like much of the ALA's work during the war, was informed by its political goals, including its desire to assist with Americanization initiatives. ALA librarians realized that scrapbooks – which privileged illustrations – were ideal for the soldiers who could not read English, including not only illiterate American soldiers but also immigrants who had not yet learned the language. Some ALA librarians therefore viewed scrapbooks as important tools in Americanization. An August 1918 ALA report on reading in hospital libraries noted that

> scrapbooks and picture books, easy readers in English, and boys' books are on hand for the uneducated and illiterate men; those who are not used to reading depend on the hospital librarians to suggest a book. She is able to furnish reading lists and books that help in Americanization.[66]

There was a paternalistic dimension to scrapbook provision. It reflected the white, middle-class concerns of the ALA's workforce and allowed librarians to shape the reading habits of the predominantly working-class immigrants for whom the scrapbooks were often intended. Educational and political motivations, then, continued to weigh more heavily in the minds of librarians than curative concerns at this stage.

The demand for scrapbooks in hospitals increased in the autumn of 1918 when the American Expeditionary Forces experienced heavy causalities in battle. Librarians believed, however, that the production of scrapbooks would need to be standardized to be effective. On 10 September 1918, the organization issued guidelines for their creation, which stressed that the 'scrapbooks are for young American men, not for children. Contents should appeal to virile, active adults with wide interests and a lively curiosity'.[67] Scrapbooks needed to be accessible for illiterate soldiers, but librarians feared this might encourage volunteers to collate childish content. The ALA deemed this unsuitable because they viewed their mission as conducive to the military effort. Its guidelines therefore framed the act of reading as integral to the maintenance of martial masculinity.

This link between reading and manliness (and by extension a man's health) also reflects how emerging notions of curative reading began to inform the ALA's policy on scrapbooks. Its guidelines warned that 'Sentimental subjects calculated to bring on "homesickness" or "the blues", must be resolutely excluded on plain therapeutic grounds'. These 'grounds', though, were perhaps not so 'plain' after all, for the therapeutic potential of reading was ill-defined at this stage. Some librarians nevertheless had strong opinions on the matter. Whereas depressing or sentimental subjects were to be avoided, the guidelines stressed that 'the bright and humorous side is always acceptable'.[68] Another set of guidelines urged its volunteers to 'avoid war and other horrors' and encouraged them instead to use 'jokes clipped from humorous magazines', among other more light-hearted reading matter.[69] In some instances, however, librarians recognized that scrapbooks were entirely unsuitable. A 1918 librarian's report from Walter Reed General Hospital quoted a private describing the other men in his hospital ward: 'We've got an architect, a graduate of Cornell, a graduate of Johns Hopkins and perhaps others that I don't know about. You can't give these men scrapbooks'.[70] This belief that reading matter should be carefully tailored to the individual – if not entirely reader-led – would become central to the ethos of bibliotherapy.

Curative Reading

Following the Armistice, the discourse of therapeutic reading began to suffuse ALA reports and promotional materials. Though the recreational and educational benefits of reading continued to inform the ALA's work, from late 1918 onwards librarians increasingly began to recognize and promote explicitly the *curative* potential of literature, something which they had only alluded to before in most publicity materials and private documents. Bibliotherapy, then, was more a product of the war's aftermath than the war itself. This development coincided with the expansion of the ALA's work in reconstruction hospitals, as the association began to focus on healing injured soldiers and preparing them for civilian life. An ALA promotional notice from December 1918 called for donations of books to the hospital libraries with the claim that 'Good reading is an aid to speedy recovery. These men need books *now*'.[71] That month, a librarian's report from the hospital at Fort Des Moines, Iowa, espoused the therapeutic potential of books and argued that 'the library should consider itself part of reconstruction, rather than an aid in helping others to do the work. Reading is just as curative as shop work and occupational therapy'.[72] Librarians who believed in the value of 'bibliotherapy' were inspired by the broader therapeutic culture within the hospitals. Books, in their eyes, were not simply educational tools but also curative in their own right.

This belief would be expressed more fervently the following year, but its prevalence should not be exaggerated. ALA promotional material still tended to emphasize the vocational rather than the therapeutic value of hospital reading. The March 1919 edition of the *War Library Bulletin*, for example, contained a large advert which stated 'There are books on all jobs at the HOSPITAL LIBRARY. Pick yours and GET BUSY'.[73] The importance of vocational reading and the political intentions that informed it are also evident in *Your Job Back Home*, published by the ALA in 1919. Adorned with large photographs, the book lists a wide range of civilian careers that men might pursue, alongside a bibliography of relevant technical and vocational works provided by the ALA. *Your Job Back Home* reproduced the idealistic language of wartime propaganda, stressing that the 'World has seen enough autocracies that control the lives and fortunes of the people'. It also reflected the growing paranoia regarding communist revolution which characterized the Red Scare, denouncing 'the plots and plans by which people hope to rise by tearing down everything else'. The alternative, according to the ALA, was 'Uncle Sam's new army of democracy', comprising 'a hundred million men working together, thinking together, planning together for the things that will make America a better place to live in'.[74] Books were part of a broader political project infused with a rhetoric that championed democratic values and the intrinsic value of hard work.

In this sense, the ALA's promotion of reading was not dissimilar to the rationale for reading advanced by Samuel McCord Crothers when he coined the term 'bibliotherapy' in his 1916 essay 'A Literary Clinic'. As Jesse Miller has demonstrated, Crothers was in fact satirizing the notion that patients could be prescribed specific books in order to cure distinct ailments and 'objected to what he perceived as the reduction of the reader-as-patient to a passive consumer of texts prescribed to him by some external, expert authority'.[75] Rather, in his words, Crothers extolled the value of 'the book which puts us in a working mood'.[76] This was precisely what ALA hospital librarians hoped to achieve when promoting the vocational value of reading.

When the ALA outlined its official responsibilities in the reconstruction hospitals in early 1919, it recognized the recreational, educational, vocational and curative benefits of reading. Its primary purposes were to relieve 'tedium', to provide 'entertainment and opportunity and inspiration for study', to facilitate 're-education, rehabilitation, and vocational education', to maintain 'libraries for the medical and nursing staff and for the enlisted men' and, finally, to secure 'the cooperation of libraries in the vicinity of the hospital in furnishing books and service'. Though this list only alluded to the curative power of books, elsewhere the report explicitly highlighted the therapeutic potential of reading. When summarizing the educational mission of the hospital libraries, the report noted that 'the A.L.A considers the library service a definite part of reconstruction, as well as an aid in helping others to do the work. Reading is as curative in many cases as shop work and educational therapy'.[77] Once more, librarians stressed that books were not solely tools with which to *facilitate* vocational therapy; they were also curative themselves.

In May 1919, the ALA also foregrounded its therapeutic mission in promotional materials. In the *War Library Bulletin*, Caroline Webster promoted the organization's work in the reconstruction hospitals, stressing that librarians were important members of staff, working alongside medical professionals and educational experts. Webster certainly underlined the vocational and educational significance of reading. She noted that the libraries in reconstruction hospitals were housed in the Educational Building and that librarians were considered 'part of the faculty', with much of their work 'similar to the work in a high school or college'. But this service, Webster implied, was not merely for educational reasons. It was also curative. The provision of specific books and magazines to patients, according to Webster, was valued by doctors who reported 'that its therapeutic value cannot be overestimated'. In an especially poignant anecdote, Webster recalled that 'In one hospital library it was the touch of a familiar volume of Shakespeare that first roused a psychiatric patient'.[78]

Exactly how books performed this function was unclear – systematic research into bibliotherapy did not yet exist – and so librarians often employed simplistic methods when selecting books for patients. At Camp Wadsworth, South Carolina, for example, they insisted that 'the nervous patient does not get too exciting a book'.[79] At Walter Reed General Hospital, meanwhile, the staff avoided prescribing books with 'unhappy endings', because these were known to 'cause lasting depression'.[80] For some librarians, the power of books lay in their capacity to stimulate and thus restore the minds of patients suffering from psychological trauma. As Annessa Stagner has shown, American understandings of shell shock during the war, unlike those which prevailed in Europe, were often imbued with a belief that wartime mental trauma could be cured.[81] Though reconstruction hospitals often catered to patients with physical disabilities, heavily promoting their work with amputees, they also dealt with soldiers suffering from various forms of mental trauma. It was for these men that books might have a curative impact. A February 1919 report from the military hospital library at Plattsburg Barracks in New York State observed that in 'institutions for neuro-psychiatric patients', many men 'display a lack of initiative, and literature provides one way of bringing it back'. The report stressed, however, that a library alone was not enough. Rather, the librarian had to provide 'a guide to interesting and helpful books' and needed to understand the 'patient's attitude and the books with which she is dealing'.[82] In other words, though readers' tastes were taken into account, librarians were expected to prescribe books to patients, drawing on their own professional expertise in order to help rehabilitate men suffering from mental trauma.

In May that year, Caroline Webster likewise asserted the curative power of books for patients with psychiatric ailments:

> The librarian with her bedside truck filled with books, magazines, and newspapers helps unconsciously to renew interest in life in the shattered boy ... it is a recognized fact that any one will get well more quickly if his mind is occupied and he does not have time to brood over himself and his troubles.[83]

Webster presented bibliotherapy in gendered terms, imbuing librarians, who were predominantly female, with a maternalistic capacity to restore men who had been seemingly infantilized and emasculated by their mental trauma. A belief that reading could help to cure psychiatric disorders through stimulation and distraction appears to have informed this emerging conception of bibliotherapy. A similar approach had informed the work of volunteer librarians in British military hospitals during the war.[84]

This ethos was not limited solely to military settings. At a similar time, librarians and medical professionals elsewhere also began to espouse the efficacy of therapeutic reading. In August 1919, in the magazine *Hospital Quarterly*, Sidney I. Schwab, a neurologist, and Elizabeth Green, the librarian, at the Barnes Hospital in St. Louis, Missouri, published an article entitled 'The Therapeutic Use of a Hospital Library'. In this article, Schwab and Green acknowledged that neither hospital libraries themselves nor the recognition of the benefits of recreational reading for patients was entirely new. Like most emerging practitioners of bibliotherapy, however, they expressed a desire to make 'a more definite and positively planned use of books', in which particular types of reading could be prescribed to patients in order to achieve specific outcomes.[85] Their article presented a more schematic approach than previous attempts to promote therapeutic reading, adding a scientific veneer to an imprecise and ill-defined process, one which had not yet been subject to rigorous empirical research.

Schwab and Green identified four categories of books, each of which was defined by the distinct benefit that it had for patients. The first of these included those books which interest the 'patient to such an extent that the long hours of convalescence or preparation might be gone through as quickly as possible'. The second category included books that 'can train the patient's attention and concentration'. The third category, which the authors conceded was 'the smallest', addressed books that might cause 'a change or alteration' in the patient's 'point of view'. The fourth and final category contained books that are 'educational and instructive' and which might add something to the 'personal asset of the patient'.[86] The first and fourth categories primarily addressed the recreational and educational benefits of books, which had been promoted by the ALA during the war without any overt therapeutic intentions. The second and third categories, however, suggest that books might have a direct effect on mental functioning and wellbeing, and in this sense are more explicitly 'therapeutic'.

Shwab and Green's belief that particular books could be prescribed in order to achieve one or more of these outcomes illustrates how the trope of the 'literary clinic' had begun to inform the promotion of hospital librarianship. It also reveals a salient point about the emerging discourse of curative reading: bibliotherapy was not solely about advancing the hitherto unforeseen medical benefits of reading; it was also about representing the long-recognized educational and recreational value of reading within new therapeutic language, in which specific books would be *prescribed* to individual patients with particular positive outcomes in mind. Despite this, Schwab and Green recognized that bibliotherapy lacked scientific precision, conceding that 'there is no way by which the influence of books as indicated can be measured'. In their view, 'the therapeutic effect of books' was 'too subtle for analysis and often too intangible to record'.[87]

Schwab and Green's article is also important because it illustrates that some medical professionals, as well as librarians, had begun to believe in the therapeutic value of books. This was not an isolated phenomenon. An ALA report, written by Caroline Webster in August 1919, asserted that doctors, rather than librarians, spearheaded the emergence of bibliotherapy in hospital libraries. Webster suggested that 'Librarians of course knew that fiction, poetry and books on the kindred arts would be popular and serve as recreation but it is the doctors who have emphasized the therapeutic value of reading'. She recalled that Dr William White, 'one of the leading psychiatrists of the country', had argued 'that it is almost impossible to overestimate the therapeutic value of reading and that we must consider it in this light as well as in its relation to occupational and recreational work'.[88] Whether all doctors held this belief is open to debate: facing the news that it might soon have to discontinue, largely due to the expense of maintaining the service, Webster needed to justify the ALA's continued work in military hospitals and arguments such as these helped to bolster her cause, not least because the endorsement of medical professionals added greater weight to her claims regarding the therapeutic value of reading.

In October 1920, however, the Committee on the Transfer of Library War Service Activities announced that, due to lack of funds, the ALA would discontinue its role in hospital libraries, with the federal government assuming responsibility for the work. The transfer to the Public Health Service was completed in July 1921.[89] The ALA's historical report, written shortly after the closure of the service, reflects the organisation's growing emphasis on curative reading. It proudly states the library service was 'looked upon as an important part of the curative and educational work'. It also celebrates other ALA activities in curative terms, noting how the 'distribution of hometown newspapers' had 'a decided therapeutic value'.[90] In 1917, ALA promotional materials rarely used such language. By 1921, the trope of the 'literary clinic' abounded in official documents. Bibliotherapy had truly come of age.

Conclusion

The roots of bibliotherapy predate American intervention in the First World War and the conflict itself. Bibliotherapy in the United States, however, did not emerge fully formed in response to the war. When the Library War Service began its work in

1917, the ALA was primarily driven by a range of political assumptions regarding the moral and educational benefits of reading. Even when the ALA began its work in military hospitals, the value of therapeutic reading was not at the forefront of librarians' minds. The discourse of therapeutic reading, in fact, did not begin to gain serious traction until after the armistice, as the ALA expanded its work in Reconstruction hospitals. In this setting, an emphasis on vocational therapy and the drive to rehabilitate convalescent servicemen encouraged ALA librarians to embrace and promote the curative potential of books. The growing faith in therapeutic reading, however, was entangled with the broader political imperatives which underpinned the ALA's work and that of the reconstruction hospitals. In January 1919, an article in *McClure's* magazine celebrated the ALA's provision of recreational and educational opportunities for soldiers. Looking ahead to their demobilization, the article's author, Harrison Rhodes, stressed that 'When Johnny comes marching home, we want him to be a better man physically, mentally, morally than when he went away'.[91] Rhodes perfectly encapsulated the mission of the ALA's Library War Service. By 1919, most librarians did indeed promote reading as integral to a man's physical and mental health. These beliefs were central to emerging notions of bibliotherapy. But they were also driven by moral imperatives and the political and ideological forces which underpinned them.

These values persisted after the termination of the Library War Service. In 1922, Carl Millam, then director of the American Library Association, wrote a bulletin for the Bureau of Education entitled *What Libraries Learned from the War*. Millam had played a major role in running the Library War Service and observed, among other things, that the ALA's work in hospitals during the war 'gave additional proof that the reading of books has in numerous cases a real therapeutic value'. But he also stressed the importance of books as political instruments, arguing that 'Libraries can help to create a national spirit'. 'The library has a part', Millam argued, 'in furnishing the means whereby every citizen may become an intelligent citizen'.[92] Millam, like many librarians during the war, presented reading as beneficial in both therapeutic and ideological terms.

Appreciating the context within which notions of curative reading developed during the war is essential to an understanding of the history of bibliotherapy in the twentieth century. Bibliotherapy was in fact the product of a broader political agenda that focused on educating, rehabilitating and 'Americanizing' men in order to transform them into productive citizens. These imperatives underscore the fact that caregiving, though ostensibly focused on patient wellbeing, is not politically neutral. The history of bibliotherapy, therefore, is not solely a concern for historians of reading or historians of medicine. It also illuminates the broader political, intellectual and cultural currents which characterized the Progressive Era in the United States, including attitudes to work, citizenship and national identity.

Notes

1 W. B. McDaniel, 'Bibliotherapy – Some Historical and Contemporary Aspects', *ALA Bulletin* 50, no. 9 (1956): 584–589.

2 The American Library Association itself had been formed in 1876.
3 Arthur P. Young, *Books for Sammies: The American Library Association and World War I* (Pittsburgh: Beta Phi Mu, 1981), 58.
4 Mary Mahoney, 'The Library as Medicine Cabinet: Inventing Bibliotherapy in the Interwar Period', in *Libraries: Traditions and Innovations: Papers from the Library History Seminar XIII*, eds. Melanie A. Kimball and Katherine M. Wisser (Berlin and Boston: De Gruyter, 2017), 104.
5 For example, see: Jonathan Arnold, '"Please Send Me Tess of the Dr. Rbyvilles (Harding)": The Reading Preferences of American Soldiers during the First World War', in *Reading and the First World War: Readers, Texts, Archives*, eds. Shafquat Towheed and Edmund G. C. King (Basingtoke: Palgrave Macmillan, 2015), 93–114; Kathryne A. Bevilacqua, 'Making U.S. Readers in the Early Twentieth Century' (PhD diss., University of Michigan, 2016); and Young, *Books for Sammies*, 1981.
6 Jesse Miller, 'Medicines of the Soul: Reparative Reading and the History of Bibliotherapy', *Mosaic: An Interdisciplinary Critical Journal* 51, no. 2 (June 2018): 17–34.
7 Koch's report was published in Britain by J. M. Dent in order to publicize the efforts of British charitable agencies in providing reading material for soldiers. See Theodore Koch, *Books in Camp, Trench and Hospital* (London: J.M. Dent, 1918).
8 Sara Haslam, 'Reading, Trauma and Literary Caregiving 1914–1918: Helen Mary Gaskell and the War Library', *Journal of Medical Humanities* 41, no. 3 (September 2020): 307.
9 Young, *Books for Sammies*, 10–14.
10 Young, *Books for Sammies*, xi.
11 Bevilacqua, 'Making U.S. Readers', 203.
12 'Let Your Idle Books Help Our Soldiers', *War Library Bulletin*, August 1917, 4.
13 'Preliminary List of Books for Soldiers and Sailors Libraries', 1917, Record Series 89/1/65, Box 1, Booklists Series 1, American Library Association Archives at the University of Illinois at Urbana-Champaign (hereafter ALAA).
14 For a discussion of the work of the War Library and the British origins of bibliotherapy more broadly, see Sara Haslam and Edmund G. C. King, '"Medicinable Literature": Bibliotherapy, Literary Caregiving and the First World War', *Literature and Medicine* 39, no. 2 (2021): 296–318.
15 'Good Reading Helps Make "Big Battalions"', *War Library Bulletin*, September 1917, 3.
16 *War Library Bulletin*, 18 September 1917, 4.
17 'News from Camp Libraries – Some Informal Reports. Do Men Read?', *War Library Bulletin*, April 1918, 12.
18 Andrew J. Huebner, *Love and Death in the Great War* (New York: Oxford University Press, 2018), 60; Chad L. Williams, *Torchbearers of Democracy: African American Soldiers in the World War I Era* (Chapel Hill: University of North Carolina Press, 2010), 93.
19 Young, *Books for Sammies*, 11.
20 The 'Progressive Era' – a period marked by widespread political reform and social activism – has been conceptualized and analysed by numerous historians. It is typically seen to encompass the period from the 1890s until the 1910s. For example, see John Whiteclay Chambers II, *The Tyranny of Change: America in the Progressive Era*, 2nd ed. (New Brunswick: Rutgers University Press, 2000) and Michael McGerr, *The Rise and Fall of the Progressive Movement in America, 1870–1920* (New York: Oxford University Press, 2003).
21 Williams, *Torchbearers of Democracy*, 94.

22 John W. D. Melvin to the Librarian at Boston Public Library, 1918, Record Series 89/1/5, Box 2, Volume 9, ALAA.
23 Williams, *Torchbearers of Democracy*, 97.
24 John W. D. Melvin to the Librarian at Boston Public Library, Record Series 89/1/5, Box 2, Volume 9, ALAA.
25 Florence W. Humphrey, report from Fort Sam Houston Base Hospital Library, August 1918, Record Series 89/1/5, Box 2, Volume 9, ALAA.
26 Samantha Ne Camp, *Adult Literacy and American Identity: The Moonlight Schools and Americanization Programmes* (Carbondale: Southern Illinois University, 2014), 85.
27 Desmond S. King, *Making Americans: Immigration, Race, and the Origins of the Diverse Democracy* (Cambridge, MA: Harvard University Press, 2000), 87.
28 Michael S. Neiberg, *The Path to War: How the First World War Created America* (New York: Oxford University Press, 2016), 144.
29 Quoted in Arthur S. Link, *Wilson: Confusion and Crises, 1915–1916* (Princeton: Princeton University Press, 1964), 36
30 J. Maud Campbell, 'Americanizing Books and Periodicals for Immigrants', *Bulletin of the American Library Association* 10, no. 4 (July 1916): 269–272.
31 H. H. Wheaton, 'An Americanization Program for Libraries', *Bulletin of the American Library Association* 10, no. 4 (July 1916): 265–269.
32 Wayne A. Wiegand, *'An Active Instrument for Propaganda': The American Public Library during World War I* (New York: Greenwood, 1989), 115.
33 George F. Worts, 'What Books Are Doing to Americanize Soldiers of Many Races', *The Outlook*, 2 October 1918, 186.
34 Worts, 'What Books Are Doing to Americanize Soldiers of Many Races', 186–87. *The Man without a Country* was published during the American Civil War to bolster support for the Union and was likely a more appropriate choice for readers in Massachusetts than it would have been in a southern camp library.
35 Ola M. Wyeth, Report from the Base Hospital Library at Camp Wadsworth, 1918, Record Series 89/1/5, Box 5, Volume 29, ALAA.
36 Young, *Books for Sammies,* 56.
37 'Historical Sketch, ALA War Service from Jan. 1, 1919 to Nov. 1, 1920', Record Series 89/1/52, Box 1, Series 21, Volume 1, ALAA.
38 Haslam, 'Reading, Trauma and Literary Caregiving', 306.
39 Young, *Books for Sammies*, 58.
40 McDaniel, 'Bibliotherapy', 584–589.
41 Young, *Books for Sammies*, 57. For more on Jones's role in developing the practice of bibliotherapy in the United States during the early twentieth century, see Sara Haslam, Jesse Miller and Laureen P. Cantwell-Jurkovic, 'The Flow of Comfort: Bibliotherapy, The History of Literary Caregiving, and the Academic Library Today', in *Intersections in Healing: Academic Libraries and the Health Humanities*, ed. Laureen P. Cantwell-Jurkovic (Lanham, MD: Rowman and Littlefield, 2024), 65–69.
42 Edith Kathleen Jones, 'The Growth of Hospital Libraries', *The Modern Hospital*, 18, no. 5 (1922): 452–453.
43 Beth Linker, *War's Waste: Rehabilitation in World War I America* (Chicago: University of Chicago Press, 2011), 2–3.
44 Linker, *War's Waste*, 5.
45 Linker, *War's Waste*, 80.
46 Linker, *War's Waste*, 7.

47 T. J. Jackson Lears, *No Place of Grace: Antimodernism and the Transformation of American Culture, 1880–1920* (Chicago: University of Chicago Press, 1994), 47–58.
48 Lears, *No Place of Grace*, 69.
49 'Program of Recreational Activities in Reconstruction Hospitals', 1918, Record Series 89/1/5, Box 5, Volume 29, ALAA.
50 'Report of the War Service Committee of the American Library Association', June 1918, Record Series 89/1/52, Box 1, Series 24, Volume 4, ALAA.
51 Report from New Haven General Hospital, 10 September 1918, Record Series 89/1/5, Box 5, Volume 29, ALAA.
52 'Your Job Back Home', *Carry On*, April 1919, 32.
53 Booklists, Record Series 89/1/5, Box 5, Volume 29, ALAA.
54 Booklists, 'Curative Shop Schedule', Record Series 89/1/5, Box 5, Volume 29, ALAA.
55 'Report on Reconstruction Work', U.S. General Hospital No. 28, Fort Des Moines, 18 December 1918, Record Series 89/1/5, Box 5, Volume 29, ALAA.
56 Ola M. Wyeth, Report from the Base Hospital Library at Camp Wadsworth, 1918, Record Series 89/1/5, Box 5, Volume 29, ALAA.
57 Theodore Koch, *Books in Camp, Trench and Hospital* (London: J.M. Dent, 1918), 12. See also Haslam, 'Reading, Trauma and Literary Caregiving', 311.
58 E. M. Dougherty to Theodore Koch, 21 March 1918, Record Series 89/1/5, Box 2, Volume 11, ALAA.
59 A. T. Poor to the American Library Association, 29 May 1918, Record Series 89/1/5, Box 2, Volume 11, ALAA.
60 Ellen Gruber Garvey, *Writing with Scissors: American Scrapbooks from the Civil War to the Harlem Renaissance* (New York: Oxford University Press, 2012), 27.
61 Garvey, *Writing with Scissors*, 51.
62 Report from Walter Reed General Hospital, 1918, Record Series 89/1/5, Box 5, Volume 29, ALAA.
63 'Dr. A. H. Shearer's Sketch – June, 1917 to Jan. 1919', Record Series 89/1/52, Box 1, Volume 1, ALAA.
64 'Memorandum RE: Hospitals', April 1918, Record Series 89/1/5, Box 5, Volume 29, ALAA.
65 Garvey, *Writing with Scissors*, 49.
66 Ernestine Rose, 'What Men Read in Hospitals', Press Bulletin, 3 August 1918, Record Series 89/1/5, Box 5, Volume 29, ALAA.
67 'Soldiers' Scrap Books: Suggestions to Volunteers Adapted from Outline Issued by the Chicago Public Library', 9 October 1918, Record Series 89/1/5, Box 2, Volume 11, ALAA.
68 'Soldiers' Scrap Books: Suggestions to Volunteers Adapted from Outline Issued by the Chicago Public Library', 9 October 1918, Record Series 89/1/5, Box 2, Volume 11, ALAA.
69 'Scrapbook Specifications Issued by the Denver Public Library', 22 September 1917, Record Series 89/1/5, Box 2, Volume 11, ALAA.
70 Report from Walter Reed General Hospital, 1918, Record Series 89/1/5, Box 5, Volume 29, ALAA.
71 'Suggested Copy for Leaflet or Bookmark', 5 December 1918, Record Series 89/1/52, Box 1, Series 16, ALAA.
72 'Report on Reconstruction Work', U.S. General Hospital No. 28, Fort Des Moines, 18 December 1918, Record Series 89/1/5, Box 5, Volume 29, ALAA.
73 *War Library Bulletin*, March 1919, 2.

74 American Library Association, *Your Job Back Home: A Book for Men Leaving the Service* (Washington, DC: Press of Judd & Detweiler, 1919).
75 Miller, 'Medicines of the Soul', 28.
76 Samuel McChord Crothers, 'A Literary Clinic', in *The Pleasures of an Absentee Landlord, and Other Essays* (Boston: Houghton Mifflin, 1916), 148.
77 'Library Service of the ALA in Hospitals', 1919, Record Series 89/1/52, Box 1, Series 23, Volume 3, ALAA.
78 Caroline Webster, 'Hospital Libraries', *War Library Bulletin*, May 1919, 9.
79 Ola M. Wyeth, 'Library Service in a Base Hospital', Camp Wadsworth, 1918, Record Series 89/1/5, Box 5, Volume 29, ALAA.
80 Report from Walter Reed General Hospital, 1918, Record Series 89/1/5, Box 5, Volume 29, ALAA.
81 Annessa C. Stagner, 'Healing the Soldier, Restoring the Nation: Representations of Shell Shock in the USA during and after the First World War', *Journal of Contemporary History* 49, no. 2 (April 2014): 256.
82 'Report on American Library Association Hospital Library', US Army General Hospital No. 30, Plattsburg Barracks, N.Y., 13 February 1919, Record Series 89/1/5, Box 5, Volume 29, ALAA.
83 Caroline Webster, 'Hospital Libraries', *War Library Bulletin*, May 1919, 9.
84 Haslam and King, 'Medicinable Literature', 304.
85 Elizabeth Green and Sidney I. Schwab, 'The Therapeutic Use of a Hospital Library', *The Hospital Social Service Quarterly* 1, no. 3 (August 1919), 147.
86 Green and Schwab, 'The Therapeutic Use of a Hospital Library', 149–150.
87 Green and Schwab, 'The Therapeutic Use of a Hospital Library', 151.
88 Caroline Webster, 'Suggestions for a Future Program for the A.L.A. in Hospital Libraries', 1 August 1919, Record Series 89/1/5, Box 5, Volume 29, ALAA. William White – the superintendent of St. Elizabeth's Hospital, a psychiatric institution in Washington, DC – was a leading psychiatrist in the United States at the time.
89 Young, *Books for Sammies*, 88–89.
90 'Dr. A. H. Shearer's Sketch – June 1917 to Jan. 1919', Record Series 89/1/52, Box 1, Volume 1, ALAA.
91 Harrison Rhodes, 'When Johnny Comes Marching Home', *McClure's*, January 1919, 44.
92 Carl H. Millam, *What Libraries Learned from the War*, Library Leaflet No. 14 (Washington, DC: United States Bureau of Education, 1922), 3–4.

References

American Library Association, *Your Job Back Home: A Book for Men Leaving the Service.*Washington, DC: Press of Judd & Detweiler, 1919.

Arnold, Jonathan. '"Please Send Me Tess of the Dr. Rbyvilles (Harding)": The Reading Preferences of American Soldiers during the First World War'. In *Reading and the First World War: Readers, Texts, Archives*, eds. Shafquat Towheed and Edmund G. C. King, 93–114. Basingstoke: Palgrave Macmillan, 2015.

Bevilacqua, Kathryne A. 'Making U.S. Readers in the Early Twentieth Century', PhD diss., University of Michigan, 2016.

Booklists, 'Curative Shop Schedule', Record Series 89/1/5, Box 5, Volume 29, American Library Association Archives at the University of Illinois at Urbana-Champaign.

Booklists, Record Series 89/1/5, Box 5, Volume 29, American Library Association Archives at the University of Illinois at Urbana-Champaign.

Campbell, J. Maud. 'Americanizing Books and Periodicals for Immigrants', *Bulletin of the American Library Association* 10, no. 4 (July 1916): 269–272.

Crothers, Samuel McChord. 'A Literary Clinic', in *The Pleasures of an Absentee Landlord, and Other Essays*, 117–149. Boston: Houghton Mifflin, 1916.

Dougherty, E. M. Letter to Theodore Koch, 21 March 1918, Record Series 89/1/5, Box 2, Volume 11, American Library Association Archives at the University of Illinois at Urbana-Champaign.

'Dr. A. H. Shearer's Sketch – June 1917 to Jan. 1919', Record Series 89/1/52, Box 1, Volume 1, American Library Association Archives at the University of Illinois at Urbana-Champaign.

Garvey, Ellen Gruber. *Writing with Scissors: American Scrapbooks from the Civil War to the Harlem Renaissance*. New York: Oxford University Press, 2012.

'Good Reading Helps Make "Big Battalions" ', *War Library Bulletin*, September 1917.

Green, Elizabeth and Schwab, Sidney I. 'The Therapeutic Use of a Hospital Library', *The Hospital Service Quarterly* 1, no. 3 (August 1919): 147–157.

Haslam, Sara. 'Reading, Trauma and Literary Caregiving 1914–1918: Helen Mary Gaskell and the War Library', *Journal of Medical Humanities* 41, no. 3 (September 2020): 305–321.

Haslam, Sara, and King, Edmund G. C. ' "Medicinable Literature": Bibliotherapy, Literary Caregiving and the First World War', *Literature and Medicine* 39, no. 2 (2021): 296–318.

Haslam, Sara, Jesse Miller and Laureen P. Cantwell-Jurkovic, 'The Flow of Comfort: Bibliotherapy, The History of Literary Caregiving, and the Academic Library Today', in *Intersections in Healing: Academic Libraries and the Health Humanities*, ed. Laureen P. Cantwell-Jurkovic, 63–82. Lanham, MD: Rowman and Littlefield, 2024.

'Historical Sketch, ALA War Service from Jan. 1, 1919 to Nov. 1, 1920', Record Series 89/1/52, Box 1, Series 21, Volume 1, American Library Association Archives at the University of Illinois at Urbana-Champaign.

Huebner, Andrew J. *Love and Death in the Great War*. New York: Oxford University Press, 2018.

Humphrey, Florence W. Report from Fort Sam Houston Base Hospital Library, August 1918, Record Series 89/1/5, Box 2, Volume 9, American Library Association Archives at the University of Illinois at Urbana-Champaign.

Jones, Edith Kathleen. 'The Growth of Hospital Libraries', *The Modern Hospital*, 18, no. 5 (1922): 452–454.

King, Desmond S. *Making Americans: Immigration, Race, and the Origins of the Diverse Democracy*. Cambridge, MA: Harvard University Press, 2000.

Koch, Theodore. *Books in Camp, Trench and Hospital*. London: J.M. Dent, 1918.

Lears, T. J. Jackson. *No Place of Grace: Antimodernism and the Transformation of American Culture, 1880–1920*. Chicago: University of Chicago Press, 1994.

'Let Your Idle Books Help Our Soldiers', *War Library Bulletin*, August 1917.

'Library Service of the ALA in Hospitals', 1919, Record Series 89/1/52, Box 1, Series 23, Volume 3, American Library Association Archives at the University of Illinois at Urbana-Champaign.

Link, Arthur S. *Wilson: Confusion and Crises, 1915–1916*. Princeton: Princeton University Press, 1964.

Linker, Beth. *War's Waste: Rehabilitation in World War I America*. Chicago: University of Chicago Press, 2011.

Mahoney, Mary. 'The Library as Medicine Cabinet: Inventing Bibliotherapy in the Interwar Period'. In *Libraries: Traditions and Innovations: Papers from the Library*

History Seminar XIII, eds. Melanie A. Kimball and Katherine M. Wisser, 100–107. Berlin: DeGruyter, 2017.

McDaniel, W. B. 'Bibliotherapy – Some Historical and Contemporary Aspects', *ALA Bulletin* 50, no. 9 (1956): 584–589.

Melvin, John W. D. Letter to the Librarian at Boston Public Library, 1918, Record Series 89/1/5, Box 2, Volume 9, American Library Association Archives at the University of Illinois at Urbana-Champaign.

'Memorandum RE: Hospitals', April 1918, Record Series 89/1/5, Box 5, Volume 29, American Library Association Archives at the University of Illinois at Urbana-Champaign.

Millam, Carl H. *What Libraries Learned from the War*, Library Leaflet No. 14. Washington, DC: United States Bureau of Education, 1922.

Miller, Jesse. 'Medicines of the Soul: Reparative Reading and the History of Bibliotherapy', *Mosaic: An Interdisciplinary Critical Journal* 51, no. 2 (June 2018): 17–34.

NeCamp, Samantha. *Adult Literacy and American Identity: The Moonlight Schools and Americanization Programmes*. Carbondale: Southern Illinois University, 2014.

Neiberg, Michael. *The Path to War: How the First World War Created Modern America*. New York: Oxford University Press, 2016.

'News from Camp Libraries – Some Informal Reports. Do Men Read?', *War Library Bulletin*, April 1918.

Poor, A. T. Letter to the American Library Association, 29 May 1918, Record Series 89/1/5, Box 2, Volume 11, American Library Association Archives at the University of Illinois at Urbana-Champaign.

'Preliminary List of Books for Soldiers and Sailors Libraries', 1917, Record Series 89/1/65, Box 1, Booklists Series 1, American Library Association Archives at the University of Illinois at Urbana-Champaign.

'Program of Recreational Activities in Reconstruction Hospitals', 1918, Record Series 89/1/5, Box 5, Volume 29, American Library Association Archives at the University of Illinois at Urbana-Champaign.

Report from New Haven General Hospital, 10 September 1918, Record Series 89/1/5, Box 5, Volume 29, American Library Association Archives at the University of Illinois at Urbana-Champaign.

Report from Walter Reed General Hospital, 1918, Record Series 89/1/5, Box 5, Volume 29, American Library Association Archives at the University of Illinois at Urbana-Champaign.

'Report of the War Service Committee of the American Library Association', June 1918, Record Series 89/1/52, Box 1, Series 24, Volume 4, American Library Association Archives at the University of Illinois at Urbana-Champaign.

'Report on American Library Association Hospital Library', US Army General Hospital No.30, Plattsburg Barracks, N.Y., 13 February 1919, Record Series 89/1/5, Box 5, Volume 29, American Library Association Archives at the University of Illinois at Urbana-Champaign.

'Report on Reconstruction Work', U.S. General Hospital No. 28, Fort Des Moines, 18 December 1918, Record Series 89/1/5, Box 5, Volume 29, American Library Association Archives at the University of Illinois at Urbana-Champaign.

Rhodes, Harrison. 'When Johnny Comes Marching Home', *McClure's*, January 1919.

Rose, Ernestine. 'What Men Read in Hospitals', Press Bulletin, 3 August 1918, Record Series 89/1/5, Box 5, Volume 29, American Library Association Archives at the University of Illinois at Urbana-Champaign.

'Scrapbook Specifications Issued by the Denver Public Library', 22 September 1917, Record Series 89/1/5, Box 2, Volume 11, American Library Association Archives at the University of Illinois at Urbana-Champaign.

'Soldiers' Scrap Books: Suggestions to Volunteers Adapted from Outline Issued by the Chicago Public Library', 9 October 1918, Record Series 89/1/5, Box 2, Volume 11, American Library Association Archives at the University of Illinois at Urbana-Champaign.

Stagner, Annessa C. 'Healing the Soldier, Restoring the Nation: Representations of ShellShock in the USA during and after the First World War', *Journal of Contemporary History* 49, no. 2 (April 2014): 255–274.

'Suggested Copy for Leaflet or Bookmark', 5 December 1918, Record Series 89/1/52, Box 1, Series 16, American Library Association Archives at the University of Illinois at Urbana-Champaign.

War Library Bulletin, 18 September 1917.

War Library Bulletin, March 1919.

Webster, Caroline. 'Hospital Libraries', *War Library Bulletin*, May 1919.

Webster, Caroline. 'Suggestions for a Future Program for the A.L.A. in Hospital Libraries', 1 August 1919, Record Series 89/1/5, Box 5, Volume 29, American Library Association Archives at the University of Illinois at Urbana-Champaign.

Wheaton, H. H. 'An Americanization Program for Libraries', *Bulletin of the American Library Association* 10, no. 4 (July 1916): 265–269.

Wiegand, Wayne A. *'An Active Instrument for Propaganda': The American Public Library during World War I.* New York: Greenwood, 1989.

Williams, Chad L. *Torchbearers of Democracy: African American Soldiers in the World War I Era*. Chapel Hill: University of North Carolina Press, 2010.

Worts, George F. 'What Books Are Doing to Americanize Soldiers of Many Races', *The Outlook*, 2 October 1918.

Wyeth, Ola M. Report from the Base Hospital Library at Camp Wadsworth, 1918, Record Series 89/1/5, Box 5, Volume 29, American Library Association Archives at the University of Illinois at Urbana-Champaign.

Young, Arthur P. *Books for Sammies: The American Library Association and World War I.* Pittsburgh: Beta Phi Mu, 1981.

'Your Job Back Home', *Carry On*, April 1919.

4 Autograph Books as Alleviation in British First World War Hospitals

A Case Study

Lindsay Davies

I've turned these pages over and over
To see what folks have wrote before
But on this secluded spot
I simply say forget me not[1]

On August 8, 1915, Private J. H. White, No. 2467 of the 7th Battalion, Durham Light Infantry, wrote this poem on one of the pages of the autograph book belonging to Gladys Forryan, who regularly visited the wounded soldiers in the military hospital in Clarendon Park, Leicester. In addition to its poignancy, there are two important things about this poem. First, it refers to the autograph book as concerning both reading and writing within a shared context – White reads intentionally, turning the pages 'over and over' to see what other soldiers have written. That is, the autograph book confers community and some public exposure. But, second, and in contrast, White's words also speak of a sense of seclusion. Jessica Meyer, in her essay on hospital journals from the First World War, has argued that such journals reflect the fact that the 'hospital was the site of negotiation of [multiple] social relationships during the war.'[2] Contributions from doctors, trained nurses, nursing and general service VADs, and orderlies, as well as wounded soldiers, 'demonstrate the breadth and complexity of the function of hospital journals as a form of wartime communication.'[3] Compared with other wartime periodicals, she continues, hospital journals 'act as a bridge across a liminal space' between the front line and the home front.[4] This chapter will explore the use of the autograph book in the hospital ward as a similar bridge, this time across the public conditions of the hospital ward and the private spaces of the soldier's mind.

As a central part of what Jeffrey Reznick has called 'the culture of caregiving,'[5] hospital journals provided a place for sharing stories, poems, cartoons, and other forms of commentary and expression: 'as curative activities that were part of [an] overall program of rehabilitation; editors anticipated that such contributions would foster camaraderie and hence boost morale.'[6] But it was understood that the hospital journal would be sold and circulated, both within the hospital and outside its walls. That is, there was a degree of public exposure built-in – not to mention a

DOI: 10.4324/9781003471561-6

maintaining of standards by editors.[7] The hospital autograph book, on the other hand, had an owner, not an editor. The owner of a hospital autograph book was usually a nurse or VAD (or a female visitor to the ward, like Gladys Forryan) and the book was hers to share as she chose. Long thought of as cultural ephemera, the autograph books of the First World War have only recently begun to receive scholarly attention.[8] Yet hospital autograph books had a similar rehabilitative function in the hospital ward as the journal. They too were sites for the sharing of literary, artistic, and comedic talents. They too served to build community. But, as Private White's poem indicates, the autograph book was a more 'secluded' practice – less exposed, more intimate, more personal, and arguably more private. The community within which the autograph book circulated was small and highly specific to the owner. It was close to what we now call 'a safe space.' Thus, within that more intimate communal space, autograph books offered a less exposed way for soldiers to come to terms with their war experience, their injuries (both physical and psychic), and the profound dismantling of their pre-war selves.

I

Autograph books have passed out of fashion, so I offer a definition for those less familiar with the genre. Sometimes called albums, autograph books are small volumes, often leather-bound, with multi-coloured pages. The book was circulated by its owner amongst different communities (family, school, church, etc.) and given to friends so that they could select a page to write or draw something on. Often the pages were used for small drawings and paintings; more commonly, the entries would be quotations from famous writers, well-known rhymes that were understood as conventional offerings, jokes, and sometimes longer poems as well. In most cases, the inscriber would sign and date the page.

Todd Gernes has noted that the autograph book, first known as an *Album Amicorum* (friendship album), 'grew out of sixteenth-century European [specifically German] scholasticism and flowered in the hothouse of nineteenth-century American sentimentality.'[9] By the late nineteenth century, responding to innovations in book manufacturing, the custom of keeping an autograph book had spread rapidly through the ranks of middle-class leisured young ladies who collected in its pages inscriptions and artwork from school friends, teachers, family members, and loved ones. The tradition continued and gradually adopted its popular form, derived from a formerly élite aristocratic practice.[10] The few scholars who have studied this form agree that by the mid-nineteenth century, the keeping of an autograph book was 'a practice' primarily engaged in by 'girls and young women during their formative years.'[11] Men, however, were willing contributors to their pages.[12]

As a cultural artefact, an autograph book is ambiguous. It is a book, but it is also a compilation of random 'entries' lacking intentional organization. The owner of the book seeks to fill its pages through her own network of association; as such, it reflects 'kinship, community, and affiliation.'[13] Usually, the owner does not prescribe the ordering of the entries and certainly she does not prescribe the content. She hands the book over to someone else who selects the page and decides what he or she will write/draw on it. Consequently, the text and images in the autograph book are not sequenced in any logical progression and juxtapositions can be dissociative. However, the shared context of different communities of circulation (school, church, etc.) creates cohesion and relation between various entries in a single book.

Autograph albums are collections. They function as evidence of the human connections in the owner's life, not dissimilar to the collection and display of friends on Facebook. However, unlike the technological message boards of social media, autograph books leave a visceral trace of the human beings involved. Each page offers a new style of handwriting or drawing or a wash of colour left by a hand-held brush. Such markings trigger keen awareness, even years later, of the human lives which are recorded there. The pages gather together in one small book rhetorical and artistic traces of people known or encountered by the book's owner. In this way, they are mnemonic devices. The intent is that the book, later in life, will trigger memories of the circumstances (personal and historical) when the book was being circulated and will evoke remembrance of people and friendship, both ephemeral and long-lasting, with fellow human beings. At the time of the book's circulation, it served as a means of contact, connection, and communication. It both established and affirmed community.

The very nature of the autograph book contains within it an acknowledgement of the flux of time: an awareness that lives weave in and out of connection with each other, creating sudden intensities and leaving long traces. Autograph books, in part, record the ephemerality and complexity of human experience in time and space, experience heightened during the First World War when the spatial experience of many people, men and women alike, grew much wider. The autograph book contributes to the increase in 'autobiographical genres,' as described by Shafquat Towheed and Edmund G. C. King, like the personal letter and the diary, that was caused during the First World War by the intersection of mass mobilization, near-universal literacy, and people being far away from home and family for the first time.[14] Autograph books were a small subset of the burgeoning culture of written communication and reading practices – books, journals, newspapers, diaries, letters, etc. – that the conditions of global warfare produced. They were circulated in war hospitals on the front lines and the home front, but also on ships and in prison camps.[15] Towheed and King note the increased demand for small and inexpensive literary volumes that could fit into a pack but could also easily pass from hand to hand, as part of a comradeship of readers.[16] Similarly, the autograph book was pocket-sized and made for sharing.

II

Considering the transition of the autograph book from its girlish associations to its role in war hospitals, as well as its exclusion from a broader exposure to public readership that the hospital journal implied, I will focus primarily on one particular book, owned by quite a young girl who had no significant links with either the military or hospital administration.[17] Mollie Ross (born in 1900) worked voluntarily

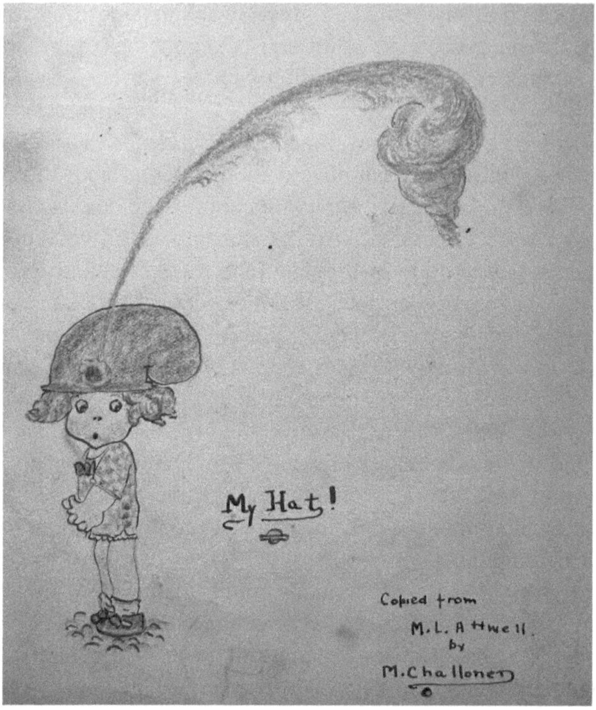

Figure 4.1 1913 illustration. Photograph owned/taken by the author.

as an auxiliary aid in the Northumberland War Hospital in Newcastle from 1915 until 1917. This hospital was the former St. Nicholas' Hospital in Gosforth, where Mollie lived, which became Northumberland's number one War Hospital for the duration of the First World War. Of the sixty-six entries in her autograph book, dating from 1911 to 1917, about half are signed by servicemen or refer to the war. There is a clear contrast in character between the pre-war and mid-war pages, reflecting two very different networks of association: school/church/family, and then, from 1914 to 1917, hospital staff and most often patients. The earlier entries made by school friends reflect pre-adolescent taste. Several of the entries imitate the style of Mabel Lucie Attwell (1879–1964), who was a very popular illustrator at the time.[18] But the childlike sweetness of that style creates a jarring juxtaposition with the contributions made by servicemen that range from satire to sadness, from patriotism to flirtation. Two pages, one from 1913 and one from 1917, both involving large hats, are exemplary of the contrast between innocence and experience characteristic of this book (Figures 4.1 and 4.2).

According to her sisters, Mollie Ross longed to be a nurse from a very young age.[19] Like many girls during the first decade of the twentieth century, she would have heard the stories about the Lady with the Lamp, Florence Nightingale.[20] And,

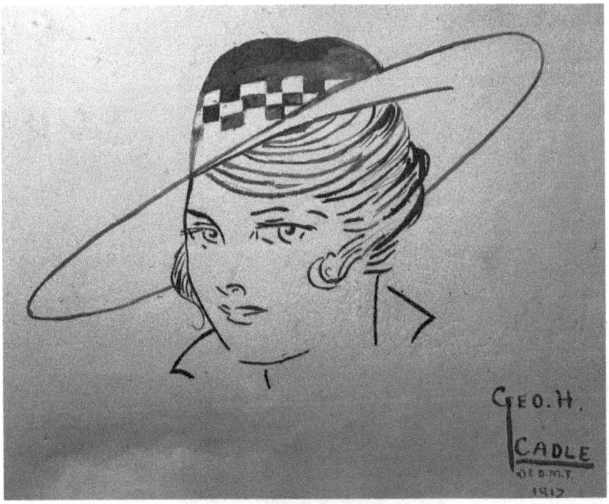

Figure 4.2 1917 illustration. Photograph owned/taken by the author.

perhaps she had read girls' fiction exploring the professional opportunities beginning to open for young women at this time.[21] The nursing profession, like teaching, represented ideals of service and nurture and thus promised to affirm, not contradict, the virtues of domestic femininity. By 1900, when Mollie was born, the efforts of Florence Nightingale and others had transformed nursing into a profession for single women of impeccable moral standards.

A photograph of Mollie, taken when she was about fourteen years old, shows her in a nurse's uniform, with a cape, starched collar, and bonnet (Figure 4.3). Mollie's serious expression is remarkable given the comedy of this picture. She cuddles her dog, which is dressed in pyjamas and has been recruited to play the role of a 'patient' for the camera. The image plays on Mollie's aspirations; the uniform seems real, as opposed to 'dress up.' Mollie, just fourteen when war broke out, was far too young to join the Voluntary Aid Detachment as an auxiliary nurse. Yet the fact that this picture was taken at all speaks to a longing inspired by what Vera Brittain describes in *Testament of Youth* as 'the sacred glamour' of nursing.[22] This longing resulted in Mollie joining youth uniformed organizations, probably before the war began – organizations such as the Girl Guides (formed in 1910) and The Church Nursing & Ambulance Brigade for Young Women & Girls (formed in 1911). While members of her family confirm she was a Girl Guide, it is unclear from surviving photographs what other groups she may have joined; she is pictured in two different uniforms between 1914 and 1917. What is clear from the evidence of her autograph book is that her enthusiasm and devotion to nursing resulted in her working in some capacity at the Northumberland War Hospital. Her book's last entries are from 1917, but it is possible that she continued working there until the end of the war.

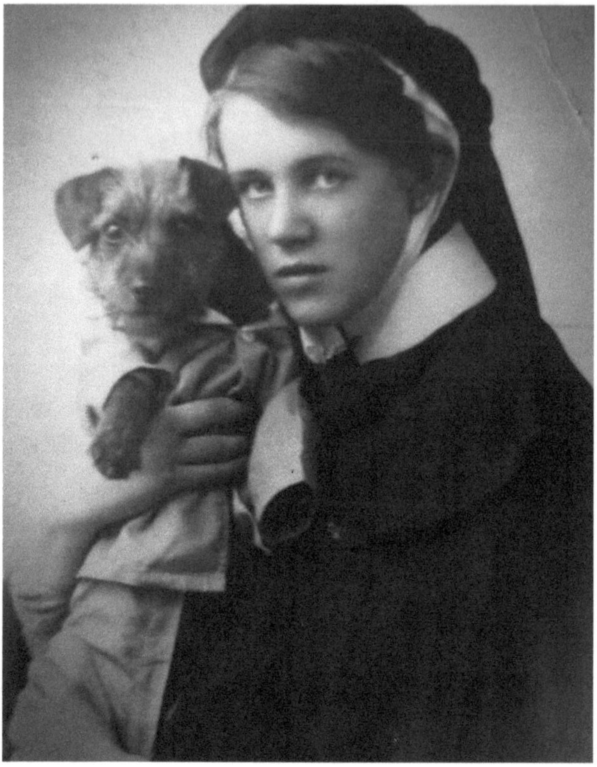

Figure 4.3 Mollie Ross aged about 14. Photograph owned/taken by the author.

There is one picture of Mollie Ross from the time when she was working at the War Hospital (Figure 4.4). She is sixteen or seventeen in this shot. She is in her uniform, standing with her two sisters and an unidentified officer. Mollie is taller than the other people in the picture, and her dark khaki double-breasted jacket and necktie give her a masculine air. Her uniform is similar to those designed for wartime female ambulance drivers; it is a militaristic outfit, not a nursing one. She has shoulder epaulettes and some kind of badge on her left sleeve. The skirt is calf-length and her shoes are dark and sensible. The large patch pockets on her jacket are bulging, inviting speculation as to what she kept in them. They are big enough, indeed, to have held the autograph book itself.

Mollie was probably fifteen when she began volunteering at the hospital. This might seem a very young age to begin such work, but it makes more sense when understood as an extension of her position as a Girl Guide. When girls began forming their own scout troops in protest at the gender exclusion of the national scouting movement, the Girl Guides were quickly established, with the initial goal of creating good wives and mothers for the Empire. But the war 'shattered

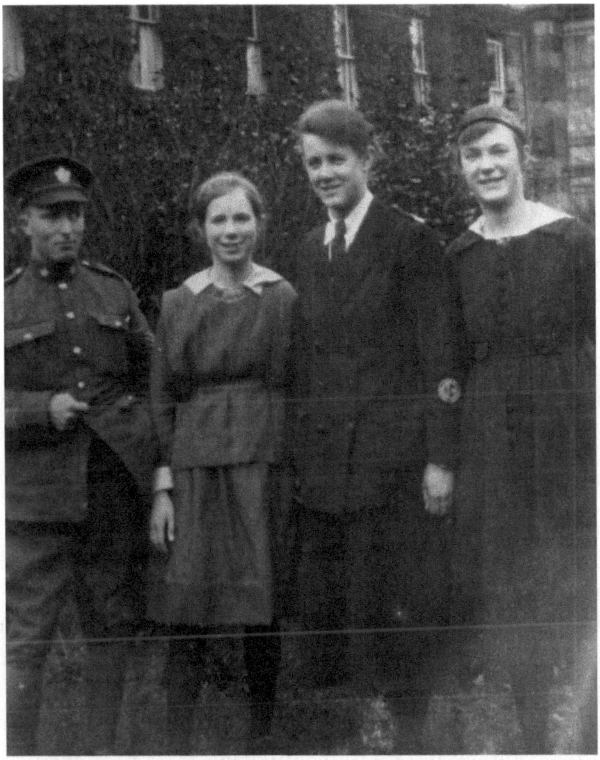

Figure 4.4 Mollie Ross and her sisters, plus an unidentified officer. Photograph owned/taken by the author.

conceptions about what constituted appropriate modes of feminine behavior' and created many more opportunities for girls to be engaged outside the home.[23] Lady Baden-Powell (who had been put in charge of the Guides by her husband) noted of girls during the war years: '[they] wanted to be out and about; and they had the war fever on them.'[24] This war fever, also known as Khaki Fever, refers to the excited behaviour of girls around young men in uniform that was thought to be a nuisance by many. With the onset of war, the Girl Guides quickly engaged with the war effort in a way that contrasted with the feckless high-spiritedness of the 'flapper' in the clutches of Khaki Fever. In May 1915, a war service badge was added to the other merit badges a Guide could earn. One way to earn this badge was for a Guide to work twenty-one days of special service for Hospitals and Nursing Institutions. 'Guides also served with the VADs … as orderlies, ward maids, messengers and laundresses.'[25] Richard Voeltz explains,

> The VADs provided auxiliary military nursing staff during the war, but the organization had originally been established as part of the Territorial Force

> before 1914 to prepare for the casualties resulting from an invasion of Britain. Prior to the war, the Guides already had very close links with the VADs.[26]

Mollie could have earned her war service merit badge in other ways, ranging from knitting socks and mittens to picking sphagnum moss for wound dressings or teaching English to Belgian refugees. The work Girl Guides did during the war was wide-ranging and ambitious. But the Northumberland War Hospital was on her doorstep in Gosforth, so it makes sense that this was the duty Mollie chose to perform. One feature of her work was to share her autograph book with the soldiers as a gesture of friendship but also as a rehabilitative intervention. The autograph book was a way to engage the patient, providing something to read and talk about, but also offering a place for the patient to participate creatively in whatever way he felt most comfortable. It might be to share a talent (like drawing or poetry), tell a joke, express gratitude (and sometimes complaint), or more directly comment on the war that led to the hospitalization in the first place.

III

The Imperial War Museum's collection holds forty-seven autograph books kept during the First World War. Despite being understood as a feminine practice, during war the autograph book became something that soldiers and prisoners also began to keep. However, the most significant number of autograph books in the collection belonged to nurses and VAD workers based in war hospitals and convalescent homes all over Britain and sometimes abroad. Sharing an autograph book as a way of building comradeship was not hard to do. They were small. They were not published (like journals) or mailed (like personal letters). They were not considered risky because they were probably assumed to have no real weight of content. They were thought of as harmless collections of signatures, drawings, and poetry. However, autograph books, in their very nature, are social things. As Santanu Das notes, they 'provide a vivid map of personal networks' between owner and contributor, and amongst contributors who examined the other entries before considering their own.[27] The context of bibliotherapy research provides an opportunity to enquire further into why the practice of keeping an autograph book grew in popularity during the war, and why in particular it became a practice of the hospital ward. Its mnemonic value, after all, could only be for the book's owner; yet it is clear to me, from researching around twenty-five nurses' autograph books in the Imperial War Museum's collection, that creating the personal entry for the book was a meaningful act to many of the contributors as well. For example, one solider at the Duchess of Westminster Hospital in Le Touquet, France, writing in the autograph book of VAD Florence Pelly on June 6, 1916, offers some barely legible script (his name is not legible at all): 'Fraid I'm not much good with my left hand yet, but let this thank you for all your kindness.'[28] With his right hand out of service, he nevertheless wanted to make the effort to leave a record of his gratitude, as well as his condition. Though some of the entries examined fall back on the well-worn rhymes and quotations that were considered standard to the practice, many more are unique and original and often take the form of detailed drawings and paintings, collages, and poetry. The sheer variety of the entries speaks of the cross-section of personalities, circumstances, and histories that filled the hospitals. The books themselves bear testimony to the many human beings who held the book, turned its pages, and, in some cases, held on to it for some time while creating an entry in it. As Santanu Das has put it so eloquently, such

> objects have a precious, living quality for they are archives of touch and intimacy – they have once been held or touched against the bodies of their possessors in their youths or in the trenches and in the hospitals, and through this intimate caress, these mute, insensate objects seem to have been touched to life.[29]

The way an entry can visually thrust before us the life of the person making it can be jarring. Lieutenant Kenneth Oakley, also recovering in Le Touquet, beautifully renders in black ink a line of musical notation across the full length of the page, with lines, bars, a treble clef, signature, and a melody. But smashing through this line, centrally and from above, he has drawn a bullet that tears the music in half. Under it, he has written 'An interrupted profession.'[30] This powerful image tells the viewer that Oakley had a life before the war that was full of possibility. He was a musician with professional ambitions. How terribly at odds this was with what he suffered on the front line. The bullet smashed through his career and his future as well as his body.

It can be assumed, from the number of contributions by soldiers, that Mollie's introduction of the autograph book into the hospital ward was not frowned upon. Amidst whatever tasks she undertook there – rolling bandages, serving meals, mopping, etc. – the autograph book suggests that value was also placed on the comfort and friendship her presence brought to these convalescent men. This is important given that it is known that there were tensions between the professional nursing staff and the auxiliary VADs during the First World War. Christine Hallett's work on 'Emotional Nursing' examines these tensions as resulting not only from different levels and standards of training and different class positioning (upper-class volunteering ladies versus the emergent middle-class working women) but also from a difference of affective disposition. Hallett explains,

> Many of these professional and class tensions were played out, particularly in the early months of the war, in the 'emotional nursing' debate. Trained nurses valued emotional containment, believing that not only was such containment important for the well-being and healing of their patients, it was also what those patients desired. VADs, by contrast, perhaps because they found themselves so often cold-shouldered by trained nurses, felt that the whole environment of the military hospital was pervaded by coldness and detachment. They believed they brought warmth, friendship, and camaraderie, crossing boundaries in the name of a unifying 'war spirit,' to this hostile environment.[31]

Trained nurses generally resisted emotional involvement because it 'could detract from the nurse's capacity to care well and effectively for all her patients,'[32] whereas the non-professional VAD focused her efforts on being a friend to the soldiers or, as one anonymous Army Nursing Reserve caustically observed, 'drivelling' over them, 'stroking their hands and smoothing their by no means fevered brows.'[33] The uniformed VADs combined a softer and more friendly demeanour with the suggestion of professionalism. This was not lost on C.H. Goulden, who also contributed to the autograph book of VAD Florence Pelly in 1916:

> Which would you rather have, M'sieur?
> Which would you rather see?
> A powdered & puffed & useless doll,
> Or a Charming VAD?[34]

The autograph book Mollie circulated amongst the patients at the Northumberland War Hospital does suggest that she was forming friendships with servicemen in the wards. Perhaps it was Mollie's considerable youth that enabled her to participate in this kind of 'emotional nursing' without attracting the hostility of the professional staff. But it also seems possible that some trained nurses welcomed, rather than resented, the kind of emotional nursing volunteer aids were able to do. Many of the hospital autograph books I have examined belonged to professional nursing staff, not auxiliaries, which suggests that trained nurses themselves created friendships with those in their charge. Thus the hospital autograph books provide evidence of friendship and engagement between servicemen and both untrained and trained nurses which somewhat contradicts the stereotypes perpetuated in VAD memoirs of cold professional nursing staff versus warm and caring volunteers. In her book *Containing Trauma: Nursing Work in the First World War* (2009), Hallett underscores this point:

> [Professional] nurses acted as surrogate mothers and sisters, offering comfort and emotional support as well as technical nursing care. They do not appear to have felt that such behavior was a crossing of professional boundaries. Rather they appear to have felt the emotional engagement with patients, within recognized limits of 'propriety,' was an essential feature of their work.[35]

Many of the autograph books I examined include entries demonstrating that the patients were quite aware of the unusual proximity between them and the female nursing staff and auxiliaries. To those on the mend, 'emotional nursing' might more immediately have meant the play of pleasurable sexual fantasy than the work of medical healing, where the crossing of boundaries occurred in the patient's imagination. This is especially well expressed in a drawing in an autograph book from the Seaford War Hospital in Sussex owned by Nurse E. Burton. The image, entered by Private G.S. Hirst (dated April 10, 1916), is a skilfully drawn depiction of a nurse kissing a patient in pyjamas. The nurse's left arm is crooked around the patient's neck, drawing his head towards hers. She, being slightly taller, seems to be kissing him, not the other way around. In her right hand, she holds a cup of medicine, which we assume she will administer after the kiss. The caption reads, 'Not in the prescription.' As if to drive home the point that this is an expression (and form of completion?) of Private Hirst's fantasy, he adds in parenthesis 'an Idyll.'[36]

In Mollie Ross's autograph book, there are several flirtatious entries from those dated between 1916 and 1917. But the unconventional proximity of access the then sixteen-year-old Mollie had to these young men, and to their vulnerable bodies, adds an element of pathos to otherwise conventional admissions of attraction. 'T.T.,' for instance, of the Durham Light Infantry, writes out in the book the hackneyed jingle, 'Mollie Ross is her name, / Single is her station / Blessed is the happy man / Who makes the alteration.' This is standard autograph album material; only the hospital context makes it particularly noteworthy. This is true, also, of another entry from 1916 by 'R.S.B.' which quotes song lyrics, "All the nice girls love a sailor," that first became popular during World War I (from a 1909 music hall number titled 'Ship Ahoy!').[37] As the song continues, the sailor is referred to as 'bright and breezy, free and easy / He's the ladies' pride and joy' – a description that awkwardly contrasts with the thought of a wounded and perhaps maimed young man in a hospital bed. Another entry, by T. Tidmarsh (possibly the T.T. of above), uses this same line in the album but customizes it to refer specifically to himself, a soldier, not a sailor: 'All the nice girls love a soldier.' One wonders what kind of friendship Mollie had with Tidmarsh, who adds a second more sobering line to the first: 'For better or for worst' [*sic*]. Indeed, the entries in the autograph book imply that this girl from 'respectable' Newcastle society was growing to like, if not love, the young men in her ward. In 1916, Mollie herself felt moved to acknowledge in her own book (quoting Thackeray) the value of love lost: 'To love and to win is the best thing. To love and to lose is the next best.' Without a doubt, some patients hoped that these friendships begun in autograph book entries would extend beyond the hospital ward. In February 1916, W.R. Broadhurst, of the 1st Gordon Highlanders, writes in Miss Pelly's autograph book 'Being 4am I simply can't write poetry. I can merely express my sincerest thanks and hope that we may meet again as civilians.'[38]

However, hospital autograph books can be considered as more than evidence of the emotional bond between the patients and the nursing staff. The practice of autograph book-keeping was one of the *means* by which the 'emotional containment' Hallett speaks of was achieved. In addition to giving convalescent soldiers a creative task to focus on, the autograph book always functioned as a way to consolidate and affirm community and communicate friendship. But, more than that, it offered a safe context for a certain kind of role-play and expression, like flirtation, amongst other things. Men such as the musician Lieutenant Oakley were thinking about who they would be if still living when the war ended. Life had been interrupted. They would be changed, perhaps physically, but definitely psychologically, by the trauma they had endured. What would it be like for them, in the future, to interact with the opposite sex, for example? The ward itself, and the autograph book circulating in that space, gave them a safe way to get used to how that would feel. The 'emotional containment' on the wards that the professional nursing staff favoured seems to imply repression or the keeping of a stiff upper lip. And it is understandable why that attitude needed to be encouraged. Nevertheless, the presence of the autograph book did allow for emotional expression in a controlled, or 'contained,' manner. It allowed for small and considered emotional release of all kinds – affection, flirtation, patriotism, satire, anger, pathos – all can be found in the pages of Mollie's book and others. In this way, the hospital autograph book became part of the processes of containment and restitution that counteracted the physical and psychic disintegrative effects of war injury and trauma.

IV

Mollie Ross' autograph book, like all the War Hospital autograph books, invites a reconsideration of the dynamic between owner and contributor in the history of this cultural practice as we determine what this genre offers to the debate about wartime bibliotherapy. In previous practice, contributors would inscribe the book specifically *for* the owner. The entries were offered to her, as the primary recipient and reader/viewer. The books, then, recorded personal relationships with the owners. We can see this in the earlier pre-war entries, contributed by Mollie's school friends, teachers, etc., which are clearly done *for* her – she is the presumed and intended audience. Marion Palmer, for example, quotes from Charles Kingsley's poem 'A Farewell' in a way that seems directed at Mollie herself: 'Be good sweet maid, let those who will be clever …' etc. However, the soldiers' entries, while sometimes addressing Mollie directly, often seem intended to garner the interest of the other servicemen in the ward, or alternatively seem entirely self-referential in a way that makes their meaning opaque. This is an interesting shift in the use of the autograph book, one that I argue here indicates the changed role of the autograph book in wartime. Its role has become more about the needs of the contributor than the entertainment or memory-building of the owner. As a rehabilitative practice, the autograph book leaves a record of how, with varying degrees of intensity and commitment, wounded and traumatized men chose to present themselves to a limited, safe, and somewhat private audience.

There is a certain performative aspect to the entries in which the servicemen choose what role they will play in the action of adding an entry to the book. Will they play the flirt or the philosopher? The patriot or the comic? Will they copy and quote from other works or will they create something of their own? Given the dissociative and disintegrative conditions of the First World War and the dependent, powerless position of being a patient, it would have been no small thing to have the chance to build an impression of self – to decide what aspect of self to reveal to the book's owner and the other people who would turn the album's pages. This is an empowering action – one that we now witness regularly in the self-constructions on social media sites. I am suggesting that the autograph book – *auto* (self) and *graph* (writing) – in the context of the wartime hospital was a self-constitutive and rehabilitative performative practice. On a modest scale, it created the opportunity for the contributor to present a 'self' to the world of the ward. The autograph book, then, offered an occasion of self-fashioning for many servicemen, whose astonishingly thoughtful, creative, and often original contributions indicate that there was value in the making of them. The evidence of the book suggests that the servicemen Mollie encountered enthusiastically contributed to her book for their own benefit, as well as for hers. Making an entry in the book was viewed as an opportunity. In the following sections, I will analyse the recuperative and reconstitutive significance of a few specific categories of entries in Mollie's book: humour, literary quotations, and those that appear to have no clear intention at all.

V

In her introduction to her book *The Politics of Humor* (edited with Patrick Merziger), Martina Kessel notes that 'humour has been interpreted, at least for the First World War, as a means of coping and as an outlet in times of disorder and friction.'[39] The many pictorial cartoons printed in the media, and especially those printed in trench newspapers, functioned this way, offering a form of 'mediation,' as Pierre Purseigle puts it, and a way 'to transcend the feelings of anxiety and insecurity produced by the war.'[40] In *Humor, Entertainment, and Popular Culture during World War One,* Clémentine Tholas-Disset and Karen Ritzenhoff assert that in addition to functioning as an 'escape valve for the stress and the fear that were inherent to trench warfare,' humour in trench newspapers had the important function of 'strengthening bonds' in the readership.[41] Similarly, in the circulation of the War Hospital autograph book, there was a readership ready to benefit from the healing effects of shared laughter. Quite a number of the servicemen in the Northumberland War Hospital chose to use Mollie's autograph book as a means to express humour.

One skilfully drawn cartoon calls attention to the disconnect between upper and lower military ranks (Figure 4.5). 'You don't seem to realise there's a war on,' barks a burly officer at a wounded and heavily bandaged Tommy. If, as Kessel argues, humour is a 'means to negotiate identity and belonging,'[42] this pictorial cartoon can be understood as a release of resentment towards an officer class that appeared to be indifferent to the suffering and trauma of the regular soldier. Those who had been on the receiving end of an officer's aggression could bond over this joke. The relative privacy of the autograph book (compared with a trench newspaper, for example) provided a safe opportunity for such an expression that deliberately addressed tension and division in the troops.

War humour also provided opportunities to bond over the faults of the enemy. As Vincent Trott reminds us, ridicule has long been understood as an assault on 'perceived inferiority.'[43] But understood in relation to the 'safety valve' theory of humour, in which it is thought to function as a release of tension and anxiety, ridicule can be seen simultaneously as an act of aggression and as a means of cathartic self-healing.

Figure 4.6 offers an interesting example of these gestures, both outward as an attack on the enemy and inward through a comforting historical reference to prior British victories. At first glance, this cartoon seems to portray Admiral Nelson,

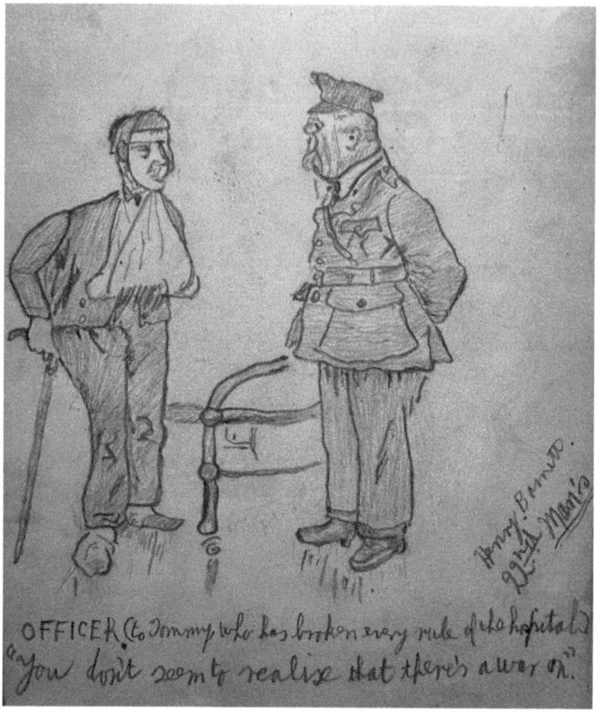
OFFICER (to Tommy who has broken every rule of the hospital)
"You don't seem to realise that there's a war on."

Figure 4.5 Cartoon. Photograph owned/taken by the author.

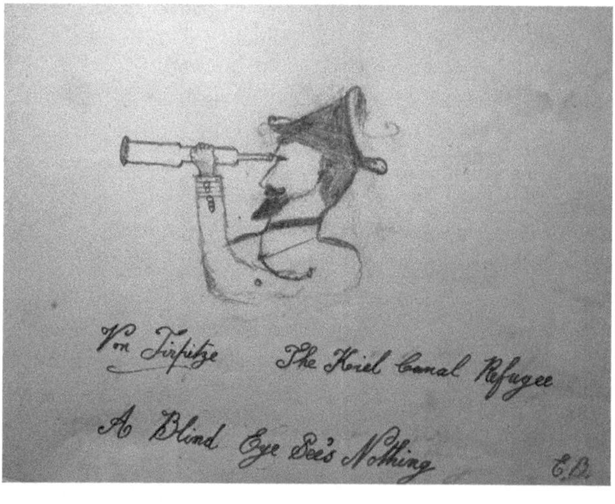
Von Tirpitz
The Kiel Canal Refugee
A Blind Eye Sees Nothing
E.B.

Figure 4.6 Cartoon: 'A blind eye sees nothing.' Photograph owned/taken by the author.

with his telescope held to his 'blind eye.' During the Battle of Copenhagen in 1801, Nelson was said to have held his telescope to his blind eye in order to deliberately ignore naval signals ordering him to discontinue action.[44] Nelson's stubbornness led to naval losses; but it was also considered a heroic stance, a refusal to be intimidated. However, the first caption on the image introduces new information that repositions it as an assault on the enemy. The caption titles the figure as 'Von Tirpitze,' a misspelling of Alfred von Tirpitz, best known for his failed attempt to boost the German fleet to compete with the British navy. Specifically, it references the failure of Von Tirpitz' Kiel Canal plan,[45] which would have enabled German battleships to access the North Sea from the Baltic. In the context of von Tirpitz, then, the 'blind eye' refers to his shortcomings as naval commander; but in the context of Nelson, it references British heroism.

The most multi-dimensional of the pictorial cartoons in the book is the page contributed by Private D.M. Carman of the Northumberland Fusiliers (Figure 4.7). This entry combines drawing and poetry. The main joke resides in the transformation of Count Zeppelin into Little Bo Peep. Referring to the vulnerability of the Zeppelin hot air balloons to ground fire, which had resulted in their frequent destruction, Carman offers a cartoon of an emasculated Von Zeppelin in a skirt, accompanied by an accented caption: 'LEAVE. THEM. ALONE. OR. DEY. VONT. KOM. OME.' Carman also invents a rhyme to accompany the image: 'Count Zeppelin in Bopeep's guise / Feels tears suffuse / His murderous eyes,' etc. The lack of poetic talent is compensated for by the sheer enthusiasm for invention. The ridicule of German technological invention is the point here; however, the infantilizing nursery rhyme reference and the effeminizing of Von Zeppelin also contribute to this morale-boosting celebration of German ineptitude. Sometimes, though, the

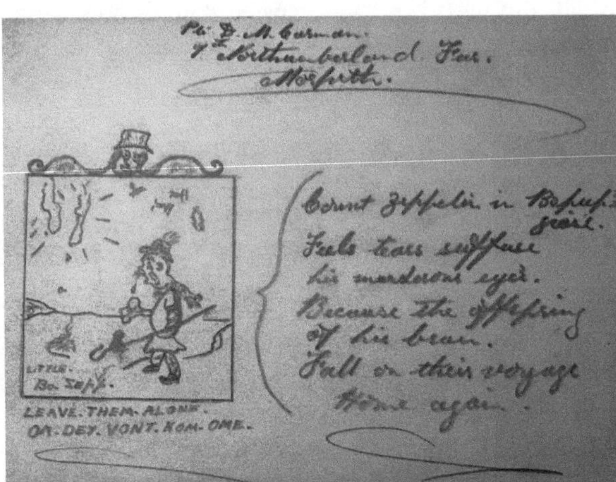

Figure 4.7 Cartoon by D. M. Carman. Photograph owned/taken by the author.

humorous entries of the autograph book struggle to translate into comedy the stress and tension that fuel them. A big blot of black ink wittily makes the 'lonely spot' on the page claimed by J. H. Gilbert of the 3rd Royal Fusiliers on November 5, 1915. Gilbert was a survivor of the Second Battle of Ypres and was possibly wounded at the Battle of Loos.[46] By also noting where he was when he made this page, 'The Northumberland War Hospital,' Gilbert undercuts the comic nature of his entry: was this place a lonely spot, for him?

VI

Whereas some servicemen turned to the satisfactions that laughter brings via acceptable forms of aggression and cathartic relief of tension, others chose to record the words of famous men and books. In these cases, the quotations, probably written from memory, emphasize heroism. J. Eric Lordman, Company Sergeant Major of the 19th Service Battalion of the Northumberland Fusiliers, wounded at the Somme, slightly misremembers some lines from Longfellow's 'The Ladder of St. Augustine': 'The heights by great men reached and kept / Were not attained by sudden flight, / But they, while their companions slept, / Were toiling upward in the night.'[47] This quotation emphasizes sacrifice and service over cowardice. Men don't become heroes by running away. The 'toiling upward' refers in the poem to St. Augustine's ladder of past vices that must be scaled and trampled underfoot to reach greatness. However, it seems possible that Lordman was reminded of the ladder he scaled on the wall of the trench to go 'up and over.'

Ernest Brown of the Durham Light Infantry, wounded at Delville Wood, also at the Somme, quotes Shakespeare ('His life was gentle and the elements / were so mix'd in him that nature might stand up / and say to all the world, "This was a man!"' *Julius Caesar* V. v. 81–83). This quotation comes from the end of the play when Anthony eulogizes Brutus as someone who committed atrocity but did so only for the good of all. But what is perhaps most striking is how these lines operate self-referentially to Brown himself. Edmund G. C. King, in his essay on soldiers reading Shakespeare during the war, writes

> To dip into the higher end of the English literary canon and retrieve something like Shakespeare was an exceptional act, although [...] one laden with a certain amount of cultural expectation. To do so – and to be seen doing so – was to distinguish oneself from one's fellow soldiers, or even, perhaps, to cast oneself as an *ideal* soldier.[48]

King goes on to note that all the examples of soldiers reading Shakespeare he discusses 'were recorded in order to be read themselves.'[49] The autograph book entries quoting Shakespeare and Longfellow create a similar record of wounded soldiers seeking to transcend their circumstances through self-identification with heroism and idealized masculinity. The fact that they could retrieve these quotations from memory, however, suggests an additional therapeutic possibility found in familiarity, or nostalgia. Lordman identifies Dunston-on-Tyne as home and Brown,

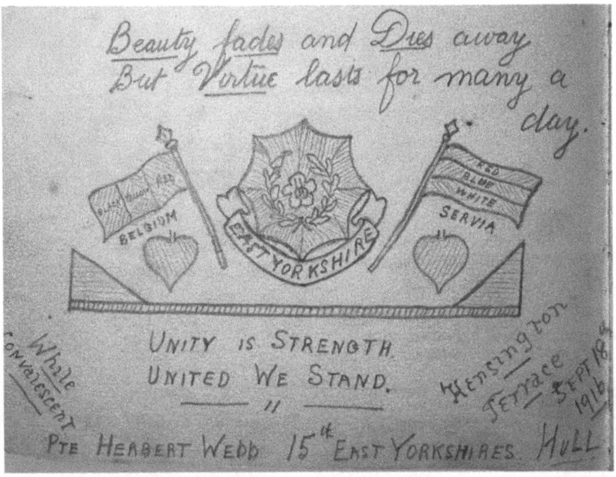

Figure 4.8 'Unity is Strength.' Photograph owned/taken by the author.

Sunderland. Being from working-class neighbourhoods, they would have had quite basic formal educations. Nevertheless, it is possible that they studied *Julius Caesar* and Longfellow at school. If so, these quotations, as King notes, 'could be a point of contact with their former, student selves – and token of the lives they hoped to resume.'[50]

However self-healing or self-bolstering the quoting of Shakespeare may have been, there is no doubt that it is reflective of how Shakespeare was mobilized during the First World War for patriotic ends.[51] Even so, there is only one entry in Mollie's book that sets about to be overtly patriotic (Figure 4.8).

Writing 'while convalescent' on September 18, 1916, Private Herbert Webb, of the 15th East Yorkshires (Hull), depicts graphically the allegiance of small nations against the German behemoth – the English Rose of the East Yorkshire Regimental badge flanked by the flags of Belgium and Serbia. In this entry, Virtue is claimed by independent small nations, and we understand that whatever Private Webb suffered, he did so gladly for this higher cause. It was this that he wanted Mollie, and the others who read her book, to know: the anguish was not for nothing.

VII

The most intriguing entries in the autograph book are those which are least easily categorized. Although inscribed in a book which exists to be circulated amongst others, these entries seem highly personal and introspective. That is, they seem at odds with the communicative function of the autograph book in their opacity of meaning. In Mollie's autograph book, there is one striking example of such an entry (Figure 4.9). Private R. March was the first person to fill two pages of Mollie's book; and he did so in spectacular style on October 28, 1915, one month

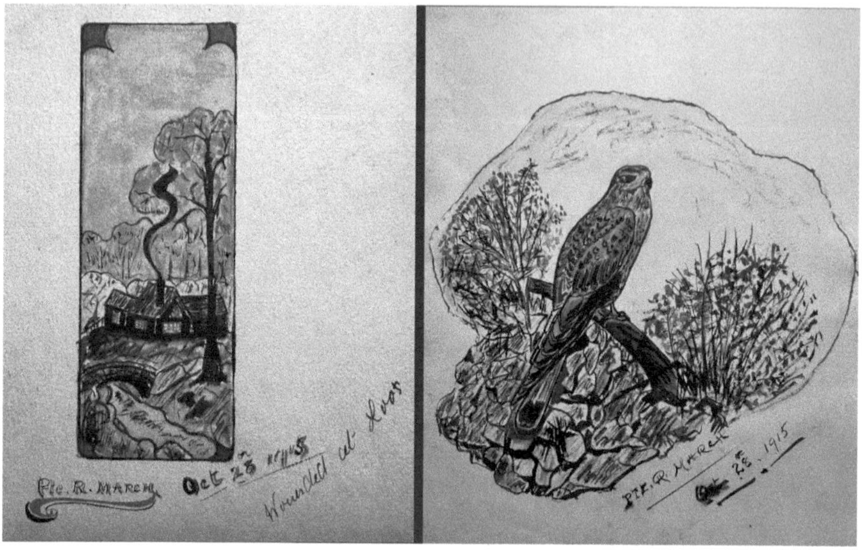

Figure 4.9 Two paintings. Photograph owned/taken by the author.

after the Battle of Loos, in which he was wounded. He notes this in small capital letters, under his first painting. The casualties at Loos had been catastrophic (60,000 or more injured, with 20,000 dead). The effort of this massive offensive, in which the British used chlorine gas for the first time, came to naught.

When leafing through the book, Private March's pages leap out for their brilliant colours and artistry. His two artworks lie side by side, on opposite pages, forming a curious dialogue. On the left side, he painted a view, as if seen through a gothic window, of a cottage in the woods by a stream. Smoke winds up from the chimney. We are left to wonder if this is a place from his imagination, a depiction of home, or a scene from his travels in France. It speaks of peace and tranquillity, and the calm of nature. Most of all, it is dream-like – an idealized vision of England. It is interesting to compare this image with a page from Nurse Burton's autograph book from Seaford, Sussex. Here, on 16 January 1917, CO McGregor had drawn in black ink a cartoon of a Tommy on the front lines having just read a letter from home, which is still in his hand. Before him is a brazier emitting light and smoke. The smoke billows above the soldier and within the fumes emerges an image of a village, with thatched cottages, a church, and trees.[52] Beneath this skilfully rendered drawing, McGregor has added the simple caption: "Reveries." McGregor gives us the soldier, his wartime context, and his dreams, all in one image. Private March, I believe, shows us only the dream.

March's second picture offers a detailed painting of a male kestrel, with its blue-grey cap and tail, sitting on a branch. The bright colours of the bird's plumage are faithfully rendered in jewelled tones. The common kestrel is a small bird of prey found widespread in Europe. And it is certainly possible that Private March was thinking of the bird he saw hovering over the English fields. However, the kestrel's preference for open habitat, lowlands, and treeless steppe ensured its presence in the landscape of trench warfare.[53] There are several references to kestrels, both in poetry from the trenches and in diaries written by soldiers from the First World War. One soldier, Private T.S. Williams of the 19th Battalion of the King's Liverpool Regiment, who served at the Somme, wrote, 'At times a kestrel hawk could be seen hovering over the desolate wastes that had once been fields.'[54] In his essay 'Birds on the Western Front' (published posthumously in 1924), Saki (pen name of Hector Hugo Munro, killed by a sniper in 1916) noted the bird's presence more emphatically: 'Kestrels hover about all day in the hottest parts of the line, not in the least disconcerted, apparently, when a promising mouse-area suddenly rises in the air in a cascade of black or yellow earth …'[55] Julian Grenfell, in his poem 'Into Battle,' draws the parallel between this particular bird of prey and the soldier, imagining the 'kestrel hovering by day' as bidding the soldier to be as 'swift and keen' as he.[56] In his evocative consideration of trench existence, Paul Fussell notes starkly,

> One saw two things only: the walls of an unlocalized, undifferentiated earth and the sky above. … As the only visible theater of variety, the sky becomes all-important. It was the sight of the sky, almost alone, that had the power to persuade a man that he was not already lost in a common grave.[57]

No wonder then that a glorious inhabitant of that sky, one with the power to stay still in the air, to hover head to the wind, one with the spirit of a warrior, should so impress himself on the imaginations of the trapped soldiers of earth.

Private March's kestrel, like his first picture of the country cottage, looks away from technological warfare to peace in the natural world. But the focus on the kestrel in particular also can propel the imagination back to the theatre of modern war. We could describe these two pages as an aesthetic processing of traumatic memory. Through his artistic talent, March is able to record the natural life that managed to impress itself on his imagination despite the terrible context. The image of the cottage appears like a dream of pre-war Britain that perhaps comforted him on the front line and was kept alive through the letters he received from home. But Private March wanted the people who look at the autograph book after him to connect his pictures with his experience as a soldier 'wounded at Loos.' He invites us to contemplate that connection, but the clue we are given to the nature of his experience is locked in the stern and dignified pose of the kestrel. It would seem, also, that Private March wanted Mollie to remember him as an artist as much as a patient. As an act of communication, these paintings resonate with effort and feeling but also suggest that they were a very private act of reconstitution. Consider us, they say, we still survive in the mind of a man who has seen into the abyss.

VIII

At the beginning of this chapter, I discussed the War Hospital autograph book in relation to War Hospital journals. In conclusion, I want briefly to consider them more broadly in relation to therapeutic reading practices in war hospitals. In their discussion of the work of British military hospital libraries, Sara Haslam and Edmund G. C. King prefer to use the term 'literary caregiving' to 'bibliotherapy' primarily because, as a term, 'it registers the affective aspects of volunteer labour in [those libraries] during the First World War (aspects which themselves were gendered).'[58] Haslam and King define literary caregiving as 'the practice of using literature, normally in volunteer-led institutions or contexts, to minister to, or alleviate the symptoms of, the sick and wounded through responsive and empathetic interactions and methods.'[59]

Describing the great desire for reading materials in the military war hospitals, Haslam and King emphasize that a guiding principle for the literary caregivers was not to try to improve or educate the patients but rather to provide a 'flow of comfort'[60] that sought to respond to their tastes and needs.[61] Beatrice Harraden, novelist and suffrage campaigner, who helped run the Endell Street Military Hospital in London, believed that librarians should 'study the temperaments, inclinations and possibilities of patients' so that they could determine how best to 'amuse, help, stimulate, lift – and heal' them through reading.[62] This method of care, which considers the patient's mind as well as his body and meets him on his own terms rather than putting further expectations of improvement or performance upon him, is precisely the kind of intervention in the War Hospital that the autograph book also offered, though on a smaller scale than the libraries. The autograph book was informal and playful enough to cater to many different talents and levels of ability and effort. It could be a site for showcasing a skill like drawing or poetry, but an entry could also be (and was more often) as simple as writing a one-line greeting. It met the men where they were in terms of their abilities and states of mind. And it was understood as a low-stakes and relatively private form of expression because the book was personally owned, and not published for distribution like hospital journals. The evidence of the significance of the autograph book in military hospital wards lies in the pages of the books themselves. These autograph books unquestionably played a role in amusing, helping, stimulating, lifting – and healing – the community within which they circulated, both as something to contribute to and something to be read. Their alleviating role should not be underestimated.

But what of the small book's owner – the young woman who brought her autograph book into the ward in the first place and introduced it as one aspect of her work as a volunteer? What must it have been like for Mollie, as she interacted with men like Private March? She was exposed to the consequences of hell without having been there herself. But she doubtless knew that life going forward would never be quite the same. She may have felt, like other young women of her generation who witnessed the suffering and loss of young men not much older than they, that hope had been stripped away in the midst of youth. 'We are left alone like old men; we should be dead / – but there are years and years in which we shall still be young,' wrote Margaret Cole in her poem 'Praematuri' (1918).[63] Mollie's world expanded in every way possible during the war years. She no doubt grew wiser than her years through the work she did, the sights she saw, the physical beings she encountered, the bodies and minds she tried to help. Her autograph book created a meeting point across gender, age, and social difference; it acted as a gesture of friendship and shared experience; it offered distraction from the pressure of circumstance and the bitterness of memory; and it provided a means of expressive release. Moreover, and perhaps most importantly, it offered an opportunity, albeit in a small way, for the soldier who had been necessarily unindividuated, uniformed, and automated in the ranks – encouraged not to think but obey – to once again imagine what kind of self he wished to rebuild by letting him decide how to perform on paper. These choices of self-projection are reflected everywhere in the highly original and strikingly individual entries found in Mollie's War Hospital autograph book. While this activity in wartime hospitals has been hidden from view and buried in archives or private collections, and while it may seem small compared to the numerous other medical advancements made in response to the injuries resulting from mechanized warfare, the sheer number of War Hospital autograph books that exist suggests that their presence in the wards was not only welcome but restorative.

Notes

1 'Kindness of Strangers: In 1909, When Gladys Forryan, of Leicester, Wrote Her Name in Her New Autograph Book She Could Not Have Imagined That Several of the Entries Would Be from Soldiers Wounded in the First World War,' *Leicester Mercury* (November 10, 2011): 16.

2 Jessica Meyer, 'Hospital Journals,' in *The Edinburgh Companion to First World War Periodicals*, edited by Marysa Demoor, Cedric Van Dijck, and Birgit Van Puymbroeck. (Edinburgh: Edinburgh University Press, 2023), 348.

3 Meyer, 'Hospital Journals,' 348.

4 Meyer, 'Hospital Journals,' 348.

5 Jeffrey Reznick, *Healing the Nation: Soldiers and the Culture of Caregiving in Britain during the Great War* (Manchester: Manchester University Press, 2004).

6 Seth Koven, 'Prisoners of Their Beds: Invalids, Injured Soldiers and Cultures of Convalescence in Nineteenth and Early-Twentieth Century Britain,' *Radical History Review* 94 (Winter 2006): 238.

7 See Edmund G. C. King, 'Networks,' in *The Edinburgh Companion to First World War Periodicals*, edited by Marysa Demoor, Cedric Van Dijck, and Birgit Van Puymbroeck (Edinburgh: Edinburgh University Press, 2023), 32–50. See also Meyer, 'Hospital Journals.'

8 See, for example, Alexandra McKinnon, 'Impressions of Empire: Autograph Books as a Historical Resource, 1899–1919' (paper presented at Researching War and Conflict through Ephemera Conference, Northumbria University, Newcastle, April 9, 2024), www.awm.gov.au/sites/default/files/impressions_of_empire_-_alexandra_mckinnon_reduce.pdf

9 Todd S. Gernes, 'Recasting the Culture of Ephemera,' in *Popular Literacy: Studies in Cultural Practices and Poetics,* edited by John Trimbur (Pittsburgh: University of Pittsburgh Press, 2001), 120.

10 See Gernes, 'Recasting the Culture of Ephemera,' and W. K. McNeil, 'The Autograph Album Custom: A Tradition and Its Scholarly Treatment.' *Keystone Folklore Quarterly* 13, no.1 (Spring 1968): 29–40.

11 Lisa Reid Ricker, '(De)Constructing the Praxis of Memory-Keeping: Late-Nineteenth Century Autograph Albums as Sites of Rhetorical Invention.' *Rhetoric Review* 29, no. 3 (June 2010): 242.

12 Gernes, 'Recasting the Culture of Ephemera,' 121; Hanna Herzog and Rina Shapira, 'Will You Sign My Autograph Book? Using Autograph Books for a Sociohistorical Study of Youth and Social Frameworks,' *Qualitative Sociology* 9, no. 2 (June 1986): 110.
13 Gernes, 'Recasting the Culture of Ephemera,' 120.
14 Shafquat Towheed and Edmund G. C. King, 'Introduction,' in *Reading and the First World War: Readers, Texts, Archives,* edited by Shafquat Towheed and Edmund G. C. King (Basingstoke: Palgrave Macmillan, 2015), 3.
15 In addition to nurses' autograph books (47 in total), the Imperial War Museum's collection has autograph books that belonged to army privates, a naval officer, several conscientious objectors in prison, and one from a troopship en route to destinations in the Mediterranean.
16 Towheed and King, 'Introduction,' 7 and 12.
17 The autograph book which belonged to Mollie Ross is in the author's possession.
18 Daniel Hahn, ed. 'Attwell, Mabel Lucie (1879–1964),' in *The Oxford Companion to Children's Literature*, 2nd ed. Oxford University Press, Inc. https://search.credoreference.com/articles/Qm9va0FydGljbGU6NDgwMjM0NQ==?aid=237298.
19 Mollie Ross was the author's maternal grandmother. Some of this information comes from other family members.
20 'Florence Nightingale: The Lady with the Lamp.' *National Army Museum*, accessed November 10, 2023, www.nam.ac.uk/explore/florence-nightingale-lady-lamp.
21 For example, *A Sister of the Red Cross*, by L.T. Meade (1901), describes the adventures of a newly trained nurse in the field hospitals of the Second Boer War.
22 Vera Brittain, *Testament of Youth: An Autobiographical Study of the Years 1900–1925* (London: Gollancz, 1935), 212. The full quotation reads: 'Every task, from the dressing of a dangerous wound to the scrubbing of a bed-mackintosh, had for us in those early days a sacred glamour which redeemed it equally from tedium and disgust.'
23 Richard A.Voeltz, 'The Antidote to "Khaki Fever"? The Expansion of the British Girl Guides during the First World War,' *Journal of Contemporary History* 27, no. 4 (October 1992): 628.
24 Quoted in Voeltz, 'The Antidote,' 633.
25 Voeltz, 'The Antidote,' 629.
26 Voeltz, 'The Antidote,' 629.
27 Santanu Das, *Touch and Intimacy in First World War Literature* (Cambridge: Cambridge University Press, 2005), 178.
28 Autograph Book, ca. 1914–1918, Documents 866, *Private Papers of Miss F.I.C. Pelly*. Imperial War Museum, London.
29 Das, *Touch and Intimacy*, 236.
30 Autograph Book, ca. 1914–1918, Documents 866, *Private Papers of Miss F.I.C. Pelly*. Imperial War Museum, London.
31 Christine E. Hallett, '"Emotional Nursing": Involvement, Engagement, and Detachment in the Writings of First World War Nurses and VADs,' in *First World War Nursing: New Perspectives,* edited by Christine E. Hallett and Alison S Fell (London: Routledge, 2013), 99.
32 Hallett, 'Emotional Nursing,' 97.
33 Quoted in Hallett, 'Emotional Nursing,' 95. From a letter to the Editor, *British Journal of Nursing*, 53 (December 19, 1914): 497.
34 Autograph Book, ca. 1914–1918, Documents 866, *Private Papers of Miss F.I.C. Pelly*. Imperial War Museum, London.

35 Christine E. Hallett, *Containing Trauma: Nursing Work in the First World War* (Manchester: Manchester University Press, 2009), 198.
36 Autograph Book, ca. 1914–1918, Documents 7700, Burton, E., *Nurse's Autograph Books Containing Contributions by the West Indian Contingent, First World War*. Imperial War Museum, London.
37 Hetty King, 'Ship Ahoy [All the Nice Girls Love a Sailor],' *Song Facts*, accessed November 10, 2023, www.songfacts.com/facts/hetty-king/ship-ahoy-all-the-nice-girls-love-a-sailor.
38 Autograph Book, ca. 1914–1918, Documents 866, *Private Papers of Miss F.I.C. Pelly*. Imperial War Museum, London.
39 Martina Kessel, 'Landscapes of Humour: The History and Politics of the Comical in the Twentieth Century,' in *The Politics of Humor: Laughter, Inclusion, and Exclusion in the Twentieth Century*, edited by Martina Kessel and Patrick Merziger (Toronto: University of Toronto Press, 2011), 6.
40 Pierre Purseigle, 'Mirroring Societies at War: Pictorial Humour in the British and French Popular Press during the First World War,' *Journal of European Studies* 31, no. 123 (September 2001): 316.
41 Clémentine Tholas-Disset and Karen A. Ritzenhoff, 'Introduction,' in *Humor, Entertainment, and Popular Culture During World War I*, edited by Clémentine Tholas-Disset and Karen A. Ritzenhoff (New York: Palgrave Macmillan, 2015), 10.
42 Martina Kessel, 'Landscapes of Humor,' 3.
43 Vincent Trott, 'Humour, Neutrality, and Preparedness: American Satirical Magazines and the First World War, 1914–1917,' *War in History*, 29, no. 1 (January 2022): 109.
44 Brendan McWilliams, 'Why Nelson Turned a Blind Eye at Copenhagen,' *The Irish Times*, April 2, 2001, www.irishtimes.com/news/why-nelson-turned-a-blind-eye-at-copenhagen-1.297163.
45 'Keil Canal, Flags, and Naval Expansion,' *Bodleian Map Room Blog*, accessed April 25, 2024, https://blogs.bodleian.ox.ac.uk/maps/2015/11/13/kiel-canal-flags-and-naval-expansion/
46 Chris Baker, *The Long, Long Trail: Researching Soldiers of the British Army in the Great War of 1914–1918*, accessed November 10, 2023, www.1914-1918.net.
47 Henry Wadsworth Longfellow, 1847, 'The Ladder of St. Augustine,' accessed April 20, 2024, www.poetryfoundation.org/poems/44636/the-ladder-of-st-augustine.
48 Edmund G. C. King, '"A Priceless Book to Have Out Here": Soldiers Reading Shakespeare in the First World War,' *Shakespeare* 10, no. 3 (2014): 241.
49 King, 'A Priceless Book,' 241.
50 King, 'A Priceless Book,' 234.
51 See Werner Habicht, 'Shakespeare Celebrations in Times of War,' *Shakespeare Quarterly* 52, no. 4 (2001): 441–455.
52 Autograph Book, ca. 1914–1918, Documents 7700, E. Burton, *Nurse's Autograph Books Containing Contributions by the West Indian Contingent, First World War* (Imperial War Museum, London).
53 Andrew Village, *The Kestrel* (London: Poyser, 1990), 21–22.
54 C.B. Purdom, ed. *Everyman at War: Sixty Personal Narratives of the War* (London: J.M. Dent & Sons, 1930), 80.
55 Carol Ann Duffy, *1914: Poetry Remembers* (London: Faber & Faber, 2013), 82.
56 Tim Kendall, *Poetry of the First World War: An Anthology* (Oxford: Oxford University Press, 2013), 110.

57 Paul Fussell, *The Great War and Modern Memory* (Oxford: Oxford University Press, 2013), 54–55.
58 Sara Haslam and Edmund G. C. King, '"Medicinable Literature": Bibliotherapy, Literary Caregiving, and the First World War," *Literature and Medicine* 39, no. 2 (Fall 2021): 299.
59 Haslam and King, 'Medicinable Literature,' 299.
60 Helen Mary Gaskell, *The Red Cross and Order of St. John War Library* (London: British Red Cross Society, 1918), 7, quoted in Haslam and King, 'Medicinable Literature,' 300.
61 Haslam and King, 'Medicinable Literature,' 305.
62 Haslam and King, 'Medicinable Literature,' 305.
63 Tim Kendall, *Poetry of the First World War*, 176.

References

Baker, Chris. 'The Long, Long Trail: Researching Soldiers of the British Army in the Great War of 1914-1918.' Accessed November 10, 2023. www.1914-1918.net.

Bodleian Library, Oxford. 'Kiel Canal, Flags, and Naval Expansion.' Accessed April 25, 2024. https://blogs.bodliean.ox.ac.uk/maps/2015/11/13/kiel-canal-flags-and-naval- -expansion/

Britannica Academic, s.v. 'Alfred von Tirpitz.' Accessed April 25, 2024, https://academic-eb-com-proxy.library.nyu.edu/levels/collegiate/article/Alfred-von-Tirpitz/72612

Brittain, Vera. *Testament of Youth: An Autobiographical Study of the Years 1900-1925*. London: Gollancz, 1935.

Burton, E. *Nurse's Autograph Books Containing Contributions by the West Indian Contingent, First World War,* ca. 1914–1918. Documents 7700. London: Imperial War Museum.

Das, Santanu. *Touch and Intimacy in First World War Literature*. Cambridge: Cambridge University Press, 2005.

Duffy, Carol Ann. *1914: Poetry Remembers*. London: Faber & Faber, 2013.

Fussell, Paul. *The Great War and Modern Memory*. Oxford: Oxford University Press, 2013.

Gaskell, Helen Mary. *The Red Cross and Order of St. John War Library*. London: British Red Cross Society, 1918.

Gernes, Todd S. 'Recasting the Culture of Ephemera.' In *Popular Literacy: Studies in Cultural Practices and Poetics*, edited by John Trimbur, 107–127. Pittsburgh: University of Pittsburgh Press, 2001.

Habicht, Werner. 'Shakespeare Celebrations in Times of War.' *Shakespeare Quarterly* 52, no.4 (Winter 2001): 441–455.

Hahn, Daniel, ed. 'ATTWELL Mabel, Lucie (1879–1964).' In *The Oxford Companion to Children's Literature*, 2nd ed. Oxford: Oxford University Press, 2015.

Hallett, Christine E. *Containing Trauma: Nursing Work in the First World War*. Manchester: Manchester University Press, 2009.

Hallett, Christine E. '"Emotional Nursing": Involvement, Engagement, and Detachment in the Writings of First World War Nurses and VADs.' In *First World War Nursing: New Perspectives*, edited by Christine E. Hallett and Alison S. Fell, 97–112. London: Routledge, 2013.

Haslam, Sara, and Edmund G. C. King. '"Medicinable Literature": Bibliotherapy, Literary Caregiving, and the First World War.' *Literature and Medicine* 39, no. 2 (2021): 296–318.

Herzog, Hanna and Rina Shapira. 'Will You Sign My Autograph Book? Using Autograph Books for a Sociohistorical Study of Youth and Social Frameworks.' *Qualitative Sociology* 9, no. 2 (June 1986): 109–125.

Kendall, Tim. *Poetry of the First World War: An Anthology*. Oxford: Oxford University Press, 2013.

Kessel, Martina and Patrick Merziger, eds. *The Politics of Humor: Laughter, Inclusion and Exclusion in the Twentieth Century*. Toronto: University of Toronto Press, 2011.

'Kindness of Strangers: In 1909, When Gladys Forryan, of Leicester, Wrote Her Name in Her New Autograph Book She Could Not Have Imagined That Several of the Entries Would Be from Soldiers Wounded in the First World War.' *Leicester Mercury* (November 10, 2011): 16.

King, Edmund G. C. ' "A Priceless Book to Have out Here": Soldiers Reading Shakespeare in the First World War.' *Shakespeare* 10, no. 3 (2014): 230–44.

King, Edmund G. C. 'From Common Reader to Canon: Memorialising the Shakespeare Reading British Soldier during the First World War.' In *Memorialising Shakespeare: Commemoration and Collective Identity 1916–2016*, edited by Edmund G. C. King and Monika Smialkowska, 35–64. Cham: Palgrave Macmillan, 2021.

King, Edmund G. C. 'Networks.' In *The Edinburgh Companion to First World War Periodicals*, edited by Marysa Demoor, Cedric Van Dijck, and Birgit Van Puymbroeck, 32–50. Edinburgh: Edinburgh University Press, 2023.

King, Hetty. 'Ship Ahoy [All the Nice Girls Love a Sailor].' *Song Facts*. Accessed November 10, 2023. www.songfacts.com/facts/hetty-king/ship-ahoy-all-the-nice-girls-love-a-sailor.

Koven, Seth. 'Prisoners of Their Beds: Invalids, Injured Soldiers, and Cultures of Convalescence in Nineteenth and Early-Twentieth Century Britain.' *Radical History Review* 94 (Winter 2006): 233–39.

Longfellow, Henry Wadsworth. 'The Ladder of St. Augustine.' *Poetry Foundation*. Accessed April 20, 2024. www.poetryfoundation.org/poems/44636/the-ladder-of-st-augustine McKinnon, Alexandra. 'Impressions of Empire: Autograph Books as Historical Resource, 1899–1919.' Paper presented at Researching War and Conflict through Ephemera Conference, Northumbria University, Newcastle, April 9, 2024. www.awm.gov.au/sites/default/files/impressions_of_empire_-_alexandra_mckinnon_reduce.pdf

McNeil, W.K. 'The Autograph Album Custom: A Tradition and Its Scholarly Treatment.' *Keystone Folklore Quarterly* 13, no.1 (Spring 1968): 29–40.

McWilliams, Brendan. 'Why Nelson Turned a Blind Eye at Copenhagen.' *The Irish Times*, April 2, 2001. www.irishtimes.com/news/why-nelson-turned-a-blind-eye-at-copenhagen-1.297163.

Meade, L.T. *A Sister of the Red Cross*. London: Nelson, 1900.

Meyer, Jessica. 'Hospital Journals.' In *The Edinburgh Companion to First World War Periodicals*, edited by Marysa Demoor, Cedric Van Dijck, and Birgit Van Puymbroeck, 338–351. Edinburgh: Edinburgh University Press, 2023.

National Army Museum, London. 'Florence Nightingale: The Lady with the Lamp.' Accessed November 10, 2023. www.nam.ac.uk/explore/florence-nightingale-lady-lamp.

Pelly, Florence Irene Clare. *Private Papers of Miss F.I.C. Pelly,* ca. 1914–1918. Documents 866. Imperial War Museum, London.

Purdom, C.B. ed. *Everyman at War: Sixty Personal Narratives of the War*. London: J.M. Dent & Sons, 1930.

Purseigle, Pierre. 'Mirroring Societies at War: Pictorial Humour in the British and French Popular Press during the First World War.' *Journal of European Studies* 31, no. 123 (2001): 289–328.

Reznick, Jeffrey. *Healing the Nation: Soldiers and the Culture of Caregiving in Britain during the Great War*. Manchester: Manchester University Press, 2004.

Ricker, Lisa Reid. '(De)Constructing the Praxis of Memory-Keeping: Late-Nineteenth Century Autograph Albums as Sites of Rhetorical Invention.' *Rhetoric Review* 29, no. 3 (June 2010): 239–256.

Tholas-Disset, Clementine and Karen A. Ritzenhoff, eds. *Humor, Entertainment, and Popular Culture during World War I*. New York: Palgrave Macmillan, 2015.

Towheed, Shafquat and Edmund G. C. King, eds. *Reading and the First World War: Readers, Texts, Archives*. Basingstoke: Palgrave Macmillan, 2015.

Trott, Vincent. 'Humour, Neutrality, and Preparedness: American Satirical Magazines and the First World War, 1914–1917.' *War in History* 29, no. 1 (January 2022): 104–136.

Village, Andrew. *The Kestrel*. London: Poyser, 1990.

Voeltz, Richard A. 'The Antidote to "Khaki Fever"? The Expansion of the British Girl Guides during the First World War.' *Journal of Contemporary History* 27, no. 4 (October 1992): 627–638.

5 Print as Caregiving in Wartime

The Role of Australian First World War Trench and Hospital Magazines

Véronique Duché and Amanda Laugesen

A 1920 edition of *Mountain Mist*, the magazine of the Bodington Tuberculosis Sanatorium in the Blue Mountains, New South Wales, Australia, that treated returned soldiers, declared that it aimed 'to speak always brightly, cheerfully and in a manly fashion to tell all that it had met of the bright sunshine that lies beyond the mist'.[1] Like many trench and hospital magazines of the war years, *Mountain Mist* was produced by and for soldiers and aimed to not only be an expression of the views, preoccupations, and experiences of the men who created and consumed it but also offer a type of comfort and caregiving to these men. The quote from *Mountain Mist* also tells us something about the typical tone and style of these publications, especially those produced by and for soldier-patients – a focus on optimism, manly stoicism despite suffering, and good cheer. Trench and hospital magazines were expressions of the times in which they were produced, but they also demonstrate the ways in which the soldier and soldier-patient were being discursively imagined and constructed.

This chapter seeks to explore the various ways in which we can understand trench and hospital magazines as a form of caregiving and as a type of bibliotherapy. What psychological and emotional benefits might soldiers and soldier-patients (and even family at home) have received from such publications? Soldiers and soldier-patients used these publications as a means of coping with the difficulties they faced; they also used them as a link to home and as a means of forging bonds of community with their fellow soldiers and patients. These types of publications could help to mediate and make sense of confusing, confronting and even life-changing experiences. Indeed, many of the key functions of trench and hospital magazines can arguably be seen to have contributed in some way to their therapeutic value for their readers.

'Bibliotherapy' was just one of a number of therapeutic movements – others included naturopathy and hypnotherapy – that emerged from the end of the eighteenth century onwards. The idea that books and reading could provide a therapeutic function took hold through the nineteenth century. By 1900, libraries 'had become a part of nearly all European mental hospitals', serving, as Claudia Cornett and Charles Cornett express it, as 'intellectual and emotional pharmacies for … patients'.[2] Libraries also became central to military hospitals, and this

DOI: 10.4324/9781003471561-7

was particularly the case during the First World War. Indeed, the British Army acknowledged the value of reading for the wounded, with an Oxford University don, H.F. Brett-Smith, 'tasked by the British Army with drawing up a "Fever-Chart" ranking the most "Salubrious reading for the wounded"'.[3] For the British and Australian armies, the Red Cross was active in setting up libraries for wounded or ill soldiers both in the theatres of war – often as part of 'recreation huts' that could also provide other means of entertaining the convalescent or ill soldier – and at home.[4]

Yet in considering the value of reading for soldiers in wartime, little attention has been paid to the therapeutic value of trench and hospital magazines. Trench and hospital magazines can be seen to have a role to play in 'literary caregiving'. Reading these kinds of publications could provide an experience of care to readers who were operating in a very particular kind of context.[5] When confronted with illness, death, or exile, literature has often been considered a remedy, an instrument bringing comfort in troubled times, and a tool to help heal individual and collective traumas. We can interpret the work of trench and hospital magazines – their production and their reading – as part of an ongoing process to work through the experiences and traumas of war. Joanna Bourke has argued that trauma is a subjective experience and that as historians we should be alert to the different languages individuals might use to package their subjective experiences of trauma.[6] Jason Crouthamel and Peter Leese add that the 'victims' of war should be understood as exerting agency through the various ways in which they shape their own narrative of trauma.[7] Magazines provided one important wartime means by which soldiers and soldier-patients could articulate and shape their personal and collective narratives of trauma and suffering both as content creators and as readers.[8]

While we seek in this chapter to assess the role and therapeutic value of such publications, we also consider the ways in which particular discourses of 'cheerfulness' could disguise the realities of suffering and shape the way soldiers and soldier-patients related to their experiences. Trench and hospital magazines arguably played a role in shaping the way soldiers and soldier-patients expressed, understood, and came to terms with their experiences. Ideas of how to deal with suffering, what it meant to be 'sick', and what it meant to be a 'man' were all constructed by and through such publications. Wartime magazines ultimately functioned to ensure that soldiers continued to fight and/or support the cause to which they were giving, or had given, their bodies.

Trench and Hospital Magazines

The First World War saw the production of a vast number of magazines written and produced by and for soldiers. These publications were produced by many of the national armies; some were written in the trenches under challenging and perilous circumstances, and some were produced behind the lines, including in hospitals. They were also produced on troopships taking men to and from war, and the tradition would continue through into veteran magazines produced after the war. According to Graham Seal, one of the foremost scholars of wartime publications, these magazines form 'a unique body of journalism, literature, art and record of events'.[9]

The production of such magazines in wartime had multiple motivations and functions. Many magazines declared that one of their key aims was to entertain the men. They therefore played an important role in sustaining morale, but they also became an important vehicle for venting complaints and expressing frustrations with military life.[10] They further had a definite psychological function: as Seal observes, they allowed soldiers to endure 'the palpable insanity to which [the men] were consigned by forces beyond their control'.[11] Stéphane Audoin-Rouzeau in his classic study of French trench publications adds that these magazines also had important functions as a means to convey information and as a record of the men's experiences.[12] They served, in Audoin-Rouzeau's words, as 'the mouthpiece of [a] common culture'.[13] Jessica Hammett, who has studied British civil defence magazines of the Second World War, argues that these kinds of magazines can 'give an unusual and rich insight into local social groups and everyday life'.[14] As collaborative productions, it is possible to use these kinds of magazines to see how 'identities and codes of behaviour were worked out'.[15]

We thus can argue that trench magazines had an important role to play in shaping and expressing identity, or more accurately, identities during the First World War. In the case of Australian trench magazines, for example, they became vehicles for shaping notions of 'Australianness', often as defined against Britishness.[16] They also helped to express an idealised identity of the 'citizen-soldier' for men who saw themselves as independent and who were reluctant to subject themselves to military structures and discipline. David Kent observes that trench magazines often paid tribute to the Australian soldier's manly virtues and rugged independence; in doing so, he argues, they helped to transform the citizen into the soldier. In turn, the work of these magazines and the broader cultural productions to which they belonged served to shape the cultural icon of the Anzac that would become so central to Australian conceptions of national identity.[17]

While trench magazines have been well-studied, there has been less focus on hospital magazines as a type of wartime publication and as an important subgenre of the soldier magazine. Australian hospital magazines were produced in a variety of locations, including overseas (and including England), at home (for soldiers who were repatriated to Australia due to the extent of their injuries), and in hospitals and convalescent homes in the years following the war. Content was typically contributed by both staff and patients. To date, Marina Larsson's study of Australian wounded and disabled returned soldiers is one of the only works to examine these publications in the Australian context. She argues that hospital magazines helped to boost morale and to give soldier-patients a positive framework within which to understand their wounds and/or disablements. She further argues that these magazines played a role in reassuring wounded men that their injuries were regarded as a 'sacrifice' to the nation – it turned their experiences into heroic narratives.[18] French hospital magazines were also produced as part of the proliferation of print during the war. While again the literature is limited, Marjorie Gehrhardt has written about *La Greffe Générale*, a hospital magazine produced for facially disfigured soldiers, arguing that it functioned as 'a platform that could be compared to modern-day therapy groups, blogs and forums' in how it dealt with the difficulties and challenges that were experienced by the wounded soldiers the magazine served.[19]

Hospital magazines performed a number of the same functions as trench magazines. They aimed to entertain their readers and to act as a record of experience. They also served to articulate a common identity, acting as the voice of the soldier-patient and the voice of those who cared for the soldier-patient. In addition, some of these magazines, especially those produced in the years that immediately followed the war, not only conveyed important information about rehabilitation efforts and government policy but could also act as a mouthpiece for soldier-patients who were demanding better support and welfare. In the most general sense, they could help to combat ignorance about illness or injury. *Mountain Mist*, produced for tubercular returned soldiers, had a professed goal of:

> engaging in combat with the tyrant prejudice that reigns against us in the minds of men. We see it persuading people to a great, more understanding charity. With its help we shall lessen the rather cruel isolation which should not be so wide and lonely. It shall show all men how they may teach us to lose that sense of ashamedness which should never have been..[20]

Mountain Mist aimed to provide 'simple and practical advice, put forward in … simple and everyday language' about the nature and treatment of the disease.[21] Such a function was invaluable in helping soldier-patients articulate a presence for themselves in postwar society.

The popularity of trench and hospital magazines attests to at least some resonance of all of this for soldier-readers. Trench and hospital magazines were eagerly read. While such reading may have been motivated by boredom for some, for many readers the multiple functions of these magazines – therapeutic, practical and diversionary – were invaluable in a time of war and change.

Entertainment, Optimism and Endurance

Trench and hospital magazines sought first and foremost to entertain their readers – this was what would guarantee a positive response, a readership and continued publication. Providing material such as entertaining stories, jokes and poems was crucial. With many contributors being 'amateurs' (although some did have professional experience in writing and illustration), it was crucial to secure quality and relevant copy wherever possible.

Editors sought out material that would be positive reading for their soldier-readers, shaping the image of the war portrayed in the pages of their publications. The editors of the trench magazine *Rising Sun*, for example, called for 'bright, short contributions' to make their publication as 'bright and interesting as possible, so that it may be equally appreciated by friends at home'. The editors of *the Kia*

Ora Coo-ee, a magazine produced for Australian and New Zealand soldiers in the Middle East, requested items that could be 'true or invented, and as humorous as possible. We have no time for sentimental gush, but there's a hearty welcome at this office for copy with a laugh in every line'.[22]

The content of trench and hospital magazines was intended to provide distraction as a form of entertainment. For example, there might be included articles on subjects such as popular entertainment, travel, sports and life at home. For readers, such articles might have offered an enticement to focus on life after the war, as well as taking soldiers' and soldier-patients' minds elsewhere, if only for a short period of time. They also offered promise to the soldiers, lifting their eyes to the horizon of postwar life. For example, *The Ghain Tuffieha Record*, a hospital magazine produced at a convalescent camp in Malta,[23] included an article for its readers on 'Opportunities after the War' and called for men to devote their energies to personal success after the war.[24]

Editors of trench magazines often explicitly discussed their role in providing entertainment. *Le Poilu* stated that its 'ambition is simply to entertain you for a moment, between two heavy mortar shells, or even between two fatigue-duties; and if we manage even for an instant to bring you pleasure, we will be only too happy to have achieved our aim'.[25] Another French trench magazine, *Marmita*, even more clearly stated that it aimed to fight off depressing thoughts:

> In your cellar or in your trench, when the hours drag, when the memory of your home or your dead friends become too sad, when depression breaks through, *Marmita* will be there to chase away *le cafard* [the gloomy mood].[26]

The *cafard* was, after the Germans, the number one enemy. A French POW magazine, *L'Anti-Cafard. Journal des Prisonniers de Tauberbishofsheim* (Baden), clearly stated this goal in its first issue, published on 20 October 1918: 'It is about fighting against the "cafard", that filthy Cockroach, more powerful, more formidable than ever, and which, if we let it happen, would end up damaging the strongest brains, the strongest minds'.[27] Another POW publication, *L'Exilé. Organe des Prisonniers du camp d'Hammelburg* (Bavaria) a weekly publication, first issued on 27 August 1916, also articulates such a mission:

> What can be our goal, if it is not to want to drive away this 'cafard' which embitters, even weakens many of our people. Rest assured, dear readers, that we are the relentless enemy of 'melancholy' and 'black'. We want to kill this 'black' and want to replace it with mirth and laughter.[28]

While the psychiatric syndrome affecting prisoners of war had been identified as early as 1918 by Swiss physician Adolf Lukas Vishner as 'barbed wire disease',[29] French soldiers were not ready yet to consider or label the *cafard* a medical condition. Yet descriptions of the *cafard* are comparable to the depression and despair felt by those who were prisoners and hinting at the fact that inertia and boredom were felt across many different conditions of war.

Many magazines argued for their role in promoting 'cheeriness' and dispelling gloom. The *Harefield Park Boomerang*, produced at the Harefield Park hospital in the UK where many Australian soldiers were sent, stated that their intent was to adopt a 'cheery tone' while another magazine, *Mountain Mist*, aimed to make its issues 'bright and gay'.[30] *La Greffe Générale: Organe des blessés de la face,* a French hospital journal, produced at the Parisian military hospital Val-de-Grâce (5th division for the wounded) and first published on 15 December 1917,[31] wrote that its goal was to fight against 'this old brother the *cafard* [the gloomy mood]'.[32] The Christmas 1918 edition of *The Jackass*, the magazine of the First Australian General Hospital, included a note from General Birdwood commenting that the magazine would 'serve as a good tonic to many of your patients, for it certainly must have a brightening effect on all who read it'.[33]

Magazines, especially hospital magazines, boasted of their apparent success in providing soldiers with emotional comfort. *Mountain Mist* insisted that the tubercular patients at Bodington Sanatorium were not 'down-hearted' and were 'a cheerful lot'.[34] The final issue of the *Harefield Park Boomerang* wrote a mock epitaph for the magazine that also emphasised its cheering role for the patients who were its readers:

In Loving Memory of Boomerang
Passed Away on Dec 31st 1918
You've been a faithful friend and true;
When times were dark and dreary,
You made us laugh when feeling blue,
And smile when very weary.
You done me good service
Told me no lies (???)[35]

Some magazines recognised the great difficulties that their soldier-patients faced. Jean-Émile Bayard, writing in the *Paris-Journal* in 1917 and exploring a series of trench and hospital magazines, examined the impact of depression on soldiers. He denounced a state of depression more dangerous than the 'neurasthenia of the area' or its first cousin the 'cafard'. This 'war work accident' slowly but surely shakes the *Poilu*. As a result, this mental disarray escalates and sometimes degenerates into 'war hypnosis'. This homesickness, this nostalgia for existence, this dis-adaptation can intensify. Also, it is up to intellectuals and leaders to fight through reason and sentimental education his organic irritability and his asthenia.[36]

Bayard therefore encouraged the soldiers to show their emotions, and he recommended the reading of *La Greffe Générale*. Indeed, the usefulness of the magazine in addressing the problems encountered by facially injured men was even acknowledged by the French government. In a letter to the editor dated 25 August 1917 and published in the first issue of the journal, the Head of the Front Journals service, stated: 'Your work [...], which will combine the useful with the pleasant, will have an excellent influence on all the soldiers [...]. It will help them to endure even better the moral sufferings of which some might feel the attacks'.[37]

Humour and Complaint

Trench and hospital magazines often employed humour as a way of entertaining the men, but also as a vehicle for complaint and self-expression. This humour served even more important functions in the context of war, however. According to Clémentine Tholas-Disset and Karen A. Ritzenhoff, humour is 'one of the most powerful instruments of psychological and political resistance on the battlefield and on the home front'.[38] The therapeutic function of humour has also been discussed by Koenraad DuPont, who argues that humour could be an 'indirect means for the soldiers to speak out about the war and its cultural implications, while at the same time emphasizing their own role in it'.[39] Humour was an indispensable coping mechanism in the context of war, and by extension, in the wartime hospital. Jacqueline Garrick has similarly emphasised the importance of humour as an essential tool for coping with the traumas of war: 'During the trauma, humor may have been a tool of survival; in the recovery process, it can be used as a tool for surviving and thriving as well'.[40]

Jane Chapman et al. in their book *Comics and the First World War* argue that the main purpose of a trench newspaper was to amuse: 'satire and irony represented an ideal vehicle for recording the human side of the Great War'.[41] They note that communal humour cemented cohesion but also acted as a prescriptive social corrective.[42] Humour, they write, is dependent on the society in which it exists, adapting and evolving with it. [43] It plays many roles in wartime, they argue, not least in alleviating the fear of death. It can create distance, release tensions, and can be used as a tool to get people to listen sympathetically to arguments and to persuade.[44]

Humour was not an inconsequential feature of trench and hospital magazines. Puns in the very titles of French trench magazines attested to their humorous orientation.[45] The names of certain Paris papers were appropriated and satirised: for example, *La Vie poilusienne* (142nd infantry regiment) [*The Soldier's Life*, a pun on *La Vie parisienne*, a weekly magazine founded in Paris in 1863] and *Le Bulletin désarmé* [*The Disarmed Bulletin*, a pun on the *Bulletin des Armées de la République*, a publication of the French Ministry of War from 15 August 1914]. If some titles showed chauvinistic triumphalism, even bellicose Germanophobia, such as *Le Bochofage* (68th infantry regiment) [German eater], *Le Vide-boche* (82nd heavy artillery regiment) [German chaser, with a pun on *vide-poche*, storage for pocket content], some clearly demonstrated their intended therapeutic quality, such as *Le Rire aux éclats*. 'Rire aux éclats' means 'to laugh out loud', but it can be literally understood as 'to laugh at shrapnels', to laugh in the face of adversity.

Humour was also a key feature of hospital magazines, some of it dark in tone. A poem in *Mountain Mist* was a play on the popular soldier song 'Parlez Vous' with words changed to reflect the experience of the tubercular soldier: 'Digger had a little cough, / It wasn't much you know, / Yet everywhere that Digger went, /

His cough it had to go'.[46] In the *Harefield Park Boomerang*, a list of hospital rules included the following introduction: 'A strict adherence to the following rules will shorten your stay here – if not they will shorten your life. Suicide is optional'.[47] The magazine also made use of the designation 'hoppy' to describe a man who had lost a leg, and this character was depicted in several cartoons showing him adapting to his disability.

Black humour was also very evident in French hospital magazines. *La Greffe Générale* claimed to offer content just as horrific as the disfigured soldiers who were treated at the hospital at which it was produced: 'the stunning fantasies, the huge jokes, the monstrous puns, all the ammunition indispensable for the fight against this old brother the Cockroach'.[48] Indeed, the Val-de-Grâce hospital treated the soldiers whose faces were mutilated in trench warfare – the men known as *gueules cassées* in France. While facially disfigured soldiers were generally cast out as social pariahs and seen as representatives of the futility of the war, *La Greffe Générale* instead demonstrated their resilience and tried to change the way these wounded combatants were regarded. It was aimed at the 'Civilian', the 'Français en veston' ['French in a jacket'] and tried to engage with him in a comic tone:

> Tell him that we do not want to excite the pity of our contemporaries, being ourselves very satisfied with our wounds. We certainly did not have, in distant days of peace, such an excuse for the flaws in our anatomy: today we can all yes, my dear – give the illusion of an ex-Adonis victim of war.[49]

A note (*petit billet*) explains the journal title and its subtitle: *La Greffe Générale [...]. Rire quand même* ['The general graft. To laugh anyway'], and explains its role as a weapon against depression. The note also offers a summary of *La Greffe Générale* as a 'heroic-comic tragedy in four acts'.[50] The set is described as 'sinister' and shows 'A corner of the hospital / where the wounded of the face are locked up. / A room, beds, horror on its stall. / Laughter and pain mixed; death passing'.[51] The characters are 'four disfigured soldiers around a table' and the atmosphere is dismal:

> Boredom oozes down the walls. Everything seems imprinted with that indefinable sadness common to the dens of suffering. The glow from the nightlights seems to pour bloody waves on the painful figures. The snoring of sleepers has the rhythm of groans. The four friends come together for a pleasant anecdote; laughter bursts out, which destroys the bad charm, goes to touch each feverish forehead, soon shaking with a strange gaiety all the ravaged faces.[52]

The characters then make the decision to create their journal and invent the pun of its title: 'Laughter will be our only master. Let us share with civilians the echoes of our laughter. [...] The ... The ... (Facial service, human graft, break from boredom ..) here we are: The General graft'.[53] This mission was admired by René Benjamin in *Le Journal*, one of the four main newspapers of the time, in an article titled 'L'esprit français. Un journal de blessés' ['French spirit. A journal of wounded soldiers']: 'To have had three quarters of the face washed away by a shrapnel, and to laugh with what remains, isn't that admirable and poignant?'[54]

Sentiment, Family and Home

While humour played an important role in coping with the horrors and challenges of war, so too did sentiment. Alongside the humour, which could be cynical, dark and ironic, sentiment thrived in trench and hospital magazines. This was especially true in the many contributions that invoked home and loved ones.

Hospital magazine, the *Harefield Park Boomerang*, included the following poem that exemplifies the kind of sentimental poetry that is featured in many trench and hospital magazines. Patient J.J. Collins wrote the following poem, 'To My Mother':

> I'm glad I came from Australia fair
> To this distant land to do my share,
> I've done my bit, and, I hope, done well!
> I'll bring home marks of a German shell.
> But what does it matter, mother dear?
> Dry from your eye that glistening tear.
> Let your heart rejoice at the pain I've borne.[55]

Invocations of mothers and sweethearts were common across soldier culture. But a link between home and the fighting front was also forged in a more 'real' fashion, through the sending of such publications to family and friends at home. *La Greffe Générale* explicitly provided a means by which the wounded soldier who would want to send a copy to 'his family, his godmother, his friends' could write, thanks to a sidebar left blank at the bottom of the last page of the magazine, 'a few words' for those loved ones at home. In this way, the therapeutic function of the trench and hospital magazine was extended to those at home, who could, through reading the magazine, gain some insight into the experiences of soldiers. But they could be reassured, thanks to the humour, cheery tones and confidence projected within the magazines, that their loved one was coping with what was happening to them.

There is much Australian evidence of trench magazines being sent home to families. One soldier from Western Australia, Patrick Lorimer, sent home copies of the *Anzac Bulletin*, *Aussie: The Australian Soldiers' Magazine*, and the publication *The Anzac Book* to his sweetheart Geraldine to give her a better, if not realistic, idea of what he was experiencing. A copy of *The Flotilla Echo* held in the Australian War Memorial has an inscription on the cover of the 1917 issue: 'Dear Dad, I hope you are keeping well also all at home. I am A1 myself. I will be writing to you as soon as I get some more news. Bert xxx'.[56]

Editors of trench and hospital magazines recognised the importance of their publication providing insight into the experience of soldiers for those at home. The inaugural edition of the *Kia Ora Coo-ee*, for instance, noted that one of the aims of the magazine was '[t]o present to those loved ones far away a reflection, however slight, of the conditions and strange surroundings in which their sons live'.[57] The *Harefield Park Boomerang* aimed to not only

> be read here in the hospital, but in France, and thousands of miles away, over in Australia, so that it may be a link between all the boys who have been here, and are now scattered, and also come as a message to your people at home of the life that they lead here at Harefield.[58]

Harefield Park was in the UK, and so it was produced by Australians who were still overseas and far from home. The July 1917 number noted: 'Remember that you can send the Boomerang home to Australia free. And there is not a person at home who would not like to see it'.[59] Readers of *Mountain Mist*, produced after the war for tubercular veterans, were frequently exhorted to lend it out and to send it to those at home to expand its readership to those outside the Bodington Sanatorium. References in some of the later issues suggest that some patients did indeed send it home and/or to those outside the sanatorium.

The forging of these links between soldier (or soldier-patient) and those at home, both at the imaginative and real level, was essential to the maintenance of morale and the forging of some kind of emotional resilience. Through sentiment, trench and hospital magazines could further their therapeutic value not only for the soldier but also for those at home.

Community and Identity

The therapeutic functions of trench and hospital magazines can also arguably be seen in the ways in which such magazines provided ways of understanding identity and forming a community. Projecting ideas of a shared experience could be a powerful way for soldiers to feel that they were united in a common struggle and that others might similarly feel, for example, disgruntlement with military life.

Some magazines explicitly touched on their role in bonding soldiers as comrades, an essential function for creating a more effective fighting force. For example, the editors of the troopship magazine *Pitch and Toss* wrote that:

> The aim and earnest desire of those interested in this publication is to strengthen every bond that shall tend to make us even better comrades than we now are, for we believe that deepest comradeship means better fighters. If, then, our purpose is effected, we shall know that 'Pitch and Toss' has done its bit.[60]

The Ghain Tuffieha Record, which was produced by both British and Australian staff, patients and convalescents, included in its January 1916 edition an article entitled 'Play the Game' that exhorted men to focus on what they needed to win the war: 'We are soldiers. We are men. We have power to restrain ourselves, power to help ourselves to fitness'.[61]

Magazines could also forge other kinds of community. As we've seen already, *La Greffe Générale* sought to create a strong community of disfigured soldiers.

It also aimed to engage with as many soldiers as possible and called for the contribution of all the wounded in France, forging an even broader sense of community: 'We need to feel with us the active crowd of our brothers in arms. Comrades, to your quills!'[62] The magazine was instrumental in the later constitution of the facially disfigured men's organisation – the *Association des Gueules Cassées*.[63] *Mountain Mist* similarly served to construct a community of soldier-patients with a common ailment: tuberculosis. The first edition noted that the editors hoped that it would 'assist TBs to a fuller understanding of one another, and a great unity of purpose between the men who have deserved well of their Country'. It was felt that tuberculosis patients were treated unfairly, and one of the functions of the magazine was to act as a voice for the community of tubercular soldier-patients and to push their cause. It sought to counter the 'tyrant prejudice' against such patients: 'With its help we shall lessen the rather cruel isolation which should not be so wide and lonely'.[64] *Mountain Mist* therefore forged a community for soldiers who were facing discrimination in postwar Australia. An association of tubercular returned soldiers was subsequently formed, and their voice was heard within the broader community of returned soldiers.

Trench and hospital magazines also served to construct masculine identity within the context of the services and war. The experience of being wounded could challenge men: it undermined their primary status as a soldier. Masculinity was proved through war service.[65] Australian trench magazines went some way to construct the ideal Australian male – self-reliant, laid-back, never entirely accepting of authority and discipline, a fearless warrior and meeting challenges with laconic humour. They contributed to the creation of the Anzac legend. But (returned) soldiers with disabilities and/or illness did not find a place within the Anzac legend.[66] Marina Larsson suggests that Australian soldiers of the First World War who were wounded or sick were reluctant to reveal their trauma, as they subscribed to Edwardian notions of manliness that did not allow for open sharing of emotion or complaining about pain. Self-control was, she argues, central to both soldierly and civilian constructions of manliness.[67] As mentioned earlier, Larsson has argued that hospital magazines transmitted heroic narratives of injury in order to allow soldier-patients to retain their manliness; this in itself, she argues, had therapeutic dimensions for the men.[68]

Conclusion

In this chapter, we have emphasised the therapeutic functions of trench and hospital magazines; indeed, we could argue that many of the primary functions of the trench and hospital magazines can be seen to have had a therapeutic effect on soldiers: the value of humour and entertainment, the links to home and the fostering of *esprit de corps*. Soldiers and soldier-patients found great value in these magazines; for those at home, these publications offered a fragile link to their loved ones and offered a means to ease their anxiety.

The principle of the usefulness of books has long been defended. Take Rabelais' *Pantagruel* (1532): In his Prologue, the first-person narrator Alcofribas Nasier (an anagram of the author) promises vigorously to his readers that they will greatly benefit from his book. He cites as evidence the famous *Great and inestimable Chronicle of the huge and mighty giant Gargantua.* Readers who 'were suffering cruelly from toothache, after having squandered all their fortune paying doctors without any profit, have found no more effective remedy than to put these Chronicles between two nice warm cloths, then apply them to the pain, after infusing them with some magic powder'.[69] This was not to mention the benefit for the readers plagued with the pox and the gout: 'their only consolation was to listen to a few pages of the book being read'.[70]

The concept of bibliotherapy has been brought up to date by Pierre-André Bonnet, a General Practitioner who defended a PhD thesis at the University of Aix-Marseille in 2009.[71] Focusing on fiction, Alexandre Gefen, a historian of ideas and literature, also makes the case for the utilitarian dimension of reading and urges us to take a fresh look at the literary tradition. Drawing on Trauma Studies which see 'literature as a form of speech in response to suffering',[72] Gefen encourages us to think of literary activity as a pragmatic linguistic activity and to 'reintegrate into the wider literary field purposeful actions (to please, to persuade, etc.) as ritual activities that a strictly aesthetic definition would have ruled out'.[73] According to Gefen, who is exploring this new interdisciplinary field of research called 'care',[74] literature has a restorative function, seeking to 'repair our conditions as victims, to correct the traumas of individual memory or of the social fabric'.[75] Indeed in French, the close connection between books and healing is reinforced by a pun: literature can both think (*penser*) and dress wounds (*panser*).[76]

We can certainly support Alexandre Gefen's argument that the recent 'therapeutic turn' has given birth to 'a literature which cares, which heals, which helps, or, at least, which "does good" '[77] and has become the default mode when all other political or societal responses prove inefficient. This therapeutic turn has also been acknowledged in the Anglophone literary world, as demonstrated by book historian Leah Price, who focusses on reading practices and the future of reading, and concedes that books have become means to medical ends.[78] However, we suggest the therapeutic value of literature can be traced back much earlier in time. Writing and reading trench and hospital journals offered soldiers an escape from hell. At a time when soldiers were looking for new ways of making sense of (and escaping) their conditions, trench and hospital journals made it possible to think about the individual, to give meaning to pluralised identities, to rewrite geography by developing a common military culture and to build a sense of community.

Notes

1 *Mountain Mist*, no. 19 (July 1921): 11.

2 Claudia Cornett and Charles F. Cornett, *Bibliotherapy: The Right Book at the Right Time* (Bloomington, IN: Phi Delta Kappa Educational Foundation, 1980), 12.

3 Jonathan Bate and Andrew Schuman, 'The Art of Medicine: Books Do Furnish a Mind: The Art and Science of Bibliotherapy', *The Lancet*, 387 (February 20, 2016): 742.

4 Amanda Laugesen, *Boredom Is the Enemy: The Intellectual and Imaginative Lives of Australian Soldiers in the Great War and Beyond* (Farnham: Ashgate, 2012), 18–22.
5 Sara Haslam, 'Reading, Trauma and Literary Caregiving 1914–1918: Helen Mary Gaskell and the War Library', *Journal of Medical Humanities*, 41 (March 2018): 6, 9.
6 Joanna Bourke, 'Why History Hurts', in *Traumatic Memories of the Second World War and After*, eds. Peter Leese and Jason Crouthamel (Basingstoke: Palgrave Macmillan, 2016): 275, 276.
7 Jason Crouthamel and Peter Leese, *Psychological Trauma and the Legacies of the First World War* (Cham: Palgrave Macmillan 2017), 3.
8 The therapeutic benefits of narrative are argued by James W. Pennebaker and Janel D. Seagal, 'Forming a Story: The Health Benefits of Narrative', *Journal of Clinical Psychology* 55, 10 (1999), 1243–54. See also Michael White and David Epston, *Narrative Means to Therapeutic Ends* (New York: Norton, 1990).
9 Graham Seal, *The Soldiers' Press: Trench Journals in the First World War* (Basingstoke: Palgrave Macmillan, 2013), 2.
10 Graham Seal, '"Written in the Trenches": Trench Newspapers of the First World War', *Journal of the Australian War Memorial* 16 (April 1990): 30.
11 Seal, *The Soldiers' Press*, ix.
12 Stéphane Audoin-Rouzeau, *Men at War 1914–1918: National Sentiment and Trench Journalism in France during the First World War*, trans. Helen McPhail (Providence: Berg, 1992), 15, 18.
13 Audoin-Rouzeau, *Men at War*, 34.
14 Jessica Hammett, '"The Invisible Chain by Which All are Bound to Each Other": Civil Defence Magazines and the Development of Community during the Second World War', *Journal of War and Culture Studies* 11, no. 2 (2018): 119.
15 Jessica Hammett, 'The Invisible Chain', 132.
16 Seal, 'Written in the Trenches', 30.
17 David Kent, 'Troopship Literature: "A Life on the Ocean Wave", 1914–1919', *Journal of the Australian War Memorial,* 10 (April 1987): 9.
18 Marina Larsson, *Shattered Anzacs: Living with the Scars of War* (Sydney: UNSW Press, 2009), 52.
19 Marjorie Gehrhardt, '*La Greffe Générale:* The Voice of French Facially Injured Soldiers', *Modern and Contemporary France* 26, no. 4 (2018): 359.
20 *Mountain Mist*, no. 2 (February 1920): 1.
21 *Mountain Mist*, no. 9 (September 1920): 1.
22 *The Kia Ora coo-ee*, no. 1 (March 15, 1918): 11.
23 Ghain Tuffieha Hospital Camp, Malta. Royal Army Medical Corps. British Army.
24 *The Ghain Tuffieha Record* (January 1916): 5.
25 *Le Poilu*, no. 1 (December 1914): 1.
26 *Marmita* (10 January 1915) quoted in Audoin-Rouzeau, 12–13.
27 *L'Anti-Cafard*, no. 1 (1918): 1. Note that *L'Anti-Cafard* gave even its English and Italian readers an opportunity to express themselves in their native language. An 'English Chronicle' followed by 'Echos and novels', and a 'Cronica Italiana' followed by 'Gilli-Morganti' occupy half a column each on the last page of the first issue of the journal (*L'Anti-Cafard*, no. 1 (1918): 4).
28

> Quel peut être notre but, si ce n'est de vouloir chasser ce 'cafard' qui aigrit, voire même affaiblit bien des nôtres. Soyez assurés, chers lecteurs, que nous sommes

l'ennemi acharné de la 'mélancolie' et du 'noir'. Nous voulons tuer ce 'noir' et le voulons remplacer par la gaieté et le rire.

(*L'Exilé,* no. 1 (1916): 1)

29 Adolf Lukas Vischer, *Die Stacheldraht-Krankheit. Beiträge sur Psychologie des Kriegsgefangenen*, in *Schweizer Schriften für allgemeines Wissen* (Heft 5, Zürich: Rascher & Cie Verlag, 1918). While an English translation was published the following year (*Barbed-wire disease- a psychological study of the prisoner of war*, London: John Bale & Danielson), this publication was never translated into French. For recent discussions of First World War hospital periodicals, see the chapter 'Hospital Magazines' in Jeffrey S. Reznick, *Healing the Nation: Soldiers and the Culture of Caregiving in Britain during the Great* War (Manchester: Manchester University Press, 2004), 65–98; Alice Brumby, 'Tommy Talk: War Hospital Magazines and the Literature of Resilience and Healing', in *The Palgrave Handbook of Artistic and Cultural Responses to War since 1914: The British Isles, the United States and Australasia*, edited by Martin Kerby, Margaret Baguley, and Janet McDonald (Cham: Palgrave Macmillan, 2019), 63–79; and Jessica Meyer, 'Hospital Journals', in *The Edinburgh Companion to First World War Periodicals*, edited by Marysa Demoor, Cedric Van Dijck, and Birgit Van Puymbroeck (Edinburgh: Edinburgh University Press, 2023), 338–51.

30 *Harefield Park Boomerang,* no. 1 (December 1916): 4; *Mountain Mist*, no. 1 (January 1920): 18.

31 The journal was dedicated to 'the Father of the mouths', Professor Hippolyte Morestin (1869–1919), one of the founders of cosmetic surgery. Eight issues were released between December 1917 and July 1918.

32 *La Greffe Générale*, no. 1 (1917): 1.

33 *The Jackass* (Christmas 1918): 7.

34 *Mountain Mist*, no. 4 (April 1920): 12.

35 *Harefield Park Boomerang*, 2, no.11 (December 1918): inside back cover.

36 Quoted in *La Greffe Générale,* no. 6 (1918): 4.

37 Pierre Chapelle, 'Messieurs les Directeurs', *La Greffe Générale*, no. 1 (1917): 3.

38 Clémentine Tholas-Disset and Karen A. Ritzenhoff, 'Introduction', in *Humor, Entertainment, and Popular Culture During World War*, edited by Clémentine Tholas-Disset and Karen A. Ritzenhoff (New York: Palgrave Macmillan, 2015), 7.

39 Koenraad Dupont, 'Nature and Function of Humor in Trench Newspapers (1914–1918)', in *Humor, Entertainment*, 116.

40 Jacqueline Garrick, 'The Humor of Trauma Survivors', *Journal of Aggression, Maltreatment and Trauma*, 12, nos. 1–2 (2006): 181.

41 Jane Chapman, Anna Hayles, Andrew Kerr and Adam Sherif, *Comics and the First World War: A Cultural Record* (Basingstoke: Palgrave Macmillan, 2015), 59.

42 *Comics and the First World War*, 10.

43 *Comics and the First World War*, 37.

44 *Comics and the First World War*, 38.

45 See Véronique Duché, 'Portraying the Enemy: Humour in French and Australian Trench Journals', in *Expressions of War in Australia and the Pacific. Language, Trauma, Memory and Official Discourse*, edited by Amanda Laugesen and Catherine Fisher (Cham: Palgrave Macmillan, 2019), 43–65.

46 *Mountain Mist*, no. 17 (May 1921): 7.

47 *Harefield Park Boomerang*, no. 8 (April 4, 1917): 4.

48 *La Greffe Générale,* no. 1 (1917): 1.
49 *La Greffe Générale,* no. 1 (1917): 1.
50 *La Greffe Générale,* no. 1 (1917): 3.
51 *La Greffe Générale,* no. 1 (1917): 3.
52 *La Greffe Générale,* no. 1 (1917): 3.
53 *La Greffe Générale,* no. 1 (1917): 1, 3. Note the pun on *Greffe / grève* (graft / strike), in reference to the strike against boredom and depression that the patients have declared.
54 *Le Journal*, no. 1 (28 September 1917), reproduced in *La Greffe Générale*, no. 3 (1918): 4.
55 *Harefield Park Boomerang*, no. 12 (June 1, 1917): 8.
56 Inside cover of *The Flotilla Echo* (December 1917) held at the Australian War Memorial.
57 *The Kia Ora Coo-ee*, no. 1 (March 15, 1918): 1.
58 *Harefield Park Boomerang,* no. 8 (April 4, 1917): 2.
59 *Harefield Park Boomerang*, no. 13, (July 2, 1917).
60 *Pitch and Toss,* no. 1 (September 9, 1916).
61 *The Ghain Tuffieha Record* (January 1916): 4.
62 *La Greffe Générale,* no. 1 (1917): 3.
63 See Marjorie Gehrhardt, *The Men with Broken Faces:* Gueules Cassées *of the First World War* (Oxford: Peter Lang, 2015).
64 *Mountain Mist,* no. 2 (February 1920): 1.
65 Jessica Meyer, *Men of War: Masculinity and the First World War in Britain* (Houndmills: Palgrave Macmillan, 2011), 83.
66 Larsson, *Shattered Anzacs,* 22.
67 Larsson, *Shattered Anzacs,* 50.
68 Larsson, *Shattered Anzacs,* 52.
69 François Rabelais. *Tout Rabelais*, Romain Menini (ed.), 13. Paris: Bouquins, 2022. (Our translation).
70 François Rabelais. *Tout Rabelais*, Romain Menini (ed.), 15. Paris: Bouquins, 2022. (Our translation).
71 See Bonnet, Pierre-André. *La Bibliothérapie en médecine générale* (Montpellier: Sauramps Médical) 2013.
72 Alexandre Gefen. *Réparer le monde. La littérature française face au XXIe siècle* (Paris: Corti, 2017), 87.
73 Alexandre Gefen. *Réparer le monde. La littérature française face au XXIe siècle* (Paris: Corti, 2017), 18. (Our translation).
74 See Alexandre Gefen. '"D'autres vies que la mienne": roman français contemporain, empathie et théorie du care', in *Empathie et esthétique*, edited by Alexandre Gefen and Bernard Vouilloux (Paris: Hermann, 2013), 279–92. Pioneered by American feminists Carol Gilligan (1982) and Joan Tronto (1993), this field of studies is now well established in France thanks to Sandra Laugier, Pascale Molinier and Patrica Paperman (2009).
75 Alexandre Gefen. *Réparer le monde. La littérature française face au XXIe siècle* (Paris: Corti, 2017), 11. (Our translation).
76 See the recent *Fictions pansantes. Bibliothérapies d'hier, d'aujourd'hui et d'ailleurs*, edited by Victoire Feuillebois and Anthony Mangeon (Paris: Hermann, 2023).
77 Alexandre Gefen, *Réparer le monde. La littérature française face au XXIe siècle* (Paris: Corti, 2017), 9. (Our translation).
78 Leah Price, *What We Talk about When We Talk about Books* (New York: Basic Books, 2019).

References

Audoin-Rouzeau, Stéphane. *Men at War 1914–1918: National Sentiment and Trench Journalism in France during the First World War.* Translated by Helen McPhail. Providence: Berg, 1992.

Bate, Jonathan and Andrew Schuman. 'The Art of Medicine: Books Do Furnish a Mind: The Art and Science of Bibliotherapy', *The Lancet*, no. 387 (February 20, 2016): 742–743.

Bonnet, Pierre-André. *La Bibliothérapie en médecine générale.* Montpellier: Sauramps Médical, 2013.

Bourke, Joanna. 'Why History Hurts'. In *Traumatic Memories of the Second World War and After,* edited by Peter Leese and Jason Crouthamel, 269–289. Cham: Palgrave Macmillan, 2016.

Brumby, Alice. 'Tommy Talk: War Hospital Magazines and the Literature of Resilience and Healing'. In *The Palgrave Handbook of Artistic and Cultural Responses to War since 1914: The British Isles, the United States and Australasia*, edited by Martin Kerby, Margaret Baguley, and Janet McDonald, 63–79. Cham: Palgrave Macmillan, 2019.

Chapelle, Pierre. 'Messieurs les Directeurs', *La Greffe Générale*, no. 1 (1917): 3.

Chapman, Jane, Anna Hayles, Andrew Kerr and Adam Sherif. *Comics and the First World War: A Cultural Record.* Basingstoke: Palgrave Macmillan, 2015.

Cornett, Claudia, and Charles F. Cornett. *Bibliotherapy: The Right Book at the Right Time.* Bloomington, IN: Phi Delta Kappa Educational Foundation, 1980.

Crouthamel, Jason, and Peter Leese. *Psychological Trauma and the Legacies of the First World War.* Cham: Palgrave Macmillan, 2017.

Duché, Véronique. 'Portraying the Enemy: Humour in French and Australian Trench Journals'. In *Expressions of War in Australia and the Pacific. Language, Trauma, Memory and Official Discourse*, edited by Amanda Laugesen and Catherine Fisher, 43–65. Cham: Palgrave Macmillan, 2019.

Dupont, Koenraad. 'Nature and Function of Humor in Trench Newspapers (1914–1918)'. In *Humor, Entertainment, and Popular Culture During World War,* edited by Clémentine Tholas-Disset and Karen A. Ritzenhoff, *I*, 107–121. New York: Palgrave Macmillan, 2015.

Feuillebois, Victoire and Mangeon, Anthony (eds). *Fictions pansantes. Bibliothérapies d'hier, d'aujourd'hui et d'ailleurs.* Paris: Hermann, 2023.

Garrick, Jacqueline. 'The Humor of Trauma Survivors', *Journal of Aggression, Maltreatment and Trauma*, 12, nos. 1–2 (2006): 169–182.Gefen, Alexandre. '"D'autres vies que la mienne": roman français contemporain, empathie et théorie du care'. In *Empathie et esthétique*, edited by Alexandre Gefen and Bernard Vouilloux, 279–292. Paris: Hermann, 2013.

Gefen, Alexandre. *Réparer le monde. La littérature française face au XXIe siècle.* Paris: Corti, 2017.

Gehrhardt, Marjorie. *The Men with Broken Faces:* Gueules Cassées *of the First World War.* Oxford: Peter Lang, 2015.

Gehrhardt, Marjorie. '*La Greffe Générale*: The Voice of French Facially Injured Soldiers', *Modern and Contemporary France*, 26, no. 4 (2018): 353–368.

Gilligan, Carol. *In a Different Voice: Psychological Theory and Moral Development.* Cambridge, MA: Harvard University Press, 1982.

Hammett, Jessica. '"The Invisible Chain by Which All Are Bound to Each Other": Civil Defence Magazines and the Development of Community during the Second World War', *Journal of War and Culture Studies* 11, no. 2 (2018): 117–135.

Harefield Park Boomerang, no. 1 (December 1916).

Harefield Park Boomerang, no. 8 (April 4, 1917).
Harefield Park Boomerang, no. 12 (June 1, 1917).
Harefield Park Boomerang, no. 13 (July 2, 1917).
Harefield Park Boomerang, 2, no. 11 (December 1918).
Haslam, Sara. 'Reading, Trauma and Literary Care-giving 1914–1918: Helen Mary Gaskell and the War Library', *Journal of Medical Humanities* 41 (2020): 305–321. https://doi.org/10.1007/s10912-018-9513-5.
Kent, David. 'Troopship Literature: "A Life on the Ocean Wave", 1914–1919', *Journal of the Australian War Memorial,* 10 (April 1987): 3–10.
L'Anti-Cafard, no. 1 (1918).
L'Exilé, no. 1 (1916).
La Greffe Générale, no. 1 (1917).
La Greffe Générale, no. 6 (1918).
Larsson, Marina. *Shattered Anzacs: Living with the Scars of War*. Sydney: UNSW Press, 2009.
Laugesen, Amanda. *Boredom Is the Enemy: The Intellectual and Imaginative Lives of Australian Soldiers in the Great War and Beyond.* Farnham: Ashgate, 2012.
Laugier, Sandra, Molinier, Pascale and Paperman, Patricia (dir.). *Qu'est-ce que le* care*? Souci des autres, sensibilité, responsabilité.* Paris: Payot, 2009.
Le Poilu, no. 1 (December 1914).
McChord Crothers, Samuel. 'A Literary Clinic', *The Atlantic Monthly* (September 1916): 291–300.
Meyer, Jessica. *Men of War: Masculinity and the First World War in Britain.* Houndmills: Palgrave Macmillan, 2011.
Meyer, Jessica. 'Hospital Journals'. In *The Edinburgh Companion to First World War Periodicals*, edited by Marysa Demoor, Cedric Van Dijck and Birgit Van Puymbroeck, 338–51. Edinburgh: Edinburgh University Press, 2023.
Mountain Mist, no. 2 (February 1920).
Mountain Mist, no. 4 (April 1920).
Mountain Mist, no. 9 (September 1920).
Mountain Mist, no. 17 (May 1921).
Mountain Mist, no. 19 (July 1921).
Pennebaker, James W. and Janel D. Seagal, 'Forming a Story: The Health Benefits of Narrative', *Journal of Clinical Psychology,* 55, no. 10 (1999): 1243–54.
Pitch and Toss, no. 1 (9 September 1916).
Price, Leah. *What We Talk about When We Talk about Books*. New York: Basic Books, 2019.
Rabelais, François. *Tout Rabelais*, Romain Menini (ed.). Paris: Bouquins, 2022.
Reznick, Jeffrey S. . 'Hospital Magazines: Writing about Wartime Recovery/Recovering Writing about Wartime'. In *Healing the Nation: Soldiers and the Culture of Caregiving in Britain during the Great* War, edited by Jeffrey S. Reznick, 65–98. Manchester: Manchester University Press, 2004.
Seal, Graham. '"Written in the Trenches": Trench Newspapers of the First World War', *Journal of the Australian War Memorial*, 16 (April 1990): 30–38.
Seal, Graham. *The Soldiers' Press: Trench Journals in the First World War.* Basingstoke: Palgrave Macmillan, 2013.
The Flotilla Echo (December 1917).
The Ghain Tuffieha Record (January 1916).
The Jackass (Christmas 1918).
The Kia Ora coo-ee, no. 1 (March 15, 1918).

Tholas-Disset, Clémentine and Karen A. Ritzenhoff, 'Introduction'. In *Humor, Entertainment, and Popular Culture During World War,* edited by Clémentine Tholas-Disset and Karen A. Ritzenhoff, *I*, 1–19. New York: Palgrave Macmillan, 2015.

Tronto, Joan. *Moral Boundaries. A Political Argument for an Ethic of Care.* New York/London: Routledge, 1993.

Vischer, Adolf Lukas. *Die Stacheldraht-Krankheit. Beiträge sur Psychologie des Kriegsgefangenen.* In *Schweizer Schriften für allgemeines Wissen*, Heft 5. Zürich: Rascher & Cie Verlag, 1918.

White, Michael and David Epston. *Narrative Means to Therapeutic Ends.* New York: Norton, 1990.

Part II

Institutional Legacies from Libraries to Hospitals, 1919–1950

6 'Return to Normalcy'

American Librarians and Bibliotherapy in the Aftermath of the First World War

Barbara Hochman

America's present need is not heroics, but healing; not nostrums, but normalcy; not revolution, but restoration.

Warren G. Harding (1920)

Introduction

A belief in the healing power of books was the logical extension of a belief in the material, moral, and aesthetic value of literature promoted by American schools and libraries in the late nineteenth- and early-twentieth centuries. As Thomas Augst has argued, 'faith in reading' became a kind of civil religion in this period.[1] Representing books as sources of nourishment, well-being, and socialization, librarians and cultural commentators agreed that literature would advance the personal development of individuals while reinforcing democratic American ideals. By the 1920s, a widely shared consensus affirmed the fundamental importance of reading, identifying it ever more firmly with social progress, especially for groups deemed in need of special guidance – children, immigrants, and African Americans. For patients, however, reading was to serve a different end: return to a former condition. What presidential candidate Warren Harding called a 'return to normalcy' in the aftermath of World War I and the flu epidemic of 1918 had particular significance for the nascent field of bibliotherapy.[2]

Hospital libraries gained many new advocates in the early twentieth century, especially after the war. As Assistant Surgeon General Lavinder of the US Public Health Service put it in 1922, a 'well conducted hospital [library] service is a therapeutic agent [… that] assists in hastening convalescence and restoration to health.' [3] This chapter argues that the goal of 'restor[ing]' patients to governing norms determined book selection in American hospital libraries of the 1920s. However, devotees of bibliotherapy were keenly aware that reading could have unpredictable effects. Indeed (unlike mainstream librarians) they often emphasized this point, using it to validate strict control of book selection.

Nineteenth-century debates about reading help explain the subsequent emphasis on both normalcy and control among early bibliotherapists in the United States.

DOI: 10.4324/9781003471561-9

During the antebellum period, as technological developments in printing, paper making, and transportation spurred the production and distribution of reading matter, a popular belief in the value of literacy evolved in tandem with a heightened sense of its potential dangers. Ministers, educators, and other commentators differentiated between valuable and perilous reading, castigating fiction for endangering social stability by stimulating fantasies, especially in women, young people, and the working class.[4] Competing claims about the benefits and hazards of reading are encapsulated in the opposition to slave literacy. Slaves were initially permitted, even encouraged, to learn their letters in order to read the Bible – an activity that was to encourage humility and obedience. However, as slaves gained access to abolitionist ideas and found justification for resistance in Biblical texts themselves, plantation owners confronted the difficulty of controlling the impact of reading. In the wake of the Nat Turner Revolt, many Southern states passed anti-literacy laws, hoping to forestall rebellion.[5]

After the Civil War (1861–1865), as Northern teachers and missionaries went South to educate freed slaves and promote Christian values, the effects of reading continued to stir hopes of transformation in some and fear of social chaos in others. By the end of the nineteenth century, however, public schools and libraries uniformly endorsed reading as both an indispensable skill and a social value. An advertisement for Charles Eliot Norton's 'Five Foot Shelf' of Classics proclaimed in 1920 that 'A Few Great Books Started Lincoln' (Figure 6.1).[6] In 1922, Ernestine Rose, head of the Harlem branch library, declared great books 'the most democratizing things in the world.'[7] Such claims about reading emphasize equality and opportunity but also endorse a pre-selected canon. The idea that book selection was 'central to the formation of character and could therefore lead to personal success or ruin' persisted well into the twentieth century.[8] Some commentators affirmed the value of all reading regardless of content – 'better bad books than no books,' Frank Norris declared in 1903.[9] Others asserted that only literature of 'quality' would serve moral, intellectual, and social ends.[10] Experts were needed to guide individual choices.

In what follows, I analyze bibliotherapy's initial aims as reflected in recommended reading for hospital patients, both before and after World War I. My first section begins by showing how nineteenth-century commentators deployed a discourse of health and illness to criticize 'unwholesome' books while arguing that good ones would 'inoculate' children against 'bad character development.'[11] Gradually, however, public schools and libraries shifted their emphasis from prevention to correction. In the wake of major demographic changes – a growing influx of immigrants and the Great Migration of free African Americans to Northern cities – librarians determined to repair so-called deficiencies of knowledge, morality, and personal habits among the children of designated populations. By the 1920s, hospital patients had become another target group for rehabilitation through reading.[12]

My second section analyzes the language of return and normalization among early bibliotherapists. As we shall see, hospital librarians and medical professionals were generally more adamant than branch librarians about the dangers of certain books, but less confident about the benefit of specific titles, and imprecise about

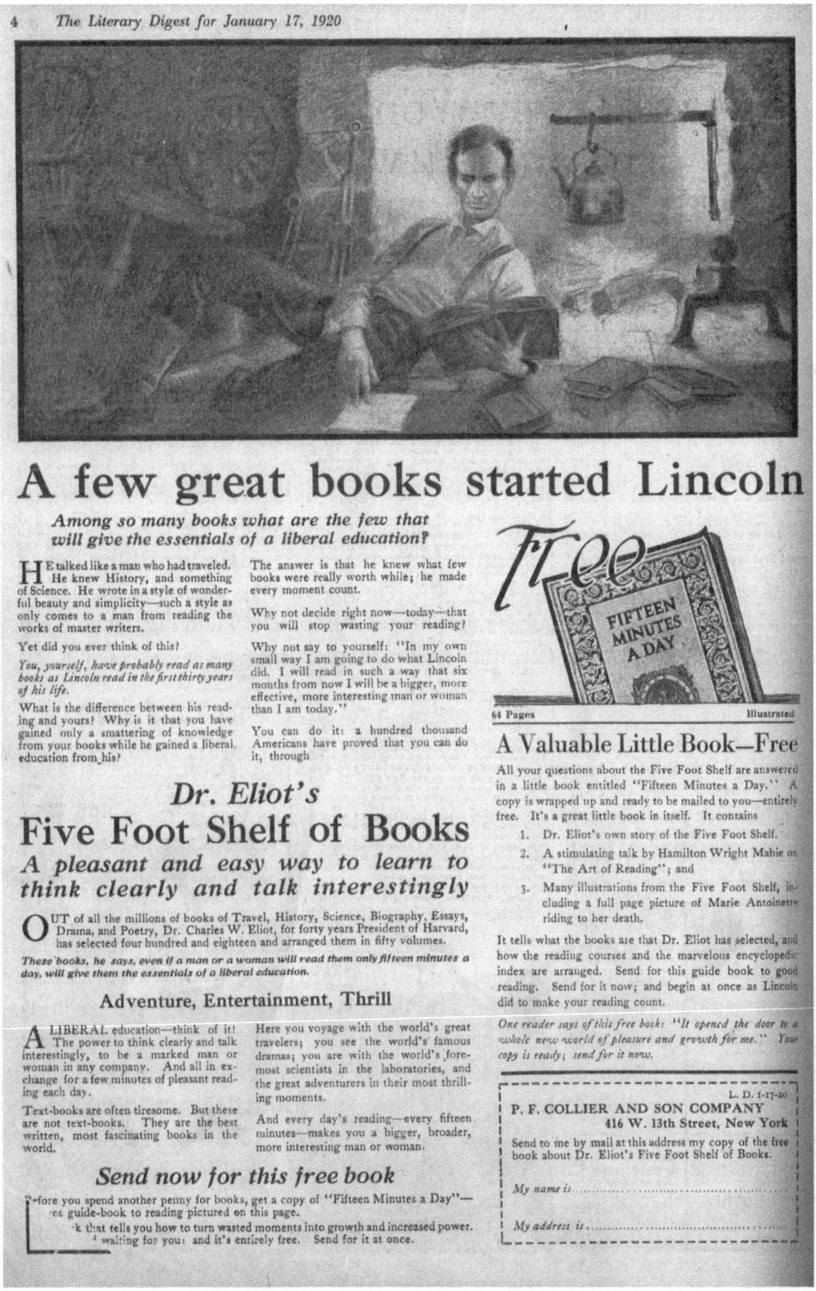

Figure 6.1 'A Few Books Started Lincoln.' *Literary Digest* (Jan. 17, 1920). Image courtesy of the New York Public Library, Astor, Lenox, and Tilden Foundation.

results. Bibliotherapists sometimes point to the hazards of reading for physical health: a heavy book may cause 'fatigue' and 'small type on shiny paper' may trigger 'a headache through eyestrain'[13] exciting 'unsanctioned' texts can cause a 'rise in temperature.'[14] But a different sort of danger appeared when mental health was the focus: practitioners overwhelmingly agreed that patients were not to read about disturbing subjects, especially anything relevant to their own condition.

By way of conclusion, I focus on three notable exceptions to the theory and practice of early bibliotherapy in the United States – librarians who pressed against the boundaries of the consensus, anticipating later developments in the field. Elizabeth Green, a librarian at Barnes Hospital in St. Louis during the 1910s and 1920s, employed a more flexible and expansive definition of reparation and normalcy than others; she also made the exceptional claim that reading could help some patients reflect upon their own disability, facilitating their re-entry into society. Sadie Peterson Delaney – an African American bibliotherapist at a Veterans' Hospital in Alabama for almost thirty-five years – provided Black patients with books by and about African Americans, acknowledging racism in the United States and defying the usual restrictions on reading material that might be distressing to patients. Ernestine Rose – head of the Harlem branch library and later a teacher at the Columbia University School of Library Service – questioned the logic of prescriptive guidelines well into the 1940s. Throughout this chapter, I assume that library history is part and parcel of a broader cultural history and that when widely circulating tropes are used to describe reading, they both shape and reflect common beliefs.[15]

Reading for Specific Groups: From Prevention to Correction

Drawing analogies between physical and moral development, nineteenth-century commentators emphasized the perils of passive, unregulated reading, especially for young people. Educators described valuable reading as both work and training: the child's intellect was a 'muscle which could be properly exercised and strengthened or improperly rested and atrophied.'[16] Teachers, librarians, and other professionals were to promote moral, intellectual, and social progress by providing children with 'wholesome reading.'[17] Conversely, there was danger in the wrong books, especially texts that challenged social norms. Fictions about seduction or crime, often compared to toxins or alcohol, were declared both disruptive and addictive. Commentators agreed that reading could have powerful effects on the mind, the spirit, and the body – for good and ill.

When Samuel Crothers coined the word 'bibliotherapy' in 1916, he drew on well-worn metaphors that represented literature not only as 'food' and 'stimulants' but also as 'counter-irritants' and 'medicine.'[18] Such images had pervaded nineteenth-century discussions of reading, but they were neither scientific nor exclusive. From the inception of the American Library Association in 1876, proponents described the work of librarians in religious terms – as a 'sacred mission' of education and uplift.[19] Literature was increasingly sacralized toward the end of the century, as Barbara Sicherman argues.[20] Yet librarians' primary goals were both pragmatic and secular. Using common library procedures, they set out not only to 'improve reading tastes' but also to form orderly, productive, responsible American citizens.[21]

Literacy was increasingly associated with 'democratic access' after the turn of the twentieth century; [22] the motto of the public library – 'Free to all' – epitomized this goal. Immigrants with no money to spare and little English language competence frequented neighborhood libraries, seeking books in their own languages. Yet in the era of legalized segregation, African Americans were often denied entry, especially in the South. Other potential readers hesitated to approach unfamiliar institutions, which were often recently built and sometimes awesomely grand.[23]

Nineteenth-century librarians claimed that those who lacked the 'healthy influences of the home' – specifically the white middle-class home – were in particular need of correction.[24] The degree of remediation for specific groups varied by age, class, race, and ethnicity. 'Without the library,' Melvil Dewey warned in 1888, 'the restless uneducated masses [... would be] left without guidance, supervision, stimulus or support.'[25] By the 1920s, a central mission of public libraries was to prepare working-class, immigrant, and African American children for inclusion in the nation by cultivating their 'love of reading' while drilling them in acceptable behavior.[26]

Indeed, the social value of literacy laid in the routines and material context of the library as much as in the books themselves. Many new library users had limited experience with either books or libraries. Middle-class adults were generally well-versed in institutional conventions (waiting in line, speaking quietly, filling out forms), but others had not yet internalized the habits required for library use. Branch librarians set out to inculcate those habits. One New York City librarian reports with satisfaction that '[d]ue to our clean hands campaign [...] dirty hands are not quite so much in evidence as they were.'[27] Or again: the 'little children stand in a long line [... .] this line, we think, is one to be proud of for it is accepted by the children as necessary and even good.'[28] As Dee Garrison notes, 'the "professionalization' of librarianship required the solemn treatment of commonplace problems.'[29]

While promoting reading and discipline, teachers and librarians of the 1920s also sought to shape 'loyal citizens.'[30] Reading had long been a technology for creating 'the right kind of American' – an exemplar of middle-class values, including civic virtue and literacy.[31] For immigrants, books were to serve the process of 'naturalization' – a telling (and enduring) concept that helped make homogeneity the standard for what counts as natural, normal, and American. African Americans, too, were considered prime candidates for such training. The Black community had become increasingly literate since emancipation – had made stupendous gains, in fact – but as late as the 1920s many African American children were the first members of their family to attend school.

Like antebellum writers and commentators, early twentieth-century librarians generally assumed that children imitate what they read.[32] Schools and libraries presented white authors and presidents as models for what Philp Fisher in another context has called 'the anticipated self.'[33] Readings, exhibits, and other library activities routinely celebrated the birthdays of famous individuals, offering examples of achievement for young people to imitate while affirming such American ideals as triumph over adversity, autonomous individualism, and self-making.[34] Such events also set limits on desire, ambition, and information, however. The presidency was open neither to immigrants – African Americans – nor women. Facts that might challenge the optimistic narrative of national progress (slavery, segregation, nativism, systemic racism, or the return of wounded soldiers) were absent in public library programs, especially for young readers, including those who might have found some of these topics pertinent to their own lives.

Choosing and Using Books in Hospital Libraries: Do No Harm

Adapting goals and methods that the public library movement had honed over decades, bibliotherapists of the 1910s and 1920s accepted not only the basic principle that reading could serve personal development and 'social improvement' but also the premise that books could be dangerous.[35] Like the groups discussed above, hospital patients, taken together, were to be reformed or re-educated. Yet the limits of the analogy are revealing. As I have been arguing, many newcomers to library use were unaccustomed to prevalent cultural norms; librarians thus promoted socialization and the work ethic along with the reading habit. Books, reading, and library decorum were to combat idleness and other undesirable conduct, especially in marginalized communities. By contrast, doctors, nurses, and hospital librarians assumed that patients had been suddenly, sometimes violently, separated from normative social behavior that they could relearn. Medical practitioners and hospital librarians concurred that library use could help patients regain access to their former selves. Those selves (not presidents or famous writers) became the model. Reading was to be a gateway to the allegedly stable and familiar past, not the future.

Many commentators took the physical space of the library as an aid to recovery by conceptualizing it as 'an environment that makes for normalcy.'[36] In this view, the library was not only a source of books, but (quite apart from the act of reading) an inviting and familiar space – 'uninstitutional and homelike' according to Edith Kathleen Jones, the first hospital librarian in the United States.[37] As Jones puts it: 'In these rooms, surrounded by the familiar backs of the books they have known and loved, they feel freer, less restrained, in a more normal atmosphere.'[38] Aided by human facilitators (not doctors and nurses in uniform), the ideal hospital library – 'a light, airy, comfortable, and homey room' – was associated with an allegedly beloved place (and time) before illness, imagined as a calm, inviting, middle-class environment.[39] Like the act of reading itself, library use was to be a prompt for recovering a lost mode of being.[40]

During the 1910s and 1920s, advocates of bibliotherapy often gave concrete and detailed attention to the bureaucratic, financial, and logistical challenges involved in establishing and running a hospital library. Yet they rarely mentioned due dates, fines, or forms.[41] Hospital librarians stress the value of order, stability, and recreation, but say little about how specific books might be used to cure the mentally or physically disabled. Commentators frequently claim that a 'well-selected library' can be 'a great factor toward recovery and health'; according to Assistant

Surgeon General Lavinder, 'a hospital library service [...] has proven to be an agency of first importance in maintaining the morale of both patients and personnel.'[42] At the same time, Lavinder acknowledges the difficulty of evaluating outcomes. Regretting the '[in]tangible' impact of books on patients, he adds that, 'unfortunate[ly...] the results obtained in a [hospital library service ...] cannot be made in exact terms.'[43] The difficulty of predicting or even describing the effects of bibliotherapy is a recurrent (and persistent) motif in lectures, commentaries, and handbooks on the subject.[44]

Samuel Crothers, who gave the 'new science' its name, may well have contributed to long-lasting uncertainty regarding methodology and results.[45] His essay 'The Literary Clinic' is a 'strange [...] point of origin' for the field, as Jesse Miller notes.[46] The ironic tone that Crothers employs throughout his sketch contributes substantially to the strangeness.[47] His central figure – Augustus Bagster, minister turned clinician – insists that books must 'do something to you.'[48] But what they do remains both elusive and comic. As Bagster describes ailments and the unlikely solutions that he often arrives at 'quite by accident,'[49] the difficulty of establishing 'the actual effect which any particular book may have' becomes amply clear.[50] 'So much depends upon the person,' Bagster explains.[51]

In real hospital libraries of the period, book recommendations were markedly cautious. Like mainstream commentators, bibliotherapists suggest 'the best books,'[52] the 'right sort of books,'[53] 'the proper books.'[54] But affirmations of literary quality were of little use in serving patients, and the material conditions of early hospital libraries were problematic. Jones notes that '[u]sually there is no system' for book selection and often no budget; many libraries relied heavily on donations.[55] What to prescribe remained unclear, but what to avoid was unambiguous. Fear of causing harm by allowing patients to read the wrong books was pervasive and persistent. The wrong books, first and foremost, were books about illness.

Hospitals served a diverse population in terms of gender, class, ethnicity, and levels of education, but they were almost entirely segregated until the early 1960s.[56] I will return to the issue of race, but here I want to emphasize that although librarians sometimes acknowledge diversity by asserting that 'foreign languages [should be] represented' in the book collection or that the library can help raise the 'mental standard' of the 'uneducated,' early discussions of bibliotherapy tend to conceptualize all hospital inmates as patients first.[57] The most consistently noted aim of book treatment is to displace the patients' concern with their own situation, and themselves. Like the material context of the hospital library, the dangers of reading were imagined differently for patients than for children, immigrants, or African Americans in ordinary libraries. The prime danger for patients was emotionally disruptive reading, especially books about disability and hospitalization. Doctors and hospital librarians thus encouraged a practice that had stirred considerable anxiety during the nineteenth century: reading for absorption and escape.

Nineteenth-century educators had frowned upon novel reading for its capacity to absorb; commentators feared that immersion in a fictional world could subvert a reader's hold on reality. By contrast, hospital librarians acknowledged that fiction will be 'much in demand' and 'should be supplied.'[58] In *A Thousand Books for the Hospital Library* (1913), more than half the list is devoted to fiction, much of it recently published.[59] Practitioners saw 'light,' entertaining literature as 'the key to temporary oblivion of [... the patient's] condition and surroundings.'[60] Librarians agreed that getting lost in a book could neutralize a patient's obsession with self and help the patient re-establish 'normal relations with the world.'[61] Paradoxically, absorption in fiction could be the first step to normalcy and wholesomeness, two terms that appear regularly in early twentieth-century discussions.[62]

The authors of *A Thousand Books for the Hospital Library* tirelessly reiterate the importance of 'wholesome, readable literature.'[63] But where mainstream librarians used the word 'wholesome' primarily to describe books that would advance the moral consciousness and socialization of young readers, bibliotherapists emphasize that the 'wholesomeness' of certain books will help prevent a preoccupation with illness by stimulating the interest of patients 'in things outside themselves.'[64] To help a patient look outward, not inward, books were to be 'bright, wholesome, [and] interesting' or again 'wholesome, not morbid, or gruesome, or depressing.'[65]

In early twentieth-century accounts of bibliotherapy, wholesomeness, like normalcy, depends upon what it displaces – anxious thoughts, idleness, and self-involvement. Speaking at the Hospital Libraries Round Table in 1923, M.P.D. Miller of the U.S. Veterans' Bureau Hospital in Little Rock, Arkansas, expresses the consensus: the book, she says, has 'therapeutic agency by stimulating the apathetic into mental activity, giving wholesome thoughts to day dreamers, by diverting morbid impulses, by providing occupation to harassed nerves.'[66] Here, not only morbid impulses but also apathy and daydreaming are framed as abnormality. The goal of treatment is 'restoration work'[67] – a return to 'the social habits acquired before the beginning of their mental disease.'[68] When Dr. Bledsoe of the Arkansas Veterans' Hospital recommends books that can bring unbalanced veterans 'back into touch with reality,'[69] the 'reality' to which he refers is emphatically not the patient's present environment or medical condition. Practitioners strongly discouraged reading about either of these.

By stressing the need to avoid painful subjects of personal significance to patients, advocates of bibliotherapy expressed a dominant but unstated assumption of mainstream, progressive-era librarians: that reading was not to engage disturbing realities – personal or social. Bibliotherapists directed patients away from stories of illness, just as teachers and branch librarians, devoted to the cultural uplift of specific groups, offered young immigrants and African Americans optimistic narratives of national progress and stories of individual success – not troubling accounts of nativism, slavery, segregation, or racism. Nevertheless, some hospital librarians questioned this ritual of avoidance, along with the reification of normalcy. Such exceptions point to the future of bibliotherapy.

Challenging the Consensus

In an essay on 'The Therapeutic Use of a Hospital Library' (1919), Elizabeth Green, librarian at Barnes Hospital in St. Louis Missouri, claims that reading is 'a means toward the restitution to the normal of a particular individual who may be handicapped permanently or temporarily by sickness.'[70] Although Green shares with other practitioners the goal of 'restitution' and return, her concept of 'the normal' is more fluid than most. The sentence I just cited may be parsed by emphasizing not 'restitution to the normal' but 'restitution to the normal of a particular individual' – to a previous way of life, whatever its norms may have been. For Green, what counts as 'normal' is likely to change from one person to another. Lest this claim seems like a stretch – lest it seem that I am reading too much into a single formulation – I will add that Green's conception of 'wholesomeness' is also unusually capacious, and more explicit: 'many and varied problems are presented to the librarian,' she writes, 'for what is a wholesome literary diet for one patient might be very unwholesome for the next.'[71]

Although some bibliotherapists note the importance of taking 'the psychology of different classes of patients [...] into consideration'[72] and even of providing 'books suited to [... the patient's] peculiarities,'[73] Green not only emphasizes the legitimate variety of individual needs and the difficulty of matching book to the patient but argues that some patients will benefit from engaging with their own disability through reading.[74] Certain books, she writes, may 'cultivate in the patient some change or alteration in his point of view and to arouse in him a stimulus toward a fresh grip on the personal situation which confronts him.'[75] She does not suggest that a patient with a particular illness should necessarily read about that illness, but neither does she reject that option out of hand. While accepting the frequently noted value of books that 'keep [...patients'] minds away from themselves' Green departs from governing assumptions by suggesting, for example, that the

> poems of [W.E.] Henley [...] have a peculiarly definite influence on the sick patient [.... .] Even if perhaps there is a touch of the gruesome, particularly about the poems of the ward and operating room, there is here a touch of reality [...] which is by far the best mental preparation for going through any kind of hospital emergency.[76]

Green suggests that the 'touch of reality' in Henley's poems may speak to a patient's complex present challenges.[77] Her comments display a rare conviction that books can do more than provide occupation, diversion, and escape: they may have an impact on the way patients understand their own circumstances.

Indeed, Green argues that books can help prepare a patient for 'the facing of the immediate thing.'[78] Recommending stories of 'courage ... and humor' she does not propose that a patient imitate heroic models but rather that narratives about difficult challenges may be individually adapted.[79] Her goal is not entertainment or distraction, but a way of seeing that may be helpful:

> [T]here is a chance for a very definite selection of books, aiming to implant in a patient's mind some particular thing which he may at that moment lack or may perhaps arouse in him the incentive to develop the necessary attitude in regard to his own problem.[80]

In addition, Green affirms (rather than regrets) bibliotherapy's lack of quantifiable rigor. 'Something remains behind' after reading, she notes, 'some small therapeutic effect too subtle for analysis and often too intangible to record.'[81] Green implies that subjectivity and even arbitrariness may be integral to treatment, embracing the librarian's 'personal predilection' as part of the process while downplaying the more typical emphasis on the practitioner's 'scientific' training and expertise.[82]

Like other practitioners, Green emphasizes restoration to health, but her definition of 'health,' like her understanding of 'normalcy' and 'wholesomeness,' is broad. Good health was a crucial value in American culture of the 1920s. Questions on the subject abound on job applications, grant applications, and recommendation forms – including those for library school. Such forms contained many specific queries about physical and emotional conditions that do not appear on application forms today. 'Have you defective sight, hearing or speech?' 'Have you any marked physical defect, such as lameness?' 'Have you ever had a nervous breakdown?'[83] As the eugenics movement gained popularity in the United States, physical fitness became an increasingly important criteria of inclusion – immigrants were screened for 'defects' before entering the country. For Green, however, health is linked neither to physical fitness nor normalcy but to more holistic and flexible notions of individual well-being. Thus, many of Green's formulations about hospital libraries point to developments that subsequently moved the field of bibliotherapy not only away from strict control of book selection and generalities about results but also away from affirmations of homogeneity and valorization of the social status quo.

In this context, the African American bibliotherapist Sadie Peterson Delaney is an exceptional example of a practitioner who pressed against the boundaries of the consensus. Chief librarian at the segregated U.S. Veterans Administration Hospital in Tuskegee from 1924 to 1958, Delaney offered her patients valuable information on a subject of intimate (and distressing) personal concern to them – not disability, but racism. Delaney thus rejected both the goal of returning Black Veterans to an idealized former life and the imperative of avoiding volatile subjects. In a rare article about Delaney, Betty Gubert notes that wounded veterans often 'did not know how to return to normal life.' But, she adds, 'for these Black veterans, normality included racial prejudice that was especially virulent after the first world war.'[84] Indeed, the cultural positioning of African Americans posed a severe challenge to recovery, and many were eager to read relevant material. 'Books about the Negro cannot be written fast enough to satisfy the insatiate desire of these veterans,' Delaney wrote in 1932; they 'long […] to know race history and facts.'[85] For Delaney, the library was to aid veterans in looking forward; books could help them 'fit themselves for life' by acknowledging (rather than evading) formidable obstacles in an 'upward struggle.'[86] Booklists in white hospital libraries rarely included texts about African American history not to speak of ongoing racism, but in the all-Black V.A. hospital of Tuskegee, Delaney was free to address these topics.

I want to conclude by turning to the work of another exceptional and neglected early advocate of bibliotherapy Ernestine Rose, whose long career combined many aspects of librarianship discussed above. In 1908, Rose was a young branch librarian on the Lower East Side of New York; in 1917, she published a discussion of her library experience with the 'foreign born.'[87] In 1920, after working for the American Library Association's Library War Service in France and Germany during the First World War, Rose became head of the 135th Street branch library in Harlem. A pro-active white integrationist, she 'hand-picked' Nella Larsen to break the color barrier that had kept African American candidates out of US library training schools.[88] Rose gradually developed an abiding interest in the 'therapeutic value of books.'[89] During the early 1920s, she was Sadie Delaney's supervisor in the Harlem branch and probably contributed to Nella Larsen's 'interest in hospital libraries' as stated on Larsen's library school application.[90] At Columbia University's School of Library Service during the mid-1940s, Rose taught courses on 'Library Work with Hospital Patients,' lobbied for student internships at hospitals, and promoted bibliotherapy as a profession, emphasizing career opportunities for 'future hospital librarians.'[91] She organized well-attended conferences and a 'Hospital Libraries Institute.' Her interest in the field, like her interest in integration, was untiring and multi-faceted.

As late as 1945, bibliotherapists tended to agree that the work of hospital libraries was to combat boredom, idleness, morbidity, and especially self-involvement; above all, patients were not to read for insight into illness or hospitalization. At a 'Conference on Hospital Library Service and Training,' which Rose organized at Columbia University in 1945, a doctor with experience in Air Force 'convalescent hospitals' expressed his skepticism about the 'curative value' of the library program, objecting particularly to the idea that patients might benefit from reading about their 'own ailments and psychology. He warned against making wide claims for [this ...] aspect' of bibliotherapy.[92] Rose urged her students to reflect upon this issue, inviting them to state their opinions for and against restricting book selection. In a summer course on 'Library Work with Hospital Patients,' her 'Final Exam' includes the following question:

> it is thought generally, in serving patients, to censor (or limit) books on some subjects, or containing certain factors. Below is a classification of patients into four groups [Neuro-psychiatric, Tuberculosis, Preoperational, Cardiac]. Answer the accompanying question for each: What type of book or subject matter would you limit if at all in the hospital?[93]

Rose repeatedly raised this question, inviting guests to speak about censorship in her classes, at a Summer Institute, and at the conference of 1945. When she invited Mary Frank Mason of *Reader's Digest* to lecture on 'the book collection in the hospital library,' Mason asked for some guidelines. In a letter of 13 July 1945, Rose responded as follows:

> I had hoped that you would discuss the question of censorship, understanding by that the necessary limitations that have to be imposed, and the use of books in any hospital and how the whole subject of restricted books might be handled.

> I think that some prospective hospital libraries are quite puzzled by this last point.[94]

Although Rose seems to accept that some limitations 'have to be imposed' on patients, she often addresses the problem of how restrictions should be defined and applied ('if at all'). Like Green and Delaney, Rose probed common assumptions about strict book control for hospital patients, expanding governing conceptions of how conflicted, socially marginalized, suffering individuals might use books to improve their lives.

Since the 1940s, the field of bibliotherapy has expanded exponentially and changed significantly. Neither normalcy nor wholesomeness dominates recent discussions. The increasingly popular idea of self-help has legitimized texts about medical or psychological problems.[95] Nevertheless, it remains difficult to establish either successful criteria for treatment or a clear line between guidance and control in bibliotherapy (as in education more broadly).[96] Thus, I want to end this discussion with a nod to the dynamic concept of 'reparative reading,' coined by the influential literary theorist and cultural historian Eve Sedgwick. Reading 'reparatively,' Sedgwick argues, opens possibilities for change by giving a subject 'room to realize [not only] that the future may be different from the past' but that the past itself might have 'happen[ed] differently.'[97] Claiming that readers may 'extract […] sustenance' from books in surprising ways that may be painful, resistant, and risky but also useful and emotionally satisfying, Sedgwick attempts to 'open a space' for reassessing the significance of reading in relation to self and society.[98] Her argument not only addresses urgent questions about reading and interpretation as practiced by literary studies but also participates in longstanding – and ongoing – debates about control, prohibition, and individual freedom in the theory and practice of bibliotherapy.

Acknowledgments

I am grateful to my enormously helpful research assistants, Uriel Rosenbloom, Michal Calo, and Tal Maletin. Many thanks to the librarians of Archives, Rare Books, and Manuscripts at Columbia University and the New York Public Library (both the Brooke Russell Astor Reading Room and the Schomburg Center for Research in Black Culture). I thank the Israel Science Foundation for its support (grant 1599/20).

Notes

1 Thomas Augst, 'Faith in Reading: Public Libraries, Liberalism and the Civil Religion,' in *Institutions of Reading the Social Life of Libraries in the United States,* eds. Thomas Augst and Kenneth Carpenter (Amherst: University of Massachusetts Press, 2007).

2 'Return to normalcy' was Warren G. Harding's campaign slogan in the U.S. presidential election of 1920: https://en.wikipedia.org/wiki/Return_to_normalcy. Harding used the

phrase 'to describe the calm political and social order to which he wished to return the United States after the idealism and commotion of the presidency of Woodrow Wilson' (E.D. Hirsch Jr., *The New Dictionary of Cultural Literacy* [Boston: Houghton Mifflin Press, 2004]: 297).

3 Levinder, C.H., 'Hospital Libraries Round Table,' *Bulletin of the American Library Association* 16, no. 4 (1922): 280.

4 For an overview of arguments for and against reading in the antebellum United States, see Scott Casper, 'Antebellum Reading Prescribed and Described,' in *Perspectives on American Book History,* eds. Casper et al. (Amherst: University of Massachusetts Press, 2002), 135–164. On cultural prohibitions and anxieties about fiction in particular, see Cathy Davidson, *Revolution and the Word: The Rise of the Novel in America* (New York: Oxford University Press, 2004); Barbara Hochman, *Uncle Tom's Cabin and the Reading Revolution* (Amherst: University of Massachusetts Press, 2011); David M. Stewart, *Reading and Disorder in Antebellum America* (Columbus: Ohio State University Press, 2011).

5 On the legal and symbolic implications of slave literacy, see Jennifer Monaghan, 'Reading for the Enslaved, Writing for the Free: Reflections on Literacy and Liberty,' *Proceedings of the American Antiquarian Society* 108, no. 2 (1998); Heather Williams, *Self-Taught: African American Education in Slavery and Freedom* (Chapel Hill: University of North Carolina Press, 2005); Hochman, *Uncle Tom's Cabin* (2011).

6 'A Few Great Books Started Lincoln,' *Literary Digest* 64, no. 4 (1920): 4.

7 Ernestine Rose, 'Books and the Color Line,' *The Survey* (Spring Book Number): 75–76.

8 Kate McDowell, 'Which Truth, What Fiction? Librarians' Book Recommendations for Children, 1876–1890,' in *Education and the Culture of Print in Modern America,* eds. Adam R. Nelson and John L. Rudolph (Madison: University of Wisconsin Press, 2010), 16. A belief in the benefits of reading persisted into the twentieth century and beyond. An NEA report of 2007 'identifies who reads as the best predictor of who exercises, plays sports, volunteers, votes and stays out of jail.' See Leah Price, 'You Are What You Read,' *New York Times* (2007).

9 Frank Norris, 'The American Public and "Popular" Fiction,' in *Literary Criticism of Frank Norris,* ed. Donald Pizer (1903), 127.

10 Carleton Washburne and Mabel Vogel, *Winnetka Graded Booklist* (Chicago: American Library Association, 1926), 6. The term 'quality' appears with characteristic frequency in Kay E. Vandergrift's account of early children's publishing and library services. See Kay E. Vandergrift, 'Female Advocacy and Harmonious Voices: A History of Public Library Services and Children's Publishing in the United States,' *Library Trends* 44, no. 4 (1996): 683–718.

11 McDowell, 'Which Truth?' (2010), 18, 17, 28.

12 Reformatories began to use literature for training and rehabilitation by 1900. Like the library, the prison reform movement promoted 'habits of order, discipline, self-control, [...] as well as respect for God, law, country, and the principles of capitalism and democracy' (Alexander Pisciotta, *Benevolent Repression: Social Control and the American Reformatory-Prison Movement* [New York: New York University Press, 1994], 4). The prison movement's flagship institution, Elmira Reformatory, was founded in 1876, the same year as the American Library Association. Similarities and differences between prison and hospital libraries deserve further exploration. See Steven Mailloux, 'The Rhetorical Use and Abuse of Fiction: Eating Books in Late Nineteenth-Century America,' *Boundary 2* 17, no. 1 (1990); Pisciotta, *Benevolent Repression* (1994).

13 Elizaeth Green and Sidney I. Schwab, 'The Therapeutic Use of a Hospital Library,' *Hospital Social Service Quarterly* (August 1919): 155.
14 Mary Mahoney, 'The Library as a Medicine Cabinet,' in *Libraries—Traditions and Innovations,* eds. Melanie A. Kimbell and Katherine M. Wissner (Berlin: De Gruyter, 2017), 105.
15 On library history as cultural history see Christine Pawley, 'Foreword,' in *Apostles of Culture: Public Librarian and American Society 1876–1920*, ed. Dee Garrison (Madison: University of Wisconsin Press, 2003). On the cultural significance of tropes for reading see Mailloux, 'Rhetorical Use' (1990); Janice Radway, 'Reading Is Not Eating: Mass Produced Literature and the Theoretical, Methodological and Political Consequences of a Metaphor,' *Book Research Quarterly* 2 (1986): 7–29.
16 McDowell, 'Which Truth' (2010), 22.
17 McDowell, 'Which Truth' (2010), 20, 17.
18 Samuel McChord Crothers, 'A Literary Clinic,' *Atlantic Monthly Magazine* 118, no. 3 (1916): 295, 294, 295, 292. On Crothers' coining of the term, see also Jesse Miller, ' "Medicines of the Soul": Reparative Reading and the History of Bibliotherapy,' *Mosaic* 51, no. 2 (2018): 17–33; Sara Haslam and Edmund G. C. King, ' "Medicinable Literature": Bibliotherapy, Literary Caregiving, and the First World War.' *Literature and Medicine* 39, no. 2 (2021): 296–318.
19 Garrison, *Apostles of Culture* (2003), 131, cf. 178.
20 Barbara Sicherman, 'Reading and Middle-class Identity in Victorian America: Cultural Consumption, Conspicuous and Otherwise,' in *Reading Acts: U.S Readers' Interactions with Literature, 1800–1950*, eds. Ryan, Barbara, and Amy Thomas (Knoxville: University of Tennessee Press, 2002), 156.
21 Garrison, *Apostles of Culture* (2003), 167.
22 Patricia Crain, 'New Histories of Literacy,' in *A Companion to the History of the Book,* eds. Jonathan Rose and Simon Eliot (London: Blackwell, 2007), 468.
23 On segregated libraries, see Cheryl Knott, *Not Free, Not for All: Libraries in the Age of Jim Crow* (Amherst: University of Massachusetts Press, 2015). In James Baldwin's *Go Tell it on the Mountain* a young black boy stands before the 'unimaginably vast' main building of the NYPL, afraid to enter (Vintage, 2013), 31. On branch librarians of the 1920s as 'forbidding authorities,' difficult for some to approach, see Janice Radway, 'The Library as Place, Collection or Service,' in *Institutions of Reading: The Social Life of Libraries in the United States,* eds. Thomas Augst and Kenneth Carpenter (University of Massachusetts Press, 2007), 248–249.
24 McDowell, 'Which Truth' (2010), 20.
25 Cited in Garrison, *Apostles of Culture* (2003), 136.
26 Vandergrift, 'Female Advocacy' (1996), 688. On the librarians' tactics for accomplishing this goal see Barbara Hochman, 'Making Americans in the New York Public Library: Fantasy and Realities,' *American Literature* 97, no. 1 (March 2025). https://doi.org/10.1215/00029831-11597539
27 Dorothy Beeken, 'Monthly Children's Room Report' (June 4, 1921), 2. Chatham Square Folder 1921–1922, Office of Children's Services, Box 7, New York Public Library Archives. The New York Public Library.
28 Dorothy Beeken, 'Monthly Children's Room Report' (April 4, 1921), 3. Chatham Square Folder 1921–1922, Office of Children's Services, Box 7, New York Public Library Archives. The New York Public Library.
29 Garrison, *Apostles of Culture* (2003), 167.

30 H.E. Fowler, 'American Literature for American Schools,' *The English Journal* VI, no. 10 (1917): 639.
31 Bernard Wishy, *The Child and the Republic: The Dawn of Modern American Nurture* (Philadelphia: University of Pennsylvania Press, 1968), 168.
32 On that principle, Lydia Maria Child, Susan Warner, Harriet Beecher Stowe, and other antebellum writers produced numerous tales of piety, good behavior, sacrifice, and literacy. From the eighteenth century onward, African Americans forged a literary canon for black children using positive models and emphasizing race pride. See Katherine Capshaw and Anna Mae Duane, *Who Writes for Black Children: African American Children's Literature before 1900* (Minneapolis: University of Minnesota Press, 2017).
33 Philip Fisher, *Hard Facts: Setting and Form in the American Novel* (New York: Oxford University Press, 1985), 157.
34 Branch libraries occasionally honored women writers and illustrators such as Louisa May Alcott or Kate Greenaway. African American models were exceedingly rare in public libraries of the 1920s. See Hochman, 'Making Americans,' (2025).
35 Vandergrift, 'Female Advocacy' (1996), 686.
36 M. P. D. Miller, 'Hospital Libraries Round Table: The Therapeutic Value of Books in a Neuro-Psychiatric Hospital,' *Bulletin of the American Library Association* 17, no. 4 (1923): 236.
37 Edith Kathleen Jones, *The Value of the Library in the Hospital for Mental Disease* (Catonsville Md: Press of Spring Grove State Hospital, 1914): 3. Library services were available to patients in some US mental health facilities from the first half of the nineteenth century. See Lisa M. Dunkel, 'Moral and Humane: Patient's Libraries in Early Nineteenth-Century American Mental Hospitals,' *Bulletin Medical Library Association*, (1983): 274–280. But when Jones became head of the patients' library at MacLean Hospital, Waverley Massachusetts, in 1904, she was the first hospital librarian with an official position. See Margaret C. Hannigan, 'The Librarian in Bibliotherapy: Pharmacist or Bibliotherapist?' *Library Trends* (1962): 184. Jones wrote prolifically on theory and practice. She became chair of the Hospital Libraries Roundtable in 1921.
38 Jones, *The Value* (1914), 3–4.
39 Dr. E. P. Bledsoe 'Hospital Libraries Round Table: The Library as a Therapeutic Agent.' *Bulletin of the American Library Association Papers and Proceedings of the Forty-Fifth Annual Meeting of the American Library Association* 17, no 4. (1923): 238. In this sense it is fitting that Crothers coined the word bibliotherapy. His central figure treats only professional white men and their wives (though these are barely mentioned); see Crothers, 'A Literary Clinic,' 291, 297, 298. In one example a 'middle-aged' man of 'middling' intelligence is sent into treatment by his friends because he is too comfortable (Crothers, 'A Literary Clinic,' 296).
40 'The library,' Hannigan writes, 'is identified with the outside world, a place where well people go; reading is one of the few hospital activities which the patient associates with his life outside the hospital. Library experience then removes him from his sickness for a short while' (Hannigan, 'The Librarian in Bibliotherapy' [1962], 195).
41 For instance, Levinder, 'Hospital Libraries,' (1922) 277–79; Perrie Jones, 'Hospital Libraries Round Table: Arousing the Library Profession to the Meet the Peculiar Needs of the Hospital Library,' *Bulletin of the American Library Association Papers and Proceedings of the Forty-Fifth Annual Meeting of the American Library Association* 17, no. 4 (1923): 236–237. The *Hospital Library Handbook* of the Library War Service notes that '[n]o borrower's card is necessary nor is any sort of list of borrowers to be kept.'

The borrower's name and location in the hospital is to be noted on the book card 'to help in locating overdues' though no penalties are mentioned (*Hospital Library Handbook,* ALA Hospital Library War Service [Jan. 1, 1919] 25). Elizabeth Green specifies 'a fine of two cents a day' for overdue books [for nurses and other hospital staff] but the 'rule does not apply to patients' who may be 'unable to come to the library and are dependent on others to see that books are returned' (Green and Schwab, 'Therapeutic Use,' (1919), 153). By contrast, institutional conventions (e.g. filling out forms, paying fines, signing pledges) became a pivotal technology for socializing children in regular public libraries. See Hochman, 'Making Americans' (2025).

42 Jones, *The Value* (1914), 1. Levinder, 'Hospital Libraries' (1922) 281.

43 Levinder, 279.

44 Describing the use of books in First World War army hospitals, W.B. McDaniels notes that 'reading matter [...] either diverted or nourished [the men] in some mysterious way' (cited in Sarah J. Jack and Kevin R. Ronan, 'Bibliotherapy: Practice and Research,' *School Psychology International* 29, no. 2 (2008): 166). In 2007, a probation officer describing the use of 'literature' in an alternative sentencing program in Massachusetts made the same point: the program 'works in mysterious ways' (Price, 'Read a Book Get out of Jail,' *New York Times*, (2009)).

45 Crothers, 'A Literary Clinic' (1916), 295.

46 Miller, 'Medicines of the Soul,'29.

47 Before his article appeared, Crothers lectured about 'bibliotherapeutics' at American Library Association conferences and elsewhere ('A Literary Clinic' [1916], 292). Professional publications such as the *Library Journal* praise his lectures but say little or nothing about his method. Instead they emphasize Crothers' charisma – his 'delightful humorous' style ('Nebraska,' *Public Libraries a Monthly Review of Library Matters and Methods* 20, no. 9 [1915]: 433). Crothers' irony is rarely noted in scholarship.

48 Crothers, 'A Literary Clinic' (1916), 292, 294.

49 Crothers, 'A Literary Clinic' (1916), 298 cf. 300.

50 Crothers, 'A Literary Clinic' (1916), 295.

51 Crothers, 'A Literary Clinic' (1916), 296.

52 Jones, *The Value* (1914), 2.

53 Jones, *The Value* (1914), 3.

54 Bledsoe, 'The Library as a Therapeutic Agent' (1923) 238.

55 Edith Kathleen Jones, *The Hospital Library, Books for the Patients: Plea for a Trained Librarian, Administration, Selection of Books, Separate Children's Library, Library Technic, Distribution of Book, the Library as an Adjunct to Other Departments* (The Modern Hospital Publishing, 1915), 6; c.f. Green 'Therapeutic Use' (1919), 152; Elizabeth Green and Elanor Gifford, 'Two Hundred Fifty Books for Ward Patients,' *The Modern Hospital* 20, no. 6 (1923): 582.

56 On key moments in the effort to integrate US hospitals, see Thomas Grillot, Pauline Peretz, and Yann Philippe, '"Wherever the Authority of the Federal Government Extends": Banning Segregation in Veterans Hospitals, (1945–1960),' *Journal of American History* 107, no. 2 (Sept. 2020): 388–410; Emily A. Largent, 'Public Health, Racism, and the Lasting Impact of Segregation on Hospital Segregation,' *Public Health Reports* 133, no. 6 (2018): 715–720.

57 Green and Schwab, 'Therapeutic Use' (1919), 155; Jones, *The Value* (1914), 1. Theorizing about patients as a group, Jones writes that 'the patients' in 'either the general or the

mental hospital' prefer 'something new'; they have 'probably [...] read and re-read' most of the books in the library 'before coming to the hospital' (Jones, *The Hospital Library* [1915b, 5). Many of the comments about the physical space of the library cited above theorize about 'patients' as though they have all been middle-class book lovers.

58 Edith Kathleen Jones, *A Thousand Books for the Hospital Library* with Additions and Annotations by Miriam E. Carey, Florence Waugh, and Julia A. Robinson, (Chicago: American Library Association Publishing Board, 1913), 3; Jones, *The Hospital Library* (1915b), 7.

59 Jones, *A Thousand Books* (1913). To be sure, fiction was quite a respectable genre by the 1920s. Successful US institutions such as The Book-of-the-Month Club helped make contemporaneous 'middlebrow' novels a cultural value. But fiction served other goals for bibliotherapists. A three-page 'Foreword' in *A Thousand Books* states that 'books in a hospital are for recreation, not for instruction, and therefore should consist principally of fiction, picture-books, travel, biography, light and popular science and outdoor books' (3). After recommending 'large, clear type' for elderly patients and 'light and simple stories' for patients who are unable to take 'initiative' (4, 3), the 'Foreword' turns to practical matters such as the price of books, noting in conclusion that the list is partially annotated to 'characterize the book and its fitness for the needs of the patient' (4–5). The 'NON-FICTION' section of the list includes 19 pages, with titles arranged in subsections such as Reference, Science, Travel, Modern History, and Literature, all further subdivided (e.g., 'Literature' includes sub-sections on Poetry and Drama, Satire, and Humor.) 'FICTION,' the final section, includes 26 pages, alphabetized by author.

60 Jones, *The Value* (1914), 1.

61 Jones, *The Value* (1914), 3.

62 The goal of 'normal living' and prevention of the patient's 'contact with harmful materials' persisted until at least the 1960s (Hannigan, 'The Librarian in Bibliotherapy' [1962)], 186). By contrast, Jack and Ronan put scare quotes around 'normal' ('Bibliotherapy' [2008] 170). More recently, 'a flexible and inclusive approach to language and conceptualization' has become a concern of medical discourse, as of the humanities. See Aurora H. Brinkman, et al., 'Shifting the Discourse on Disability: Moving to an Inclusive, Intersectional Focus,' *American Journal of Orthopsychiatry* 93, no. 1 (2023): 50–62.

63 Jones, *A Thousand Books* (1913), 3.

64 Jones, *A Thousand Books* (1913), 4.

65 Jones, *A Thousand Books* (1913), 3.

66 Miller, 'Therapeutic Value' (1923), 236.

67 Miller, 'Therapeutic Value' (1923), 235.

68 Bledsoe, 'The Library as a Therapeutic Agent' (1923), 239.

69 Bledsoe, 'The Library as a Therapeutic Agent' (1923), 239.

70 Green and Schwab, 'Therapeutic Use' (1919), 148.

71 Green and Schwab, 'Therapeutic Use' (1919), 154.

72 Levinder, 'Hospital Libraries' (1923), 278.

73 Edith Kathleen Jones, 'On Books and Reading: Outline of a Course of Lectures for Nurses in Hospitals,' *American Journal of Insanity* (October 1915): 297.

74 Sara Haslam argues that H. G. Wells' popular novel *Mr. Britling Sees It Through* (1916) enabled British soldiers 'to process their own loss and trauma' ('Reading, Trauma, and Literary Caregiving: Helen Mary Gaskell and the War Library,' *Journal of Medical Humanities* [2020]: 316). On reading as 'caregiving' in the British context of the First World War, see also Haslam and King, 'Medicinable Literature.'

75 Green and Schwab, 'Therapeutic Use' (1919), 149.
76 Green and Schwab, 'Therapeutic Use' (1919), 150–151.
77 In 1939, Alice Bryan notes the importance of encouraging readers 'to face their situation realistically,' making it an 'objective' for the field (cited in Jack and Ronan 'Bibliotherapy' [2008], 167). This approach has become increasingly common (Jack and Ronan, 168, 171–172).
78 Green and Schwab, 'Therapeutic Use' (1919), 150–151.
79 Green and Schwab, 'Therapeutic Use' (1919), 150. For some recent bibliotherapists 'a key step in the bibliotherapeutic process' is inviting patients to 'identify with [fictional] characters and situations.' See Paula McMillen and Dale Elizabeth Pehrsson, 'Bibliotherapy for Hospital Patients,' *Journal of Hospital Librarianship* 4, no. 1 (2004): 76–77.
80 Green and Schwab, 'Therapeutic Use' (1919), 150.
81 Green and Schwab, 'Therapeutic Use' (1919), 151.
82 Green and Schwab, 'Therapeutic Use' (1919), 150; Bledsoe, 'The Library as a Therapeutic Agent' (1923), 238; Jones, P. 'Arousing the Library Profession' (1923), 237.
83 Cited in Barbara Hochman, 'Filling in Blanks: Nella Larsen's Application to Library School,' *PMLA* 133, no. 5 (2018): 1177, 1181. In a lecture on 'Opportunities in the Library Field' at Columbia University's School of Library Service, Ernestine Rose explains that 'good health' is a perquisite for library service in a hospital. 'Course Related Materials,' Box 1, Columbia University Rare Books and Manuscripts.
84 Betty K. Gubert, 'Sadie Peterson Delaney: Pioneer Bibliotherapist,' *American Libraries* 24, no. 2 (Feb. 1993): 127.
85 Cited in Gubert, 'Sadie Peterson Delaney', 127.
86 Cited in Gubert, 'Sadie Peterson Delaney', 127.
87 Ernestine Rose, 'Bridging the Gulf Work with the Russian Jews and Other Newcomers,' in *Work with the Foreign Born*, ed. John Foster Carr (Immigrant Publication Society, 1917).
88 George Hutchinson, *In Search of Nella Larsen: A Biography of the Color Line* (Cambridge, MA: Harvard University Press, 2003), 8. While Green and Delaney are neglected figures, Rose has gained attention over the past twenty years, not for her espousal of bibliotherapy, but for her work in the Harlem branch library. See S. A. Anderson, 'The Place to Go: The 135th St. Branch Library and the Harlem Renaissance,' *Library Quarterly* 73, no. 4 (2003); Hutchinson, *In Search*; Ann Sandford, 'Rescuing Ernestine Rose (1880–1961): Harlem Librarian and Social Activist,' *Long Island History Journal*, 22, no. 2 (2011); Barbara Hochman, 'Investing in Literature: Ernestine Rose and the Harlem Branch Public Library of the 1920s,' *Legacy: A Journal of American Women Writers* 31, no. 1 (2014); Shauntee Burns-Simpson, Nichelle M. Hayes, Ana Ndumu, Shaundra Walker, *The Black Librarian in America: Reflections, Resistance, and Reawakening* (Lanham, MD: Rowman and Littlefield, 2022).
89 Ernestine Rose, Letter to Karl A. Menninger (January 24, 1946). Ernestine Rose Collection, 'Correspondence.' Box 1, Columbia University Rare Books and Manuscripts.
90 Cited in Hochman, 'Filling,' 1187.
91 Letter to Menninger, 'Correspondence.' Yet Rose rarely used the word 'bibliotherapy' itself. In an 'Outline' for a course on 'Library Work with Hospital Patients' (1946), she writes: 'Bibliotherapy is in its beginning. Perhaps it hardly deserves that name as yet.' 'Course Related Materials' (1946), Box 1, Ernestine Rose Collection, Columbia University Rare Books and Manuscripts.

92 Ernestine Rose, 'Minutes of the Conference on Hospital Library Service and Training' (1945), Box 2, Ernestine Rose Collection, Columbia University Rare Books and Manuscripts.
93 Ernestine Rose, 'Final Exam.' 'Course Related Materials' (1946), Box 1, Ernestine Rose Collection, Columbia University Rare Books and Manuscripts.
94 Rose, Letter to Mary Frank Mason (July 13, 1945). 'Course Related.'
95 Self-help books 'have become bestsellers' in recent decades (Jack and Ronan, 'Bibliotherapy' [2008] 172). On 'positive outcomes using self-help books with adults to address health-related problems,' see McMillen and Pehrsson, 'Bibliotherapy for Hospital Patients' [2004] 77, 78.
96 Twenty-first century commentators note that the field 'must continue to strive toward more systematic research and evaluation' (Jack and Ronan, 'Bibliotherapy' [2008] 178). A recent dissertation argues that much confusion remains as to 'what is and what is not bibliotherapy, who it is meant for, and what kind of materials should be used in the practice' (Maria Wideman, 'Bibliotherapy in the Public Library; An Analysis of the Concept and Recommendations for Practice,' MSc diss., University of Strathclyde [2019]: ii).
97 Eve Kosofsky Sedgwick, 'Paranoid Reading and Reparative Reading, or, You're so Paranoid You Probably Think This Essay Is About You,' in *Touching Feeling* (Durham: Duke University Press, 2002), 146, 137.
98 Sedgwick, 'Paranoid Reading and Reparative Reading,' 150, 124.

References

'A Few Great Books Started Lincoln.' *Literary Digest* 64, no. 4 (1920).

Anderson, S.A. 'The Place to Go: The 135th St. Branch Library and the Harlem Renaissance.' *Library Quarterly* 73, no. 4 (2003): 383–421.

Augst, Thomas. 'Faith in Reading: Public Libraries, Liberalism and the Civil Religion.' In *Institutions of Reading the Social Life of Libraries in the United States*, edited by Thomas Augst and Kenneth Carpenter, 123–148. University of Massachusetts Press, 2007.

Baldwin, James. *Go Tell It on the Mountain.* Vintage, 2013.

Beeken, Dorothy. 'Monthly Children's Room Report (April 4, 1921).' Chatham Square Folder 1921–1922, Office of Children's Services, Box 7, New York Public Library Archives. The New York Public Library: 1–4.

Beeken, Dorothy. 'Monthly Children's Room Report (June 4, 1921).' Chatham Square Folder 1921–1922, Office of Children's Services, Box 7, New York Public Library Archives. The New York Public Library: 1–3.

Bledsoe, E. P. 'Hospital Libraries Round Table: The Library as a Therapeutic Agent.' *Bulletin of the American Library Association Papers and Proceedings of the Forty-Fifth Annual Meeting of the American Library Association* 17, no. 4 (1923): 238–239. Available online: www.jstor.org/stable/25686180?seq=1#metadata_info_tab_contents

Brinkman, Aurora H. et al. 'Shifting the Discourse on Disability: Moving to an Inclusive, Intersectional Focus.' *American Journal of Orthopsychiatry* 93, no. 1 (2023): 50–62.

Capshaw, Katherine and Anna Mae Duane, eds. *Who Writes for Black Children: African American Children's Literature before 1900.* Minneapolis: University of Minnesota Press, 2017.

Casper, Scott E. 'Antebellum Reading Prescribed and Described.' In *Perspectives on American Book History,* edited by Casper et al., 135–164. Amherst: University of Massachusetts Press, 2002.

Crain, Patricia. 'New Histories of Literacy.' In *A Companion to the History of the Book,* edited by Jonathan Rose and Simon Eliot, 467–470. London: Blackwell, 2007.

Crothers, Samuel McChord. 'A Literary Clinic.' *Atlantic Monthly Magazine* 118, no. 3 (1916): 291–301.

Davidson, Cathy. *Revolution and the Word: The Rise of the Novel in America.* New York: Oxford University Press, 2004.

Dunkel, Lisa M. 'Moral and Humane: Patient's Libraries in early Nineteenth-Century American Mental Hospitals.' *Bulletin Medical Library Association* (July 1983): 274–80.

Fisher, Philip. *Hard Facts: Setting and Form in the American Novel.* New York: Oxford University Press, 1985.

Fowler, H.E. 'American Literature for American Schools,' *The English Journal* 6, no. 10 (1917): 637–644.

Garrison, Dee. *Apostles of Culture: Public Librarian and American Society 1876–1920.* Madison: University of Wisconsin Press, 2003.

Green, Elizabeth and Sidney I. Schwab, M.D. "The Therapeutic Use of a Hospital Library." *Hospital Social Service Quarterly* (August 1919): 147–157.

Green, Elizabeth and Eleanor Gifford. 'Two Hundred Fifty Books for Ward Patients.' *The Modern Hospital* 20, no. 6 (June 1923): 582–583.

Grillot, Thomas, Pauline Peretz, and Yann Philippe. ' "Wherever the Authority of the Federal Government Extends": Banning Segregation in Veterans Hospitals, (1945–1960).' *Journal of American History* 107, no. 2 (Sept. 2020): 388–410.

Gubert, Betty K. 'Sadie Peterson Delaney: Pioneer Bibliotherapist.' *American Libraries* 24, No. 2 (Feb. 1993): 124–125, 127, 129–130.

Hannigan, Margaret C. 'The Librarian in Bibliotherapy: Pharmacist or Bibliotherapist?' *Library Trends* 11, no. 2 (Fall 1962): 184–198.

Haslam, Sara. 'Reading, Trauma, and Literary Caregiving: Helen Mary Gaskell and the War Library,' *Journal of Medical Humanities* 41, no. 3 (2020): 305–321.

Haslam, Sara, and Edmund G. C. King. ' "Medicinable Literature": Bibliotherapy, Literary Caregiving, and the First World War.' *Literature and Medicine* 39, no. 2 (2021): 296–318.

Hirsch Jr., E.D et al. eds. *The New Dictionary of Cultural Literacy.* Boston: Houghton Mifflin Press, 2004.

Hochman, Barbara. *Uncle Tom's Cabin and the Reading Revolution.* Amherst: University of Massachusetts Press, 2011.

Hochman, Barbara. 'Investing in Literature: Ernestine Rose and the Harlem Branch Public Library of the 1920s.' *Legacy: A Journal of American Women Writers* 31 (2014): 93–107.

Hochman, Barbara. 'Filling in Blanks: Nella Larsen's Application to Library School.' *PMLA* 133, no. 5 (2018): 1172–1190.

Hochman, Barbara. 'Making Americans in the New York Public Library: Fantasy and Realities.' *American Literature* 97, no. 1 (March 2025): 121–154. https://doi.org/10.1215/00029831-11597539

Hospital Library Handbook. ALA Hospital Library War Service, Jan 1, 1919.

Hutchinson, George. *In Search of Nella Larsen: A Biography of the Color Line.* Cambridge, MA: Harvard University Press, 2003.

Jack, Sarah J. and Kevin R. Ronan. 'Bibliotherapy: Practice and Research.' *School Psychology International* 29, no. 2 (2008): 161–182.

Jones, Edith Kathleen. *A Thousand Books for the Hospital Library.* Chicago: American Library Association Publishing Board, 1913.

Jones, Edith Kathleen. 'The Value of the Library in the Hospital for Mental Disease.' Catonsville Md: Press of Spring Grove State Hospital (1914): 1–6. Reprinted from the

Maryland Psychiatric Quarterly, (July 1914): 8–13. Available online: https://archive.org/details/valueoflibraryin00jone/mode/2up?view=theater

Jones, Edith Kathleen. *The Hospital Library, Books for the Patients: Plea for a Trained Librarian, Administration, Selection of Books, Separate Children's Library, Library Technic, Distribution of Book, the Library as an Adjunct to Other Departments.* St. Louis: The Modern Hospital Publishing, 1915.

Jones, Edith Kathleen. 'On Books and Reading: Outline of a Course of Lectures for Nurses in Hospitals.' *American Journal of Insanity* 72, no. 2 (October 1915): 297–303.

Jones, Perrie. 'Hospital Libraries Round Table: Arousing the Library Profession to the Meet the Peculiar Needs of the Hospital Library.' *Bulletin of the American Library Association Papers and Proceedings of the Forty-Fifth Annual Meeting of the American Library Association* 17, no. 4 (1923): 236–238.

Knott, Cheryl. *Not Free, Not for All: Libraries in the Age of Jim Crow.* Amherst: University of Massachusetts Press, 2015.

Largent, Emily A. 'Public Health, Racism, and the Lasting Impact of Segregation on Hospital Segregation.' *Public Health Reports* 133, no. 6 (2018): 715–720.

Levinder, C.H. and Caroline Webster. 'Hospital Libraries Round Table: Hospital Library Service.' *Bulletin of the American Library Association* 16, no. 4 (1922): 276–281. Available online: www.jstor.org/stable/i25686016.

Mahoney, Mary. 'The Library as Medicine Cabinet.' In *Libraries—Traditions and Innovations*, edited by Melanie A. Kimbell and Katherine M. Wissner, 100–107. Berlin: De Gruyter, 2017.

Mailloux, Steven. 'The Rhetorical Use and Abuse of Fiction: Eating Books in Late Nineteenth-Century America.' *Boundary 2* 17, no. 1 (1990): 133–157.

McDowell, Kate. 'Which Truth, What Fiction? Librarians' Book Recommendations for Children, 1876–1890.' In *Education and the Culture of Print in Modern America*, edited by Adam R. Nelson and John L. Rudolph, 15–33. Madison: University of Wisconsin Press, 2010.

McMillen, Paula S. and Dale Elizabeth Pehrsson. 'Bibliotherapy for Hospital Patients.' *Journal of Hospital Librarianship* 4, no. 1 (2004): 73–81.

Miller, Jesse. 'Medicines of the Soul: Reparative Reading and the History of Bibliotherapy.' *Mosaic* 51, no. 2 (2018): 17–33.

Miller, M. P. D. 'Hospital Libraries Round Table: The Therapeutic Value of Books in a Neuro-Psychiatric Hospital.' *Bulletin of the American Library Association* 17, no. 4 (1923): 235–236.

Monaghan, E. Jennifer. 'Reading for the Enslaved, Writing for the Free: Reflections on Literacy and Liberty.' *Proceedings of the American Antiquarian Society* 108, no. 2 (1998): 308–340.

'Nebraska.' *Public Libraries: A Monthly Review of Library Matters and Methods* 20, no. 9 (1915): 433.

Norris, Frank. 'The American Public and "Popular" Fiction.' Reprint. *Literary Criticism of Frank Norris*, edited by Donald Pizer, 126–128. 1903; New York: Russell and Russell, 1976.

Pawley, Christine. 'Foreword.' In *Apostles of Culture: Public Librarian and American Society 1876–1920*, xvii–xxxiv. Madison: University of Wisconsin Press, 2003.

Pisciotta, Alexander W. *Benevolent Repression: Social Control and the American Reformatory-Prison Movement.* New York: New York University Press, 1994.

Price, Leah. 'You Are What You Read,' *New York Times* (23 December 2007). www.nytimes.com/2007/12/23/books/review/Price-t.html

Price, Leah. 'Read a Book Get out of Jail,' *New York Times* (26 February 2009). www.nytimes.com/2009/03/01/books/review/Price-t.html

Radway, Janice. 'Reading Is Not Eating: Mass-Produced Literature and the Theoretical, Methodological and Political Consequences of a Metaphor.' *Book Research Quarterly* 2 (1986): 7–29.

Radway, Janice. 'The Library as Place, Collection, or Service.' In *Institutions of Reading the Social Life of Libraries in the United States*, edited by Thomas Augst and Kenneth Carpenter, 231–263. Amherst: University of Massachusetts Press, 2007.

Rose, Ernestine. 'Bridging the Gulf Work with the Russian Jews and Other Newcomers.' In *Work with the Foreign Born*, edited by John Foster Carr. New York: Immigrant Publication Society, 1917.

Rose, Ernestine. 'Books and the Color Line,' *The Survey* 48 (Spring Book Number 1922): 75–76.

Rose, Ernestine. Letter to Mary Frank Mason (July 13, 1945). 'Course Related Materials,' Ernestine Rose Collection, Box 1. Columbia University Rare Books and Manuscripts.

Rose, Ernestine. 'Final Exam' (1946–1947). 'Course Related Materials.' Ernestine Rose Collection, Box 1. Columbia University Rare Books and Manuscripts.

Rose, Ernestine. Letter to Karl A. Menninger. Correspondence (January 24, 1946). Box 2. Ernestine Rose Collection. Columbia University Rare Books and Manuscripts.

Rose, Ernestine. 'Minutes of the Conference on Hospital Library Service and Training (1946).' Box 2. Ernestine Rose Collection. Columbia University Rare Books and Manuscripts.

Rose, Ernestine. 'Opportunities in the Library Field.' (1946) 'Course Related Materials,' Ernestine Rose Collection, Box 1, Columbia University Rare Books and Manuscripts.

Rose, Ernestine. 'Outline. Library Work with Hospital Patients.' (1946) 'Course Related Materials' Box 1, Ernestine Rose Collection, Columbia University Rare Books and Manuscripts.

Sandford, Ann. 'Rescuing Ernestine Rose (1880–1961): Harlem Librarian and Social Activist.' *Long Island History Journal* 22, no. 2 (2011).https://lihj.cc.stonybrook.edu/2011/articles/rescuing-ernestine-rose-1880-1961-harlem-librarian-and-social-activist/

Sedgwick, Eve Kosofsky. 'Paranoid Reading and Reparative Reading, or, You're So Paranoid You Probably Think This Essay Is About You.' In *Touching Feeling*, 123–151. Durham, NC: Duke University Press, 2002.

Sicherman, Barbara. 'Reading and Middle-class Identity in Victorian America: Cultural Consumption, Conspicuous and Otherwise.' In *Reading Acts: U.S Readers' Interactions with Literature, 1800-1950*, edited by Ryan, Barbara, and Amy Thomas, 137–159. Knoxville: University of Tennessee Press, 2002.

Stewart, David M. *Reading and Disorder in Antebellum America.* Columbus: Ohio State University Press, 2011.

Vandergrift, Kay E. 'Female Advocacy and Harmonious Voices: A History of Public Library Services and Children's Publishing in the United States.' *Library Trends* 44, no. 4 (1996): 683–718.

Washburne, Carleton and Mabel Vogel. *Winnetka Graded Booklist.* Chicago: American Library Association, 1926: https://babel.hathitrust.org/cgi/pt?id=mdp.39015033640940&view=1up&seq=9

Wideman, Maria. 'Bibliotherapy in the Public Library; an Analysis of the Concept and Recommendations for Practice.' MSc diss., University of Strathclyde, 2019. https://local.cis.strath.ac.uk/wp/extras/msctheses/papers/strath_cis_publication_2761.pdf

Williams, Heather A. *Self-Taught: African American Education in Slavery and Freedom.* Chapel Hill: University of North Carolina Press, 2005.

Wishy, Bernard. *The Child and the Republic: The Dawn of Modern American Nurture.* Philadelphia: University of Pennsylvania Press, 1968.

7 Can There Be a Science of Bibliotherapy?

Imagining Bibliotherapy and Its Uses in a Modern Hospital

Mary Mahoney

On a 2014 episode of the Royal College of Physicians podcast, bibliotherapist Jennifer Strickland offered the following description of bibliotherapy. 'It has the word therapy in it, but it isn't therapy like counseling', Strickland noted, 'it's a bit of a stupid sort of American word that we're stuck with'. Though a casual remark, Strickland's assessment accurately describes efforts by Americans to create a science called bibliotherapy based on therapeutic uses of reading during the First World War. When these professionals returned from the war, they imagined an entirely new specialty called 'bibliotherapy' over which they might hold dominion. For them, the word itself signaled the importance of professionalism to their work. Only bibliotherapists, they would argue, could practice bibliotherapy. Readers might stumble on a book that offered comfort or read a poem suggested by a friend and feel helped, but that was not a therapeutic encounter. Even librarians offering suggestions to patrons in public libraries as part of early readers' advisory service could not claim to be offering literary cures. What set these practitioners apart in the interwar period was a dedication to making their work a science. They believed there was a truth of what effect reading could have on the mind and body which could be captured, categorized, and prescribed. This could only happen, they claimed, if the work was done by trained librarians who themselves were a 'therapeutic agent' in distributing books expected to serve as a 'psychological aid'.[1] This set them apart from their British peers, whose war work relied on volunteer distribution of books to soldiers in hospital.[2] While they set out to their work with great confidence, American inventors of bibliotherapy were quickly humbled by the lack of support for their 'science', though they never wavered in their belief in the healing power of reading.

At the end of the war, librarians serving in the Library War Service – particularly those who had served in hospitals and experimented in applying books therapeutically – believed there was a new field before them. As one librarian who had worked in a military hospital overseas put it:

> Those of us who had experience with the nervous and mental patients in camp hospitals, and those of us who continued to work among them long enough to see results, realized that a new field of work was before us. Doors were opened

DOI: 10.4324/9781003471561-10

to us, which had never been open before, and possibilities for service presented to us that we had not even suspected.[3]

Faced with challenges in obtaining government funding in veterans' hospitals and in creating public acceptance of this new field in civilian hospitals, librarians and physicians had to create a workable system for applying books as medicine, and in creating a story of the science itself. They had to shape a narrative that normalized the place of bibliotherapy in hospitals, made hospital libraries and librarians appear valuable, and reimagined hospital patients as subjects whose health could be assessed and improved upon by imagining their lives as readers. To do so, they began to describe their work immediately following the war as central to the notion of modern hospital care. 'I am amply satisfied that the modern hospital will be compelled to adopt a hospital library service', Assistant Surgeon General C.H. Lavender argued in 1922, 'as one of its essential activities'. Hospital library work, and the promise of bibliotherapy, Lavender argued, were essential as part of a modern hospital's new focus on the psychology of patients, what he described as 'a matter of paramount importance'. Hospitals now had to treat the whole person, no matter the specific diagnosis or disease in need of attention. Books were uniquely equipped to do this, yet librarians and physicians struggled to explain the value of their work to peers in terms medical experts could understand. In a line, Lavender articulated the challenge that would face those who believed in bibliotherapy in the years ahead. 'The things achieved are not such tangible things as can be weighed, measured or estimated in columns or figures', Lavender stated, 'and yet they have a value none the less important'.[4]

The incorporation of bibliotherapy into modern hospitals in the interwar period began with the use of the word 'bibliotherapy' itself. Dating back to lectures Boston minister Samuel McChord Crothers first delivered on the therapeutic value of books in 1914, 'bibliotherapy' began its life as a word coined as a playful critique of Americans' alleged turn away from the counsel of religion to treat life's ills in favor of the more morally suspect world of literature.[5] The story recounted a visit by a minister to a physician friend who'd taken up residence in an abandoned church he'd repurposed as a 'Bibliotherapeutic Clinic', prescribing novels as plasters for common illnesses. After the war, librarians and veterans in military hospitals coopted this word as an earnest moniker for this emerging field. 'I know not the lucky person who coined the term *bibliotherapy*', American veteran Frank Kane reflected in 1923, 'It may be of recent circulation … Matters not who coined it. We have the thing itself, and in the many disabled men's hospitals throughout the nation it has been given local habitation and a name'.[6] For American librarians, the word helped inscribe a greater importance to their work. They were not just stewards of a hospital library; instead, bibliotherapy was something they could practice – a positivist science that could determine the effect of reading on readers and be manipulated in the name of health by experts. 'It is being more and more generally declared that a physician should know books as well as he knows drugs and symptoms and that a nurse ought to be trained to give her patient not only baths and shots in the arm but first aid in his reading', librarian Fairfax Downey noted.

'Bibliotherapy they call it, for the medicos like words like that, and it deserves a resounding label. It's a science'.[7]

This was a 'science' that librarians believed could be incorporated into every modern hospital. The war had been a laboratory for medical experimentation, and other specialties emerged after the war to become departments in hospitals across the nation, including nutrition, orthopedics, and occupational therapy.[8] These new emerging specialties catered to the needs of the individual, a focus that was part of an early twentieth-century shift in cultural notions of selfhood that had ramifications in social science, medicine, and psychology, all of which shaped the standards of modern hospital care and the place of bibliotherapy within it. These specialties were grounded in a contemporary idea of a 'mutable' or changeable self that could be influenced by culture and environment, making social and individual intervention invaluable.[9]

This reorientation of medicine and hospitals in the interwar period around the individual coalesced with the emergence of personality as a new notion of self-hood. Historian Elizabeth Lunbeck noted its essential quality to the emergence and development of psychiatry, replacing the symptom in the mid-twenties as 'the discipline's main unit of analysis'. Personality, she argued, 'offered psychiatrists a dramatically broadened investigatory field, as they saw it, both its ubiquity (everyone had one) and its separability from the core of the self (its malleability) invited their attention'.[10] Personality offered multiple points of intervention and assessment for experts in psychology, and healthcare broadly welcomed the expertise of specialists to intervene in social and environmental factors to improve health.

The location of these debates within hospitals, expanding in number after the war due to federal investment, presented sites where experts continually negotiated the definition of health and of the specializations developed in its service. This set the stage and created the stakes for the development of bibliotherapy in the interwar period. Like dietetics, occupational therapy, and medical social work, its development had to suit the needs of modern hospitals, serving large populations. It also had to meet the standards of science, its subjectivities encouraging the skepticism of physicians and others who measured occupational therapy and bibliotherapy not by its demonstrated results, but by its ability to express itself in the language of objective science, measured in metrics grounded in the lab, not the library.

Before detailing how librarians created a science of bibliotherapy in their hospitals, it is important to note that this insistence on 'bibliotherapy' as a descriptor of their work and on the expertise of librarians and physicians as its chief practitioners set American practice apart from its British and European counterparts. 'In contrast to England', Marjorie Roberts wrote in a history of The British Red Cross Society and Order of St. John Hospital Library, 'the paid librarian with training and status is a prominent feature in America'.[11] In most libraries documented by the Hospital Library Committee of the International Federation of Library Association, the schemes varied not in terms of funding and public/private involvement, but in terms of labour. Most hospital libraries were volunteer-driven. At the Library Association's Annual Conference in Cambridge in 1930, participants extolled the virtues of hospital libraries and their reliance on volunteer workers to make them possible. By comparison, American librarians spoke at the same conference specifically on the value of trained librarians.[12]

Americans' preference for professional librarians supervising hospital library work and bibliotherapy stemmed in part from the development of institutional librarianship that predated the war. Systems varied by state, but the advent of professional librarianship coincided with the creation of positions to oversee libraries in state schools for orphans, prisons, tuberculosis sanatoria, and, significantly for the development of bibliotherapy, mental health hospitals. Edith Kathleen Jones is emblematic of this pre-war evolution in institutional librarianship.

At Massachusetts General Hospital in 1904, Edith Kathleen Jones, the first full-time librarian, established bedside service to patients. In so doing, she made herself the first point of contact and authority figure on what patients should read. While various authority figures in and outside of Boston in this period had their own ideas of what books could heal, how that worked, and what books made the best medicine, librarians quietly established themselves as authorities in this evolving debate simply by delivering books to the patients' bedside. The invention of a mobile book cart in 1910 at Mass General further provided an apparatus to professionalize their work and contribute to their appearance at patient bedsides alongside doctors and nurses as 'natural'.

Edith Kathleen Jones left Massachusetts General Hospital to organize and run the hospital library at the nearby McLean Hospital from 1904 to 1918. Publishing articles and pamphlets on her work in this period, she imagined that hospital libraries could do more than provide patients with a space to browse shelves and books to entertain during hospitalization.[13] She, like other librarians working in hospitals, believed that there could be methods of applying books to patients to make reading therapeutic. In 1913, she published a list of a thousand books appropriate for hospital libraries with annotations of select books.[14] Her selections, with broad guidelines as to moral suitability, resulted from collaborations with librarians across the country working to create standards for library work in hospitals and other institutions. Jones, like her colleagues, believed standards were necessary to professionalize their work and provide the highest level of care. 'Anyone can give out books', she explained in a 1912 article in the *American Journal of Insanity,* 'but not everyone can give them out intelligently'.[15] As a librarian at a mental hospital, she knew that the collections she organized for that population of patients differed from the needs of tuberculosis patients, for example, or of those in a general hospital. While all books should be 'wholesome'[16] for all readers, she explained, the selection of fiction allowed to mental patients or prisoners should be more highly censored than the 'morbid' books kept from a general hospital's fiction collection, for example. Those in mental hospitals or prisons should not read anything that might further any possible delusions or promote bad behavior.[17]

Jones and her peers wanted a national system of administering books in institutions. It proved difficult to suggest best practices when each state was subject to different funding mechanisms and organizational schemes. State hospitals were difficult to use as points of experimentation due to the lack of funding most states faced. Iowa and Minnesota were pioneers in hiring a professional librarian through their state board of control or library commission who then curated libraries for state institutions. However, this was more exceptional than common practice. The war proved instrumental here in presenting an occasion and population on which to experiment and create a more widely adopted set of practices. In 1918, Jones herself resigned as head of the library at McLean Hospital to serve as a field representative at hospital libraries in the Library War Service. The service, organized to provide reading material to troops serving at home and abroad during the First World War, became the impetus for the organization of a 'science' to use books as medicine. After the war, veterans' hospitals and state hospitals would serve as the main sites of experimentation for hospital librarians hoping to establish bibliotherapy as a field.

So how did librarians and physicians practice bibliotherapy in American hospitals in the interwar period? How did they turn library shelves into medicine cabinets? For this first generation of bibliotherapists, it was important to present themselves, not just books, as 'therapeutic agents'.[18] To do this, they adopted outward signs of professionalism, making rounds in white coats with their book carts and prescribing at the bedside. A former patient profiled hospital librarian Elizabeth Reed in *American Magazine* to publicize the work of bibliotherapists. Published with a portrait of Reed in her white coat prescribing from her book cart at a patient's bedside, the piece (entitled 'She Takes Her Patients' Literary Pulse') articulated the imagined mission of these early bibliotherapists: to read their patients and know how best to match the right book to the right patient.[19] In this work, librarians could offer a therapy not unlike other new technologies in a modern hospital that made the individual patient 'calculable and knowable', like the x-ray, blood type testing, and personality test. By 'taking a literary pulse', the librarian could gather information on a patient's personality of use to the physician, and, in collaboration with physicians, make adjustments to it using medicine drawn from the hospital library. 'A scientific approach to the choice of the right reading for a given patient', Dr. Gordon Kamman, an early advocate for bibliotherapy, explained,

> involves knowing the patient's personality type, – introvert, extravert or paranoid; his intelligence level; his educational and social background; his special aptitudes and interests; previous reading; illness from which he is suffering; how long he will be incapacitated; the prognosis; whether he will be a handicapped.[20]

Librarians and physicians with whom they worked enshrined this practice with the trappings of a science by creating their own prescription forms.[21] These forms tell us much about how librarians and physicians believed books could heal and the 'first do no harm' approach they devised. By offering physicians the chance to prescribe specific genres, for example, librarians demonstrated the belief that some genres held particular therapeutic values. Travel books could distract a patient during a long convalescence, for example, while biographies of figures who had overcome challenges might inspire a newly disabled veteran.[22] Travel, biography, history, poetry, and curated fiction were universally prescribed. 'There should be short stories, love stories, adventure tales, happy and enjoyable verse and light magazines of special interest to both men and women', one librarian directed.[23] Inspirational biographies were also used to inspire patients. Librarians frequently suggested *I Begin Again* by Alice Bretz as a book that might inspire adult patients disabled by injury or illness in adulthood as a source of inspiration, along with *The World at My Fingertips*, Karsten Ohnstad's memoir of going blind in high school.[24] These books and others like it suggest that therapeutic reading consisted of books that might entertain and offer some form of escape.

Librarians aspired to edify with their work, not just entertain.[25] As a profession, librarianship emerged from a progressive movement 'convinced humankind could be much improved – if not perfected'. To do this, librarians insisted it was their job to provide readers with culturally uplifting and educating books. They believed education and character were two areas they were qualified to develop in readers through carefully chosen collections. This meant they also had to save readers from themselves, advising readers on what they should read, and, when readers rebelled, censoring books they held to be morally suspect.[26] This created some tension when patients requested mysteries or Zane Grey westerns and librarians hoped to encourage the reading of 'good' books. Edith Kathleen Jones and her peers aspired to use librarianship to improve society through a reliance on efficiency, organized systems, and fields of expertise. In so doing, they hoped to improve society by extending access to books: symbols of citizenship, education, and uplift. By presenting themselves as needed experts, they also reframed commonly held beliefs about reading into new technologies over which they might hold dominion. 'Librarians are the apostles of the obvious', Miriam Carey claimed. 'They are forces advocating what the world takes for granted'.[27] Although some historians view the war as the end of the progressive movement, this desire to solve society's problems through solutions of their own design drove prescription in interwar hospital work. A librarian might interview a patient and learn they are a new parent in addition to their reading tastes. In suggesting books to fill their recuperation, they might include lighter fare as a helpful distraction and a book on parenting. Librarians in some cases offered instruction on literacy, or more commonly delighted in educating their patients about free public libraries and the lifelong source of reading they could provide. Some librarians also drew on war work to offer books on occupational training or prescribe classics to improve the taste of their patients, no matter how often they were disappointed in these efforts. As one librarian described it,

> They are not interested in Sir James Jean's idea of the universe nor in the causes of the World War; books on old coins or how to keep bees do not stir the imagination. Travel in Africa or Byrd's Expedition to the South Pole hold no allure for them. They want a story. A story! What treasure it holds.[28]

While prescription offered librarians a chance to match book to patient, their published research on these efforts reveals that for most librarians, prescription functioned as proscription. These guidelines of what must be kept from patients of different diagnoses stemmed from the real effects librarians and physicians believed books could have on the mind and body.[29] Primarily, librarians believed in the dangers of suggestibility, or the idea that illness or injury made readers more vulnerable to the suggestion of their reading materials. It was this fear that led librarians during the war to ban political propaganda. It also meant most materials about the nature of a patient's disease or disability were banned as well for returning a reader's gaze back on themselves. The *Journal of Outdoor Life*, which reviewed the latest research in treating tuberculosis, was banned from a veterans' tuberculosis hospital, for example, despite patients' desire to read it. Any reading that might excite pulse rates or elevate temperatures was also prohibited.[30]

In mental hospitals, any materials that might further a patient's delusions were strictly banned. One librarian recalled that a patient was banned from reading a biography of Commodore Vanderbilt. Though the genre was harmless and mostly deemed helpful as a distraction from hospital life, in this case it only further convinced the patient that he was in fact reading his own life story.[31] This tells us much about the authority librarians and physicians assumed the printed word carried. 'The printed page appeals with authority', one physician noted. 'If anything is printed in a book, it must be so! With almost no effort on the part of the mind, a message comes home'.[32] Librarians imagined themselves standing between book and reader, using their knowledge of the therapeutic values of reading to prevent them from harm. 'The practice of giving just any book to a patient is obsolete', one librarian noted in an article to fellow professional librarians.[33]

The dangers reported by librarians and physicians in journals functioned in part as a performance of their skill – only they could discern a healing from a dangerous book. So much relied on their professional ability to 'read' patients and both know their preferences and what they needed based on the state of their health. In making these considerations, however, some librarians bristled at the accusation that they were supporting censorship. In 1929, Louise Sweet, a librarian at a veterans' hospital treating patients with tuberculosis, published her own standards of what books should be allowed in hospital libraries which she hoped would be widely adopted. Her work is a perfect case study of the complicated considerations guiding the rules of prescription. She banned 'depressing' books and books that depicted medical staff in a negative light which could adversely affect the trust patients invested in their caregivers. Further fearing the suggestibility presented by illness, she warned against 'religious or ethical propaganda', using Upton Sinclair's *Boston* as an example. 'It is the rare individual who is not emotionally biased in his convictions and when ill he is peculiarly vulnerable to bombardments of this nature', she argued. Sinclair's examination of the Sacco and Vanzetti trial would then make 'poor hospital reading for either sympathizers or disparagers of the much-exploited Sacco and Vanzetti', she reasoned.[34]

Biography, travel, and poetry were all encouraged, as were 'authors with an assured and reasonable philosophy that sees purpose and compensating satisfactions in life', such as Marcus Aurelius. Sweet could appreciate the value of fiction but restricted any fiction with references to suicide, using Oscar Wilde's *Picture of Dorian Gray* as an example of a book that 'sparkles with brilliance' but that nonetheless was unacceptable as a therapeutic book. As evidence, she cited an anonymous newspaper article that described 'a suicide that beside him was found a copy of *Dorian Gray*, opened at a page where suicide was discussed'. This distinction between literature of cultural value and books suitable to be used therapeutically was important to a librarian who did not want bibliotherapy to get confused with rote censorship. 'Therapeutic disqualification' was not the same as 'censorship', she argued.[35] She struggled to communicate this to peers among the hospital staff who were puzzled by the sight of a librarian voluntarily restricting books. 'The public library can and should be broadly inclusive in its book selection since literary quality so predominantly decides its choice', she explained, but not so in hospital libraries.

> It frequently happens that when the circulation of a book of deserved reputation but of hospital disability is discouraged within the latter precincts, uninitiated partisans of the book accuse a 'Puritan of lurking behind the cloak of the alleged therapeutics'.[36]

As librarians struggled to explain these evolving systems that helped them match the right book to the right patient, they also encountered challenges in explaining what happened when a reader encountered a book and felt healed by it. To record this process in real time in the hopes of understanding patient experiences and to create guidelines that might be broadly applied, some librarians started to keep case files. These files allowed librarians to contribute to the overall narrative of a patient's care of which they hoped to be a part in a modern hospital.

Patients reticent or perhaps unaware of their own unconscious issues driving ill health might be induced to reveal them through a conversation about their lives as readers. Librarians analyzed these disclosures in case files, mining them for significance. Case files kept at Bloomingdale Hospital in New York in the early 1930s are emblematic of this trend. One patient, a seventeen-year-old girl diagnosed as having a 'psychopathic personality', requested books on pioneer life. The librarian believed the way she spoke about her reading revealed an internalized conflict over gender. 'She said to her physician', the librarian noted, 'my temperament and my desires clash. I have my mother's temperament and my father's desires. I would like to be a rough frontiersman; that is a masculine desire'. This facet of her personality revealed itself in her book selection. 'She had often expressed the wish to be a boy', the librarian explained. 'She "liked to read stories that boys read – cowboy and explorer stories"'.[37] The librarian and physician in charge of her care kept her under observation over multiple years, keeping a careful record of her reading from 1931. The increased diversity in the genres of books she requested became for the librarian a sign of recovery, and the case record a mechanism to define what a successful treatment in bibliotherapy might look like.

Even as they experimented out of their libraries, librarians and physicians struggled to explain their new science. Instead of relying purely on experiments grounded in statistical analysis of reading in hospitals, or controlled studies testing the application of different genres to different diseases, the 'science' of bibliotherapy reported by self-proclaimed experts in the field was built mostly on language. When Sigmund Freud was attempting to articulate psychoanalysis in its earliest phases, he spoke of a kind of longing for a language to explain the meaning of his new science and its uses.[38] Similarly, bibliotherapists reported on their work in hospitals by employing language to describe a process for which there was still no exact science. Mainly, these writings show a great reliance on metaphor and anecdote to authenticate this new therapeutic practice of 'matching book to patient'. Metaphor and anecdote provided librarians and physicians with 'a way of visualizing the as yet undiscovered phenomena' of the healing power of books.

Bibliotherapists made frequent use of the metaphor of books as food, for example, in which they were charged with monitoring a patient's literary diet. Noting an analogous rise in the field of nutrition, doctors and librarians invested in gaining respect for bibliotherapy within medicine used the language of food to explain the science of bibliotherapy and their role as its experts. In doing so, they built on common elisions of the language of eating to describe the act of reading. The notion of 'devouring' a book, for example, was a familiar phrase. In a speech before a conference of the American College of Surgeons, Dr. Gordon Kamman of the University of Minnesota defined bibliotherapy as 'a form of psychological dietetics' and claimed that librarians must be allowed to serve as its chief experts. 'To allow patients to read without expert supervision', he claimed, 'is analogous to allowing a diabetic to eat indiscriminately'.[39]

Similarly, to hospital administrators looking to cut costs by letting volunteers distribute books or allowing patients to select their own materials, bibliotherapists imagined the danger of indiscriminate reading by comparing books to poison. Dr. G. O. Ireland warned about the dangers posed to patients allowed to select their own books in a 1929 article in the *Medical Bulletin of the Veterans Administration*. Speaking of mentally ill patients, he said, 'If the ward surgeon and the librarian cooperate properly we can have the assurance that his interest will be directed along proper channels… We never allow drugs to be given indiscriminately', he argued. 'No sane man would prescribe strychnine in unlimited doses for insomnia. Then why books?'[40]

The key to success, according to experts, appeared to be attention to the individual needs of each reader:

> The hospital librarians must give individual diagnosis to the reading prescription, and thought, not only to the general symptomology and the causes responsible for it, but also the particular needs, and fancies of each patient, preventing, as does the pharmacist, the indiscriminate use of what might be poison in some instances, yet have therapeutic value in others'[41]

one hospital librarian noted. This proved a problem for librarians tasked with overseeing the reading lives of a large patient population where resources were scarce. It would be easier to operate as if *I Begin Again* was the ideal prescription for all newly disabled adult patients, for example, than to assess each reader to determine the appropriate literary treatment.

Sadie Delaney met these challenges as a pioneering bibliotherapist at Tuskegee Veterans Hospital in Alabama. There, in a career spanning thirty years, she managed to make the value of such a subjective science legible in a medical space where funding and credibility were tied to objective results. She also provided individual attention to patients in a large patient hospital. Delaney became an influential figure in the field despite facing challenges of being a black librarian in a white profession. She'd started her career at Harlem Public Library and had been recruited to create a bibliotherapy pilot program at Tuskegee in the early 1920s. There she used her library as a laboratory for experiments in therapeutic reading, developing programs to treat a diverse range of health issues with attention to issues of accessibility. She projected books on the wall for disabled readers and incorporated talking books for blind patients, for example. In so doing, she provides a counter to the medical experimentation for which Tuskegee is most known, the contemporaneous syphilis trial.

Significantly, she incorporated issues of identity into her therapeutic program, prescribing works by black authors, and surrounding her library with portraits of black leaders. This imbued her bibliotherapy program with greater meaning. Books held therapeutic value to heal the mind and body and served as a source for racial uplift in the segregated south. She was working in an era in which public libraries in the south were themselves heavily segregated, so just the physical space of an inclusive library that centered on Black experiences was itself therapeutic. Health and identity were inextricably linked for Delaney, who believed the library was a place where a man might find healing books, and in the process 'find himself'.[42]

Delaney wrote prescriptions and kept case files, adopting the technologies used by peers – but she also created a bibliotherapy group and library press club to encourage patients to create community and discussion around books, a process she believed led to therapeutic results. As she wrote in one case file of a mentally ill patient:

> (B) This man was uncommunicative; was almost mute. It was difficult to have him respond, even to questioning. He sat and stared blankly, dully. He was brought to the library with the Bibliotherapy group each day. He was given books of poetry to read. Late he began copying poems. Daily, poems were selected from his copies for circulation to bed patients. He was given selected editorials and essays to read at each Library Press Club meeting. This gave him a chance to talk. Also he would read aloud to other patients. Gradually, by reading aloud, he has become communicative for periods and it is felt that with continued treatment, he may become normal.[43]

This case in many ways demonstrates the ways bibliotherapy offered patients in the interwar period the ability to identify with what they read, and in so doing, find a language for their own experience and even catharsis. It also models the inextricable link between reading and writing as both necessary parts of any history of bibliotherapy. In this instance, patients copied poetry to share with peers.

In a New York hospital in the 1930s, patients gathered to read poetry and then attempted to write their own.[44]

We might read Delaney's case file and others as stories, and, in fact, narrative was an essential means of communicating the value of bibliotherapy. Indeed, this improvised science was not the fruit of lab research or even broad statistical analysis of patients. Anecdote was the chief technology used by librarians and physicians in their published research to describe best practice and express some sense of what bibliotherapy could do. Most of the published 'research' consisted of anecdotes of individual patient experience that librarians presented with the implication that they might offer universal application.

In many ways the greatest mystery remained how bibliotherapy actually worked; whether its methods could be evaluated objectively and replicated broadly. So much of the research notes the importance of the personality of individual librarians and their ability to 'read' patients and 'match' the right book to the right patient. By the end of the interwar period, pioneers in the field called for more standardization and experimentation in order to invest their work with greater authority and professionalization.

In 1939, librarian and psychologist Alice Bryan published an article in the *Library Journal* entitled 'Can there be a Science of Bibliotherapy?' In this piece, she set the stakes for the importance of the field and presented a broader vision of its future. First, she reimagined the terms and potential beneficiaries of bibliotherapy. For most of the interwar period, professionals spoke of bibliotherapy as a therapeutic practice mainly for use with patient populations in hospitals. However, Bryan suggested that bibliotherapy might serve instead not as a means of treatment of a preexisting disease, but rather as a preventative measure 'to develop emotional maturity and nourish and sustain mental health'. With this redefinition, the field could also be 'a preventative agent to keep people well'.[45] Bryan considerably broadened the appeal of this burgeoning science by making it accessible to and recommended for every reader who valued his or her health.

In order to meet these heightened stakes, Bryan called for greater experimentation and higher standards of research. Simply put, a science built on anecdotes was not viable. 'If we are to have a science of bibliotherapy', she argued, 'we must pass beyond the anecdotal stage in formulating principles and proceed to scientific experimentation. Anecdotes drawn from practical experience may serve as illustrations of principles or as suggestions for formulating hypothesis. They cannot be made the basis for valid generalizations'.[46] Bryan wanted the research on bibliotherapy to read more like scientific literature and less like storytelling. In her anxiety that bibliotherapy would not receive the respect or acceptance it deserved if it lacked the credibility of methodology, broad testing, and double-blind experiments, Bryan echoed Sigmund Freud in his early case studies. Describing his early findings in psychoanalysis, Freud worried that his work read more like 'short stories' and that they lacked 'the serious stamp of science'.[47]

Alice Bryan was not the only professional skeptical of the field for its lack of scientific authority. In 1937, Perrie Jones, a pioneering hospital librarian who had served in the war, refused to use the word 'bibliotherapy' to describe the field. Under an article subheading labeled 'What We Don't Know', she explained,

> you may have noticed that I have not used the word 'bibliotherapy'. I have deliberately avoided it as I felt that we are not yet sufficiently skilled in our handling of reading as an aid to convalescence to term ourselves bibliotherapists.[48]

Almost two decades after the First World War, when hospital librarians of Jones' generation imagined a system of therapeutic reading in modern hospitals, its leaders hesitated to claim ground in the form of linguistic signifiers of expertise. Similarly, those willing to use the word 'bibliotherapy' debated whether it was a 'science' or 'art'.[49]

Bibliotherapy survived, as we can well note with the contemporary programs that practice therapeutic reading both in the UK and around the world, though it did not become a department in every modern hospital as this first generation of bibliotherapists dreamed. Perhaps the closest modern attempts to prove the value of bibliotherapy objectively rely on MRI machines, as some research teams hope the brain might reveal the secrets of how certain books hold such therapeutic power. One recent study, for example, measured the effects of novel reading on the resting brain.[50] Today, most bibliotherapy programs thrive on the subjective nature of this work – that individual readers may identify with texts for the purpose of self-help or development. As W. H. Auden once wrote, 'It is not so much I read a book as that the book reads me'.[51] This trajectory – from taking a literary pulse to using books to provide readers with a language for their own experiences – began with these first experiments at turning library shelves into medicine cabinets during World War I and in the early practice of bibliotherapy in a modern hospital.

Notes

1 'Hospital Libraries: Cambridge Conference', *The Lancet* 216 (October 4, 1930): 777. See also: Perrie Jones. 'The Mutual Interests of the Medical Social Worker and the Hospital Librarian'. *Hospital Social Service* 11 (1925): 84. Scrapbook 2. University of Minnesota Archives.

2 Marjorie Roberts noted the contrast between American service and the British Red Cross Society and Order of St. John Hospital library, for example, noting 'the paid librarian with training and status is a prominent feature in America'. See *The British Red Cross Society and Order of St. John. Hospital Library (Reg. under War Charities Act, 1916) Its Origin, Aim and Development* (1930).

3 Ruth Bradley Drake, 'An Experiment in Library Work in a Hospital for Mental Disease', *Mental Hygiene* 5 (1921): 133.

4 C.H. Lavender, Assistant Surgeon General, US Public Health Service, 'Hospital Library Service' Delivered June 27, 1922. American Library Association Archives. University of Illinois Urbana-Champaign (hereafter ALA Archives). Health and Rehabilitative Library Services Division. Institutional Libraries Committee. Institutional Libraries Committee Publications, 1920–1924. Box 1. Folder1920–1929.

5 Samuel McChord Crothers. 'The Therapeutic Value of Books', *Pennsylvania Library Notes* 7, no. 4 (October 1914): 108.

6 Frank Kane, *The Bookman* 58, no. 4 (December 1923): 491.

7 Fairfax Downey, 'Dose: Books as Needed' *The American Legion Monthly* 12, no. 3 (1932): 8.

8 Katie Wright, *The Rise of the Therapeutic Society: Psychological Knowledge and the Contradictions of Cultural Change* (New Academia Publishing. 2015).

9 Greg Eghigian, Andreas Killen, and Christine Leuenberger, 'Introduction: The Self as Project: Politics and the Human Sciences in the Twentieth Century', *Osiris* 22 (2007): 9.

10 Elizabeth Lunbeck, *The Psychiatric Persuasion: Knowledge, Gender, and Power in Modern America* (Princeton, NJ: Princeton University Press, 1996), 69.

11 *The British Red Cross Society and Order of St. John. Hospital Library (Reg. under War Charities Act, 1916) Its Origin, Aim and Development.*

12 'Hospital Libraries: Cambridge Conference', 777.

13 See for example: Edith Kathleen Jones, *Libraries for Patients in Hospitals for the Insane* (Baltimore: Johns Hopkins University Press, 1911).

14 Edith Kathleen Jones, *A Thousand Books for the Hospital Library*. Selected from the shelf-list of the Library of the McLean Hospital, Waverly, Massachusetts. With additions and annotations by Miriam E. Carey, Supervisor of Institution Libraries, Minnesota State Board of Control; Florence Waugh, Librarian for State Institutions, Nebraska Library commission, and Julia A. Robinson, Secretary, Iowa Library Commission. (Chicago: American Library Association Publishing Board, 1913).

15 Edith Kathleen Jones, 'State Control of State Hospital Libraries', *American Journal of Insanity* 69 (April 1912): 712.

16 Edith Kathleen Jones, *A Thousand Books for the Hospital Library*, 3.

17 Edith Kathleen Jones, 'State Control of State Hospital Libraries', 712.

18 Perrie Jones, 'The Mutual Interests of the Medical Social Worker and the Hospital Librarian', *Hospital Social Service*, XI, 1925, 84. Scrapbook 2. University of Minnesota Archives.

19 Fairfax Downey, 'She Takes Her Patients' Literary Pulse', *American Magazine* 344 (April 1932): 71–72.

20 Dr. Gordon R. Kamman, 'The Role of Bibliotherapy in the Care of the Patient', *The Bulletin of the American College of Surgeons* 24 (1939): 183.

21 G. O. Ireland, 'Bibliotherapy – The Use of Books as a Form of Treatment in Neuropsychiatric Hospital', *Medical Bulletin of the Veterans Administration* 5 (1929): 442.

22 Isabel DuBois, 'Biography and Travel Have Large Place in Naval Hospital', *Hospital Management* 29 (1930): 46.

23 Emma Tevis Foreman, 'Carefully Chosen Books Have Therapeutic Value', *The Modern Hospital* 41 (November 1933): 70.

24 Perrie Jones, 'Hospital Libraries – Today and Tomorrow', *Bulletin of the Medical Library Association* 32 (1944): 474.

25 Wayne A. Wiegand, *Part of Our Lives: A People's History of the American Public Library* (Oxford: Oxford University Press, 2015), 53–105.

26 Wiegand, *Part of Our Lives*, 50–65. For example, in order to read books labelled by some as 'immoral' at Boston Public Library in the 1880s, patrons had to request their book using a form that asked their age, occupation, the contact for a character reference, and reason for requesting the book.

27 Miriam Carey, 'Organized Library Service in State Institutions', *Wisconsin Library Bulletin* 22 (February 1926): 51.
28 Dorothy Coachman, 'The Therapeutic Value of Light Fiction in Hospital Libraries', *The Medical Bulletin of the Veterans Administration* 9 (1932): 98.
29 Gordon R. Kamman, 'The Role of Bibliotherapy in the Care of the Patient', *The Bulletin of the American College of Surgeons* 24 (1939): 183–184. See also: E. D. Clarke, M.D., 'The Mental Hygiene of Reading', *New York Libraries* 14 (1934): 98–101.
30 Louise Sweet, 'Amenities of Library Work in a Hospital for the Tuberculous', *The Modern Hospital* 19 (December 1922): 527–528.
31 Sadie P. Delaney, 'The Library – a Factor in Veterans Bureau Hospitals', *United States Veteran's Bureau Medical Bulletin* 6 (1930): 332.
32 Dr. Josephine A. Jackson, 'The Therapeutic Value of Books', *The Modern Hospital* 25 (August 1925): 50.
33 Emma Tevis Foreman, 'Carefully Chosen Books Have Therapeutic Value', 70.
34 Louise Sweet, 'Prescribing Books for the Sick', *Library Journal* 54 (September 1929): 970.
35 Louise Sweet, 'Prescribing Books for the Sick', 971.
36 Louise Sweet, 'Prescribing Books for the Sick', 971.
37 Mary Morrissey, Case #6. 'Notes on the Reading of Mental Patients' Hospital Libraries Round Table, March 26, 1934, 10. Perrie Jones and Family Papers. Minnesota Historical Society.
38 Josef Breuer and Sigmund Freud, *Studies on Hysteria*, translated by James Strachey and Anna Freud (New York: Basic Books, 1895), 160.
39 Gordon Kamman, 'The Role of Bibliotherapy in the Care of the Patient', *Bulletin of the American College of Surgeons* 24 (1939): 183.
40 G. O. Ireland, 'Bibliotherapy – The Use of Books as a Form of Treatment in Neuropsychiatric Hospital', 442.
41 Catherine Povas Walker, 'When the Doctor Prescribes Books', *American Journal of Public Health* 22 (1932): 177.
42 Sadie P. Delaney, 'The Library – a Factor in Veterans Bureau Hospitals', 332–33.
43 Sadie Delaney, 'The Place of Bibliotherapy in a Hospital', *Library Journal* 63 (1938): 307.
44 Jack Leedy, M.D., ed. *Poetry Therapy: The Use of Poetry in the Treatment of Emotional Disorders*. Philadelphia: J.B. Lippincott Company, 1969.
45 Alice Bryan. 'Can There Be a Science of Bibliotherapy?', *Library Journal* 64 (1939): 774.
46 Bryan, 'Can There Be a Science of Bibliotherapy?', 776.
47 Breuer and Freud, *Studies on Hysteria*, 160.
48 Perrie Jones, 'Mental Patients Can Read', *Modern Hospital* 49 (September 1937): 75.
49 Fairfax Downey, 'Dose: Books as Needed', 8.
50 N. P. Canty, 'Bibliotherapy: Its Processes and Benefits and Application in Clinical and Developmental Settings', *Logos* 28, no. 3 (2017): 32–40.
51 W.H. Auden, quoted in *Psychobook: Games, Tests, Questionnaires, Histories* (New York: Princeton Architectural Press, 2017), 74.

References

Bryan, Alice. 'Can There Be a Science of Bibliotherapy?', *Library Journal* 64 (1939): 773–776.

Canty, N. P. 'Bibliotherapy: Its Processes and Benefits and Application in Clinical and Developmental Settings', *Logos* 28, no. 3 (2017): 32–40.

Carey, Miriam. 'Organized Library Service in State Institutions', *Wisconsin Library Bulletin* 22 (February 1926): 47.

Clarke, E. D. 'The Mental Hygiene of Reading', *New York Libraries* 14 (1934): 98–101.

Coachman, D. F. 'The Therapeutic Value of Light Fiction in Hospital Libraries', *The Medical Bulletin of the Veterans Administration* 9 (1932): 97–99.

Crothers, Samuel McChord. 'The Therapeutic Value of Books', *Pennsylvania Library Notes* 7, no. 4 (October 1914): 107–108.

Delaney, Sadie P. 'The Library – a Factor in Veterans Bureau Hospitals', *United States Veteran's Bureau Medical Bulletin* 6 (1930): 331–334.

Delaney, Sadie P. 'The Place of Bibliotherapy in a Hospital', *Library Journal* 63 (April 15, 1938): 305–308.

Downey, Fairfax. 'Dose: Books as Needed', *The American Legion Monthly* 12, no. 3 (1932): 8–9.

Downey, Fairfax. 'She Takes Her Patients' Literary Pulse', *American Magazine* 344 (April 1932): 71–72.

Drake, Ruth Bradley. 'An Experiment in Library Work in a Hospital for Mental Disease', *Mental Hygiene* 5 (1921): 130–138.

DuBois, Isabel. 'Biography and Travel Have Large Place in Naval Hospital', *Hospital Management* 29 (1930): 45–48.

Eghigian, Greg, Andreas Killen, and Christine Leuenberger. 'Introduction: The Self as Project: Politics and the Human Sciences in the Twentieth Century', *Osiris* 22 (2007): 9.

Foreman, Emma T. 'Carefully Chosen Books Have Therapeutic Value', *Modern Hospital* 41 (November 1933): 69–70.

Freud, Sigmund, and Josef Breuer. *Studies on Hysteria*. Translated by James Strachey and Anna Freud. New York: Basic Books, 1895.

'Hospital Libraries: Cambridge Conference'. *The Lancet* 216 (4 October 1930): 777–778.

Ireland, G. O. 'Bibliotherapy – The Use of Books as a Form of Treatment in Neuropsychiatric Hospital', *Medical Bulletin of the Veterans Administration* 5 (1929): 442.

Jackson, Dr. Josephine A. 'The Therapeutic Value of Books', *The Modern Hospital* 25 (August 1925): 50–51.

Jones, Edith Kathleen. 'State Control of State Hospital Libraries', *American Journal of Insanity* 69 (April 1912): 712.

Jones, Edith Kathleen. *A Thousand Books for the Hospital Library*. Chicago: American Library Association Publishing Board, 1913.

Jones, Edith Kathleen. *Libraries for Patients in Hospitals for the Insane*. Baltimore: Johns Hopkins University Press, 1911.

Jones, Perri. 'Hospital Libraries – Today and Tomorrow', *Bulletin of the Medical Library Association* 32 (1944): 467–478.

Jones, Perrie. 'Mental Patients Can Read', *Modern Hospital* 49 (September 1937): 72–75.

Jones, Perrie. 'The Mutual Interests of the Medical Social Worker and the Hospital Librarian', *Hospital Social Service* 11 (1925): 84

Kamman, Gordon R. 'The Role of Bibliotherapy in the Care of the Patient', *The Bulletin of the American College of Surgeons* 24 (1939): 183–184.

Kane, Frank. 'Letter to the Editor', *The Bookman* 58, no. 4 (December 1923): 491.

Lavender, C. H. 'Hospital Library Service'. Delivered June 27, 1922. American Library Association Archives. University of Illinois Urbana-Champaign. ALA Archives.

Health and Rehabilitative Library Services Division. Institutional Libraries Committee. Institutional Libraries Committee Publications, 1920–1924. Boc 1. Folder 1920–1929.

Leedy, Jack, ed. *Poetry Therapy: The Use of Poetry in the Treatment of Emotional Disorders*. Philadelphia: J.B. Lippincott Company, 1969.

Lunbeck, Elizabeth. *The Psychiatric Persuasion: Knowledge, Gender, and Power in Modern America*. Princeton, NJ: Princeton University Press, 1994.

Perrie Jones and Family Papers. Minnesota Historical Society.

Roberts, Marjorie E. *The British Red Cross Society and Order of St. John. Hospital Library (Reg. under War Charities Act, 1916) Its Origin, Aim and Development*. London: 1930.

Rothenstein, Julian, ed. *Psychobook: Games, Tests, Questionnaires, Histories*. New York: Princeton Architectural Press, 2017.

Sweet, Louise. 'Amenities of Library Work in a Hospital for the Tuberculous', *The Modern Hospital* 19 (December 1922): 527–528.

Sweet, Louise. 'Prescribing Books for the Sick', *Library Journal* 54 (1929): 969–971.

Walker, Catherine Povas. 'When the Doctor Prescribes Books', *American Journal of Public Health* 22 (1932): 174–178.

Wiegand, Wayne A. *Part of Our Lives: A People's History of the American Public Library*. Oxford: Oxford University Press, 2015.

Wright, Katie. *The Rise of the Therapeutic Society: Psychological Knowledge and the Contradictions of Cultural Change*. Washington, DC: New Academia Publishing, 2015.

8 The Curative Value of Reading

Hospital Libraries and Literary Therapeutics in Britain, 1919–1946

Edmund G. C. King

The 11 am armistice on 11 November 1918, representing the end of the First World War, produced spontaneous celebrations around the world, but it was also marked by a sense of uncertainty about what the immediate future would bring. Writing in her diary at around 11.25 that morning, Virginia Woolf recorded that the sirens that had gone off to mark the end of hostilities were still 'hooting' along the River Thames, just north of her house in the West London suburb of Richmond.[1] Later, venturing into the streets herself, Woolf found them thronged with people out celebrating, but, she observed, there seemed to be 'no centre, no form for all this wandering emotion to take'. The crowd's collective euphoria was, she wrote, accompanied by a certain 'restlessness' and 'inability to settle down'.[2] The rhythms of wartime had been suspended, but it was not yet clear what kind of peacetime regime would replace them. At Surrey House in Marble Arch, about eight miles northeast of where Woolf was living, Helen Mary Gaskell (1853–1940), the founder of the British Red Cross Society and Order of St. John War Library, experienced Armistice Day with a similarly mixed suite of emotions. With the rest of the staff out celebrating 'with the crowd', Gaskell found herself 'alone in the silent rooms' of the War Library's headquarters that evening. Surrounding her were the shelves and tables bearing the 300,000 books and magazines still waiting to be sent out as part of the War Library's ongoing operations. The Armistice, however, posed some immediate and existential questions about the relevance of a wartime charity in a post-war world. 'What next?', Gaskell remembered asking herself that night. 'Is all our work to cease?'[3]

Founded in the war's first week, the War Library was one of about 18,000 British charities established between August 1914 and November 1918 – a number that reflects the sheer scale of voluntary activity that accompanied the conflict.[4] Formally affiliated with the British Red Cross from August 1915 onwards, the War Library aimed to supply reading material to the sick and wounded members of Britain's fighting forces.[5] Using funds supplied by the British Red Cross, it bought (on average) around 100,000 books, novelettes, and magazines each month.[6] By the war's end, the War Library had purchased 1,237,246 books for its operations and received a further 2,889,233 items as donations, as well as distributing over 36 tons of weekly papers.[7] In 1917, its regular recipients included over 1,900 hospitals

DOI: 10.4324/9781003471561-11

and medical units and 56 naval hospitals and hospital ships. The War Library endeavoured to supply every British-operated 'Hospital, Casualty Clearing Station, Ambulance Train, Flotilla, Rest Station, Convalescent Camp, Isolation Camp, and Hut, etc.' in France with between one and three book parcels (depending on the size of the unit) every three weeks. Further book parcels were sent that year to British military hospitals and medical units in Malta, Salonika, Egypt, Mesopotamia, India, Corfu, East Africa, and Italy.[8]

An average day at the War Library brought roughly 100 written requests in the form of letters, in addition to telegrams, telephone calls, and in-person visits at its London offices.[9] Staff monitored this traffic to ensure that the books being sent out were what readers in the field were demanding. Describing the tone of the War Library's inbound correspondence, Gaskell wrote that 'books were *asked* for, *cabled* for, *demanded, implored*'. One letter-writer stressed that wounded soldiers were especially keen to receive the latest detective novels – 'any good murder cases or excitements'.[10] Writing about what he had witnessed in hospitals in the Mediterranean, a British Red Cross volunteer informed the War Library that 'I am sure it would delight you and your fellow workers to see ward after ward where the patients are kept interested and happy by the books and magazines which you send out with such splendid regularity'.[11] Based on feedback in the correspondence they received, the War Library accordingly sought to provide for 'every taste, from the "Smart Set" or a penny novelette, to Montaigne's "Essays" and Wordsworth's "Prelude"' in their weekly shipments. 'The man who got the book he needed', Gaskell wrote, 'was the man who really benefited by our Library, physically and mentally'.[12]

Gaskell's Armistice Day fears that the War Library's work would soon have to cease did not come to pass. Letters from hospitals, soldiers, and the War Office sent to Gaskell in the weeks following the end of the war implored her not to wind up the charity. 'Don't stop sending books', she was told. 'Increase supplies. Idleness and lack of excitement are telling badly on the sick and wounded'.[13] However, Gaskell was adamant that any post-war afterlife that the charity had would need to represent more than a simple continuation of existing services. As far as Gaskell and the War Library Trustee and Honorary Secretary, Charles Hagberg Wright (1862–1940), were concerned, the success of the War Library provided proof of concept for a much more ambitious and extensive future project. Describing their thinking, Gaskell wrote that 'Civilian patients suffer as acutely from lack of occupation as War wounded. We felt therefore that now was the moment to start organising libraries and librarians in Home hospitals'.[14]

Focusing on the period between 1919 and 1946, this chapter will describe how the War Library became the postwar, civilian-focused British Red Cross Society and Order of St. John Hospital Library. In doing so, it will trace some of the wider sociocultural and institutional contexts that shaped the contours of the new project. It will examine how the Library drew on the memory of wartime operations to justify its mission and assert the healing potential of reading. Finally, it will consider how the British Red Cross Society and Order of St. John Hospital Library might be reconciled with the wider histories of bibliotherapy. How accurate would it be to claim that British hospital librarians during this period were practising bibliotherapy as it was then being defined by American librarians?

Describing the financial constraints under which hospital libraries in England and Wales operated between the world wars, the library historian Ronald Sturt has argued that patient libraries in the 1920s and 1930s succeeded in providing 'a better organized *supply* of books and papers', but that the 'same could seldom be said about *service* the bedside help to individual patients in their reading'.[15] Sturt's caveats are important reminders not to exaggerate what services like this were able to achieve, given their very real limitations. However, I will suggest that British hospital librarians *did* succeed in developing their own distinctive forms of literary-therapeutic rhetoric and practice in the interwar period. These ideas centred upon mobilising what they called 'the curative potential' of books through the mediating, bedside interventions of 'informed' (though typically voluntary) librarians.[16] The ethos of service in British hospital libraries expressed itself as the supply of 'the right book' to a hospital patient at just 'the right time' to aid recovery.[17]

Reading, Recovery, and Reconstruction

In the years following the First World War, both state and voluntary institutions in former combatant nations engaged in large-scale projects of reconstruction. The bodies of disabled veterans represented some of the most visceral and enduring evidence of the war's destructive legacies, and large amounts of resources were devoted to their postwar rehabilitation.[18] By the late 1920s, Weimar Germany was spending nearly 20% of its annual budget on pensions for war-disabled soldiers.[19] However, the postwar ethos of reconstruction was not solely material, nor was it devoted entirely to repairing what the war had damaged or destroyed. Reconstruction also had significant social, cultural, and metaphysical dimensions. Postwar reform movements encouraged nation-state populations to feel a sense of connection with national pasts and national identities. Matters of health, fitness, education, and the general improvement of postwar societies, meanwhile, began to preoccupy reform-minded policymakers.[20]

Reading and literature came to play pivotal roles in postwar reconstruction discourses.[21] In Europe, the disruption of book-trade networks and the corresponding inability of intellectuals to buy books due to scarcity and postwar inflation encouraged cross-border humanitarian 'book relief' efforts to supply them with new titles. Significant funds were also devoted to rebuilding libraries destroyed during the war and securing new collections for them.[22] In Britain, meanwhile, with the publication of the 1921 Newbolt Report, the teaching of English Literature was made central to the school curriculum. As Christopher Lawrence and Anna-K. Mayer write, the 'mission' of English Literature thereby became 'explicitly social, moral, and political' – part of a 'new programme of national regeneration' directed towards the creation of a 'new, emerging England'.[23]

Postwar developments in the British public library system also bore the imprint of these ideas. Even in the midst of the financial crisis that engulfed the sector immediately after the war, public library advocates represented the expansion of library access to under-served communities – particularly in rural areas – as an urgent matter of social 'revitalisation'.[24] Vividly illustrating how a wartime programme could be extended to serve a postwar civilian population, the YMCA took the book stocks from wartime soldiers' hut libraries and redistributed them to village clubs in Britain.[25] As the YMCA official Basil Yeaxlee put it, 'the development of the hut-habit' among serving soldiers thereby 'pointed the way' to a postwar programme of social improvement in Britain's rural areas. During the war, Yeaxlee told a Library Association audience, YMCA volunteer librarians had encouraged soldiers 'to find friends among books' and 'take up definite lines of reading'. This, he said, was just 'the kind of service I covet for the villages'. The postwar 'revival of village life' that Yeaxlee envisaged involved village reading groups connecting – via their collective engagement with books and newspapers – to the nation's wider communications circuits and thereby becoming part of what he called 'an educated democracy'.[26]

The need to extend the War Library into a permanent programme for civilian patient-readers was argued in similar terms. The aim of doing so, advocates suggested, would be to apply the lessons learned during wartime to the social problems facing postwar civilian populations. In his January 1919 Scheme outlining the proposed programme for the British Red Cross, Hagberg Wright stated that:

> The need for providing our Military and Civil Hospitals with a constant supply of literature does not now require any demonstration. No one disputes the fact that convalescence is accelerated if the mind of the patient can be kept interested and occupied, and that books are essential for the sickroom.[27]

A 1919 appeal to the British Red Cross in support of the Scheme elaborated on these points. It claimed that the wartime experiences of medical personnel had 'convinced' them that patients needed 'distraction and occupation' of the kind that could be brought about through reading, both in hospital and during their convalescence. Noting its 'dismay' that there was no such programme yet in operation during peacetime, the appeal observed that 'disabled soldiers will be inmates, or needing treatment in Hospital for years'. However, it continued, 'we take a wider view and feel that one of the lessons learnt in this War is, that no Hospital should be without a suitable library for the patients'.[28]

These appeals were successful. In 1919, the British Red Cross awarded the Library an initial sum of £22,316 (equivalent to £1,295,000 in 2023 terms) to support operations for five years.[29] This was sufficient time, it was thought, to assess how popular the scheme would be and whether it would succeed in obtaining 'the approval of the hospitals which it intended to benefit'.[30] However, any wider ambitions to make libraries a feature of *all* British hospitals were (initially at least) tempered. The British Red Cross provided its funding on the understanding that the programme would prioritise libraries in *military* hospitals, as well as those operated by the Ministry of Pensions for the care of disabled veterans.[31] When the new scheme's organisers registered under the War Charities Act in April 1920, the final wording they settled on for 'the precise objects of the Charity' reflected this mixture of initial priorities. According to the completed form, the British Red Cross Society and Order of St. John Hospital Library would aim:

> To supply free books and magazines to naval, military and civil hospitals and hospital ships and homes and similar institutions for the care of sick or wounded within the United Kingdom (but more especially to hospitals, hospital ships, homes or institutions, treating or having the care of persons injured in the war).[32]

These objectives indicate the challenging nature of the Hospital Library's initial mission. It was tasked with simultaneously performing the kinds of duties fulfilled by the War Library and with extending those services into new territory – the complex landscape of voluntary, municipal, and Poor Law civilian hospitals and private infirmaries and asylums that provided medical treatment in pre-NHS Britain.[33] In doing so, its staff would need to convince a new range of stakeholders – doctors, nurses, matrons, and hospital administrators – of the value of hospital library services, as well as the putative benefits of allowing a new category of hospital visitor (the voluntary hospital librarian) into the wards.

The 'Curative Value' of Reading

War Library publicity material had made measured (but suggestive) claims for the healing powers of reading. These claims relied in turn on eyewitness testimonials sent in from wards and hospital ships, which imbued the appeals with a sense of immediacy and authenticity. In a fundraising address for the War Library in 1918, the Liberal Party politician Augustine Birrell drew on letters sent from the field to demonstrate the effectiveness of the charity's work. One letter described a wounded Scottish private at the 55 General Hospital in France who was provided by the War Library with a copy of 'a book … called "Scottish Recitations"'. After spending the day reading it and reciting bits aloud to his ward mates, it was reported that the soldier 'said he had had a beautiful day, and composed himself to sleep, hugging his book'.[34] In Birrell's account, this soldier's bodily gestures – physically embracing the War Library's book as he slept – testify to an affective (and implicitly healing) connection between reader and book more visceral than verbal testimony could convey. Another of Birrell's wounded soldier-witnesses sent the War Library a short, but highly charged, letter. 'I would have gone mad but for the books', he wrote.[35]

Throughout the 1920s, the British Red Cross Society and Order of St. John Hospital Library continued to deploy this form of suggestive testimonial to promote its activities. In its annual reports, the Library included a regular section entitled 'Notes of Appreciation', in which it extracted comments from letters sent in by hospital staff and volunteer librarians. In 1920, the Matron of the East End Mothers' Home in London wrote to thank the Library, saying 'The books and magazines you have so kindly sent are a great boon to my mothers. Nothing gives them more pleasure than an interesting book. It takes their minds from their many cares and worries and gives them a better convalescence'.[36] A volunteer librarian at the Royal National Orthopaedic Hospital, London, described how one timely textual intervention had brought about a decisive change in a patient's approach to treatment: 'One man was very terrified and gloomy and thought he would die and asked for "a book on Religion". So I gave him "Things to Live For", by [James Russell] Miller. He kept it two weeks, and now reads detective stories quite happily'.[37] The County Mental Hospital, Newport, wrote to assure the Library that 'literature … is indeed a means of forwarding the recovery of some of our patients'.[38] The Manor Hill Hospital for Disabled Soldiers and Sailors in Birkenhead, meanwhile, remarked that 'as our patients are all suffering from some form of paralysis and have been with us for long periods (two of them for nine years) you will understand what a boon your gifts are'.[39] Illustrating the Hospital Library's credo that the book a patient specifically requested to read was the title 'that will help him recover in body and mind', a staff member at the Croydon Borough Tuberculosis Sanatorium wrote to say that:

> One of the men here, a gardener, has asked for a book on 'Kitchen Gardens'. I should be so much obliged if you could get it for him. The Library gives the greatest joy to the patients, particularly the cot cases. It was delightful to see the men's faces light up when I appeared with the books, and nearly all of them seem to like really good reading. Thank you ever so much for the splendid supply of books – they cheer so many sad lives.[40]

The inclusion of these vivid anecdotal snapshots in the Hospital Library's annual reports reflects long-established rhetorical strategies in charity work.[41] Complemented by the numerical evidence contained in each report (the number of books purchased, donated, and distributed each year to hospitals), they act as mobilising examples, providing proof of the charity's effectiveness and testimony to the work still to be done. In doing so, they convey the kinds of striking 'details' of 'healing truth' necessary for generating empathetic responses among readers and encouraging further support for its therapeutic mission in return.[42]

By October 1933, the British Red Cross Society and Order of St. John Hospital Library was supplying books and magazines to 2065 of the approximately 3030 hospitals and public assistance institutions in Britain.[43] However, growing challenges in the funding environment had by this time compelled the Library to reassess the way it conducted its business. Applying for funding to the newly formed grant-making charity the Pilgrim Trust in July 1933, the Library claimed that 'the realisation of the value of reading in illness, and the consequent demand for books has far exceeded the scope of the income derived from the capital sum given in 1923' by the British Red Cross.[44] Since it was now running an annual budget deficit of £800 (equivalent to £60,240 in 2023 terms), its current operations were manifestly unsustainable. Were it not able to reduce its overheads, the Hospital Library Chairman, Lord Balniel, told the Pilgrim Trust, the 'only alternatives' would be 'either to seriously curtail the service; or to close down the organisation … before we have had time to create a permanent hospital library service on a national basis'.[45]

Rather than shrinking its operations, however, the Library proposed a second course of action – an ambitious programme of organisational transformation designed to secure its financial position and make a nationally comprehensive and 'permanent hospital library service' in Britain a reality. Part of this programme entailed raising annual hospital subscription rates and asking hospitals to assume the costs of freight for book parcels.[46] The main avenue of transformation, however, involved a policy that the Library called 'decentralisation'. Under decentralisation, local authorities would be asked to extend public library services to municipal hospitals in their regions, thereby assuming the costs of staffing and book supply for hospital libraries themselves.[47] In other cases, voluntary organisations (such as women's institutes and Toc H) would be approached to operate hospital services on a cooperative basis.[48] This would enable the British Red Cross Society and Order of St. John Hospital Library to focus their efforts on those hospitals that had no other likely sources of book supply, such as tuberculosis sanatoria, psychiatric hospitals, military and veterans' institutions, and voluntary hospitals.[49] Drawing on the lending collections of local authority libraries would also enable hospital libraries to meet particular community needs and sentiments more closely, such as the demand in Wales for books in Welsh.[50]

The plans that Balniel outlined to the Pilgrim Trust were the product of several years of organisational rethinking within the Library itself.[51] After a meeting held on 10 March 1930, the Trustees expressed a sudden and 'strong opinion' that the Library's long-standing Librarian, Cecil Hewetson, be asked to resign. Simultaneously, a new member of staff, Marjorie E. Roberts, was appointed as Secretary to Gaskell, a position raised in seniority to Organising Secretary three months later.[52] What, other than a desire to give Roberts free rein to reorganise the Library, led to Hewetson's dismissal is unclear. However, the stipulation (in the next meeting) that any cheques drawn on the Library's accounts in the future be additionally signed by one of the Trustees may provide a clue. Hewetson, who had been with the Library since its inception, responded to his dismissal by establishing a rival charity, The National Hospital Library Society.[53] He was found guilty in 1937 of 'making collections without authority' for his Society 'in the streets' and fined £2. At his trial, he admitted that only about £20 of the Society's £893 in annual earnings had been spent on books during its most recent year of operation and that the vast bulk of the charity's money went to cover salaries and organisational costs instead.[54] Marjorie Emmeline Roberts (1892–1964), meanwhile, came to play a pivotal role in the growth of the British Red Cross Society and Order of St. John Hospital Library. Roberts had worked as a VAD (Voluntary Aid Detachment) nurse, quartermaster, and commandant between October 1914 and December 1918, caring for wounded soldiers at the Furzedown Auxiliary Hospital in Limpsfield, Surrey, and at Charing Cross Hospital in London.[55] She was awarded an MBE in recognition of her service in 1920.[56] Jokingly (but accurately) described by a colleague as a 'relentless propagandist' for the cause of hospital librarianship, Roberts quickly brought her leadership and organisational skills to bear on the Library. Her ideas – and talents for public outreach and professional networking – decisively shaped the direction British hospital librarianship would take during the interwar years.[57]

No matter how ambitious its plans were, the Library realised that making them work at scale would require a sustained programme of publicity, one that could raise the Library's profile, extol the healing powers of books, and convince funders that hospital libraries were essential public services. While the Library might have had a presence of *some* sort in thousands of British medical institutions by this time, its position could nonetheless feel precarious. British hospital libraries were sometimes little more than cupboards shared with 'brooms and cleaning materials'.[58] Moreover, there could be some resistance to the idea of patient libraries from hospitals themselves, both at the level of upper management and among ward staff.[59] Guaranteeing more permanence would therefore entail the Library demonstrating the benefits of its services more explicitly to the medical and library professions. It would also involve mobilising key allies within those groups to advocate on its behalf. Moreover, this publicity campaign demanded a new *rhetoric* of textual therapeutics that could communicate the idea of the healing book to professional audiences in a compelling and accessible way.

Beginning in 1930, British Red Cross Society and Order of St. John Hospital Library publicity and outreach activities focused on enhancing the visibility of hospital libraries and representing them as an indispensable healthcare intervention. Led by Roberts, the Library engaged in a systematic programme of professional networking, with staff attending, presenting at, and sponsoring panels at both library and medical conferences. This form of professional networking had three main functions. It raised awareness of hospital librarianship as its own branch of library work, deserving of recognition and support; it provided a means of sharing key terms and discourse; and it was a way of recruiting existing professional networks and associations (both library and medical) into the wider campaign for hospital libraries in Britain.

Giving a paper in support of the Library at the Royal Institute of Public Health annual congress at Portsmouth in June 1930, the physician Sir Bruce Bruce-Porter (1869–1948) argued that the 'supply of good literature of all types' in hospitals was 'as essential – indeed in my considered opinion much more essential – than most of the drugs commonly prescribed'.[60] According to Bruce-Porter, British medicine had hitherto taken an 'ultra-conservative' approach to new curative treatments, especially those that 'act[ed] through the mind'. However, a new understanding of the psychological aspects of healing was now developing. Were the 'mind' of the hospital patient not 'supplied with material for healthy thought', he wrote, 'it will become a prey to introspection'. Bruce-Porter suggested that all hospitals should therefore set aside 'a really good room' with 'proper bookcases' for specialist patient libraries. These, he counselled, should be staffed by librarians – 'sympathetic, cultured folk who love humanity and books' – who could 'after a few minutes conversation with a patient … suggest the sort of book which would interest and be practical', considering the nature of the patient's medical condition.[61]

After Bruce-Porter delivered his paper, a resolution was passed at the congress 'urging that all hospitals should have libraries as part of their curative treatment'.[62] The previous month, a similar resolution – 'expressing the conference's approval of the principle of reading as a part of curative medicine' – was passed at the

Empire Red Cross conference in London after an address by Hagberg Wright.[63] In 1930, the Library Association established a special committee to help the British Red Cross Society and Order of St. John Hospital Library coordinate its work with public libraries.[64] At the Library Association annual meeting in Cambridge that year, a resolution was passed '[urging] upon Hospital Authorities the therapeutic and social importance of providing properly chosen libraries for patients'.[65]

The insistence in these statements that reading had a specifically 'curative value' was part of a wider international trend. As Jennifer J. Connor has shown, and as Mary Mahoney further demonstrates in her chapter in this volume, American hospital librarians and medical practitioners were deploying similar metaphors based on the idea that literature was 'curative' at much the same time (and for similar reasons).[66] In the same year that Bruce-Porter delivered his paper, the tuberculosis specialist Gerald R. Webb addressed the Association of American Physicians with a lecture entitled 'The Prescription of Literature'. Webb recommended that medical practitioners look for advice on suitable patient reading in Robert Haven Schauffler's 1925 anthology, *The Poetry Cure*.[67] This traffic of bibliotherapeutic metaphors across national borders was enabled by the internationally networked nature of the hospital library movement in this period. One consequence was the circulation of new ideas and terminology via the conference circuit and periodicals, a form of traffic in turn underpinned by the founding of new associations like the International Guild of Hospital Librarians.[68] It was also, however, a reflection of the international dominance and prestige of curative medicine in the early twentieth century. By representing books as 'curative', the hospital library movement could argue that libraries were natural additions to hospitals, which had been (by the late nineteenth century) decisively reimagined as specifically 'curative' spaces for their patients, rather than infirmaries where the sick were simply quarantined.[69]

Given weight by congress resolutions and medical authorities like Bruce-Porter, the assertion that reading had 'curative value' quickly became something of a catchphrase in the British Red Cross Society and Order of St. John Hospital Library's external communications – a way of crystallising the essential core of the charity's mission.[70] Writing to the King Edward's Hospital Fund in July 1931, for instance, Roberts observed that 'the principle that there is curative value in reading is taking root'.[71] However, the Library was also keen to stress that the mere *presence* of books in hospitals was not enough to perform this curative function. The relationship between hospital patients and their books could not, it insisted, be a wholly unsupervised one. For its full 'curative potential' to be realised, patient reading had to be *mediated* by empathetic literary dispensing agents – Bruce-Porter's 'sympathetic, cultured folk' – who could find 'the right book' at the 'right time' for each individual patient.[72]

First World War hospital library workers situated the healing potential of books in the context of what Sara Haslam has termed 'literary caregiving' – that is, 'responsive and empathetic interactions' between sick and wounded readers and the volunteer literary aid workers who 'ministered' to them through books, a form of care that was in turn highly female-gendered.[73] For the wartime volunteer librarian and novelist Beatrice Harraden (1864–1936), for instance, books could only perform their therapeutic function if there were 'direct personal intercourse' between patient and librarian. Providing the precise book that would 'amuse, help, stimulate, lift – and heal' depended on an awareness of 'the temperaments, inclinations and possibilities' of individual patients that only sustained bedside conversation could provide.[74] The publicity that the British Red Cross Society and Order of St. John Hospital Library produced from the early 1930s onwards represented *its* work in the same sorts of terms while positioning the Library's activities as a natural development of earlier wartime practice.[75] In their emphasis on 'interpersonal work', interwar representations of British hospital librarianship also bear comparison with the wider ethos of what the social worker Constance Braithwaite (1904–1985) termed 'voluntary citizenship'. As Braithwaite's 'voluntary citizens' did, hospital-based literary caregivers consciously mobilised the philanthropic sector's traditional, feminine-coded 'adeptness' at fostering a 'personal attitude towards clients' in order to give a modern social service an approachably human face.[76]

Sketching out the Library's mission in a 1930 pamphlet, Roberts began by locating the scheme's origins in the War Library before describing how the postwar Library conducted its activities. These, she explained, were based on the 'principle of a well selected library, from which the books are distributed to the patients in the wards, with understanding and sympathy'. The provision of books in hospital, she wrote, had to 'be suited, as far as possible, to the tastes and needs of each reader', and to bring *this* about, 'the right type of person must act as librarian and distributor' in the wards. 'By this method', she wrote, putting the Library's new catchphrase into use, 'there is curative value in reading'.[77] Other forms of Hospital Library publicity produced at this time expanded on the 'sympathetic' qualities, emotional skills, and literary expertise of the ideal volunteer hospital librarian. Addressing a British nursing audience in *The Nursing Mirror and Midwives' Journal* in 1930, Roberts identified reading for the sick 'as an important part of occupational therapy' and argued that 'the time is overdue for the curative powers of reading to be recognised universally as part of the science of healing'.[78] However, she wrote, the effectiveness of hospital libraries was 'less than halved unless the books can be distributed individually to the patients'. What volunteer librarians needed, she wrote, was 'a knowledge of books' and 'an intuitive understanding of human nature', which would enable them to 'fit the book to the patient, according to his natural tastes and his illness'.[79] Expanding on her theme, she observed that:

> It is not always easy … to turn a mind in a morbid condition towards a cheerful story; or to content an over-excited condition with literature that is soothing rather than stimulating. The librarian in these cases needs great tact, patience and understanding, and with these she can usually win through.[80]

The role of the librarian was to carefully select the book that would enable the patient's mind to 'be carried away outside the ward walls and away from his own pains and worries'. Without this personalised and selective element, books were 'little more than useless pastimes'.[81] Writing in more thumbnail fashion in a later issue of the *Nursing Mirror*, Roberts summarised 'the essential qualifications' of the volunteer hospital librarian as 'an understanding of human nature, a love of books, tact, regularity, and about two spare afternoons a week'.[82]

The experiences of one volunteer hospital librarian illustrate the range of therapeutic interventions this work involved and the kinds of personal qualities that individual volunteers could bring to it. Mona E. Going (1910–2003) contracted polio when she was nineteen, putting her in hospital for three months and forcing her to drop out of secretarial college. Looking for an alternative career that would suit her disability, she settled on librarianship, eventually completing her ALA and FLA certificates part-time. Beginning in 1938, she worked as a volunteer librarian for the British Red Cross Society and Order of St. John Hospital Library at Kent and Sussex Hospital in Tunbridge Wells.[83] The medical professions and disability were both significant factors in Going's own backstory. Her father had been a surgeon before a serious stroke disabled him; her brother lost a leg during the Second World War. Going's mother (a nursing matron) and her sister (a physiotherapist) found themselves having to act as caregivers for their whole family.[84] Going's volunteer work with the British Red Cross gave her an entry point into the library profession – she ultimately retired as Hospitals Librarian for the county of Kent in 1975.[85] However, Going regarded hospital librarianship as more than simply an occupation. She believed that her own experiences of living with disability helped her empathise with patients and gain their trust. 'If someone sees you with a disability', she told an interviewer, 'they realise that you speak the same language'.[86] Going evidently brought the longstanding ethos of 'direct personal intercourse' with patient-readers to her professional work. As Hospitals Librarian for Kent, she regarded it as her 'job to talk to the different patients and find what their interests were. You didn't just take a clump of books; you tried to find the interests of people all the way through'.[87]

Hospital Librarianship *versus* Bibliotherapy?

In 1939, the British librarian Louis Stanley Jast (1868–1944) concluded his book *The Library and the Community* with a chapter subtitled 'The Future'. Acknowledging that 'reading has a definite therapeutic value', Jast predicted that in the future:

> The term 'literary doctor' may yet designate a new profession, or a new aspect of one profession, that of the physician-librarian, whose drugs will be books, and whose prescriptions will be authors and titles. A [P. G.] Wodehouse perhaps for paralysis of the facial muscles, a [W. W.] Jacobs for confirmed melancholia, and, on the inoculation principle, the tales of Edgar Allan Poe for recurring nightmare.[88]

Thirty-five years earlier, Jast had joked about the British library profession's fascination with American librarianship. 'Perhaps the two most valuable and satisfactory products of American civilisation', he quipped at a 1904 library conference, 'are the librarian, on one hand, and the cocktail on the other'.[89] Just as British bartenders adopted the most recent American cocktail recipes, so too would British librarians import the latest American library trends as they appeared. Jast's gesture towards the bibliotherapist (in his imagined figure of the 'physician-librarian') was one of many apparent references to American bibliotherapeutic practice in British journalism and library discourse in the late 1930s. Some of these references implied that there were no equivalent programmes being undertaken in Britain.[90] One story, initially reported by the British *Library Association Record* and then excerpted by *The Lancet* in 1938, recorded how an American librarian at Ann Arbor University Hospital had discovered that a polio patient was fascinated by cathedrals. The librarian then collaborated with an occupational therapist to enable the patient to create her own cathedral in needlepoint, thereby giving her a unique 'means of self-expression'. *The Lancet* generalised from this report to conclude that 'the value of books to patients does not yet seem to have received the same recognition here' – in other words, in Britain – 'as in some other countries'.[91]

Many British hospital librarians, however, resisted suggestions that their practice could be wholly absorbed under the classificatory heading of 'bibliotherapy' (as they understood it), just as they (understandably) resented insinuations that they were not providing adequately for their own patient-readers. Roberts responded to the *Lancet*'s report with a forthright letter, stating that 'I cannot agree with your statement … that the value of books to patients has not received the same recognition in this country as in some others. Actually', she wrote, 'it has received more, but here the *method* of establishing the libraries has been different'.[92] Due to Britain's complex administrative web of voluntary, municipal, military, and for-profit hospitals and asylums, any attempt to impose, top-down style, a standardised or utopian system of library provision across all of them was impractical. Instead, Roberts observed, the British Red Cross Society and Order of St. John Hospital Library had focused on giving patients *access* to books across the full range of hospital types, rather than trying to establish model or experimental therapeutic projects in a smaller number of locations.

In a September 1945 letter recounting her experiences organising hospital libraries in bombed-out English cities during the Second World War, Roberts returned to this theme. In doing so, she extolled the benefits of the British voluntary approach to interwar hospital library labour in contrast to the professionalised model that operated in the United States.[93] Watching volunteers disregarding their own safety to deliver books during the Blitz had reaffirmed Roberts's conviction that hospital librarianship was 'a great human work'. While a 'certain degree of efficiency and training' might be 'essential', she wrote, '[o]verstep that degree by even too rigid suggestions, and the healing and educative power of the right book for the patient who needs it is endangered; and the librarian tends to become a small part of a theoretical undertaking'.[94] Focusing on libraries in psychiatric hospitals, Roberts observed that 'one school of thought … teaches that patients' reactions to various types of books should be carefully watched and recorded'. However, she continued:

> The other school, and the one that really holds good today in England … feels that too watchful an attitude, too highly trained and supervised librarians, are apt to increase the uphill task of achieving success in mental hospitals … Success depends on having very well-read librarians, with a reasonable amount of technical training, and a special kind of sympathy. Over-train, or over-theorise, and the very slender threads of sympathy between librarians and patients will almost certainly become damaged.[95]

Roberts's letter more or less explicitly distinguishes an English or British 'school' of hospital librarianship from the overly 'theoretical', scientistic, and surveillant ('too watchful') approach she evidently associated with the emerging, American-led institution of bibliotherapy. In making these distinctions, she returned once more to the mechanism that she believed generated 'success' – the interventions of self-aware and 'well-read' (as opposed to 'over-trained') librarians who could stage beneficial personal encounters with patients through the medium of books. To put it in more comparative terms, Roberts's model of hospital librarianship was clearly triadic, in that it involved a three-way relationship between reader, literature, and librarian. However, the librarian did not act (as in later, interactive or client-centred forms of triadic bibliotherapy) as a *facilitator* for the reader's feelings and responses, but only as an *informed mediator* who could 'fit the book to the patient'.[96] What Roberts called 'the healing and educative power' of literature was secured by the appropriateness of that fit and finally realised in the (implicitly private and beneficial) reading experience it enabled.

In the 1945–1946 lecture series that supported Britain's first professional certification programme for hospital librarians, lecturers displayed a similar desire to present a positive image of British hospital librarianship as contrasted against the emerging bibliotherapeutic model, while emphasising those 'threads of sympathy' that ideally connected patients and librarians. In her lecture on 'Psychology', the Royal College of Nursing academic Norah Mackenzie acknowledged the 'therapeutic value of reading', but observed that 'to degrade reading to the status of being useful from a therapeutic point of view seems to me an abuse of one of our greatest privileges and joys'.[97] Describing 'The Approach to the Patient', Barbara Paget-Cooke (the Librarian of St. Bartholomew's Hospital in London) wrote that 'the up-to-date hospital librarian must be a person of books and a person of profound human sympathy, without bias on either side'.[98] 'What is the function of the hospital librarian?', she asked. 'Is it to broaden and improve the patients' literary outlook'; was it 'to distract the mind from the sufferings of the body, thus rehabilitating by rest'; or could, she asked, 'certain books in themselves have a definite therapeutic value, and be prescribed by the librarian in certain cases?'[99] Expanding on this latter possibility, she cautioned that: 'Librarians do not know enough of the doctor's work or doctors of the possible scope of the work of the librarian to justify the hospital librarian being designated as bibliotherapist'. Instead, she wrote, patients should 'be supplied with as many of the sorts of books they like as possible', considering their specific medical conditions, and 'the librarian should appear to be interested in giving them', without betraying any snobbishness. Patients awaiting major surgery, for instance, could be distracted 'with books so gripping' that they temporarily 'forget what is in store' for them in the operating theatre.[100] The key, Paget-Cooke concluded, was 'to try and realize the patient's point of view, and to see things as he or she sees them, not only in sickness but in ordinary life'. It was only through establishing this empathetic connection on the individual level, she suggested, that the hospital librarian could be 'that perfect combination of literary guide, friend, and so often the comforter, whose visits mean so much to the suffering and the convalescent'.[101]

Conclusion

Any new professional group seeking to establish itself faces three main challenges. It must prove that it possesses a unique form of expertise; it must stake out a definable territory as its own jurisdiction; and it must demonstrate its legitimacy – that is, its fundamental connection to the wider values of the culture within which it operates.[102] For the British hospital library movement between the First and Second World Wars, expertise lay in the ability of hospital librarians to stage informed and beneficial 'interpersonal encounters' with patient-readers through the provision of books.[103] By combining their literary knowledge with an empathetic awareness of individual patients' needs, tastes, and medical conditions, librarians could select 'the right book at the right time' and thereby activate the 'curative potential' of reading. To carve themselves out a distinct jurisdiction, British hospital librarians represented patient libraries as essential public services, positioning reading as a uniquely valuable therapeutic intervention within the wider system of curative medicine. By emphasising the movement's proximate origins in the War Library, patient library advocates sought to represent their work as a culturally legitimate enterprise, one sanctioned by an historical connection with the national war effort and which reflected postwar convictions that literature had a peculiarly regenerative power.[104] Finally, while acknowledging developments in American and continental European bibliotherapy, British hospital librarians during the interwar period consciously asserted possession of their own distinct forms of professional practice and expertise. It was these, they believed, that enabled them to mobilise the 'special kind of sympathy' linking patient and hospital librarian and allow the curative potential within literature to perform its healing work.

Acknowledgements

I am grateful to Stephen Noble and Karim Hussain at the British Red Cross Archives, London, for their advice and assistance, as well as to the Interloans team at The Open University Library. I would also like to thank Siobhan King, whose genealogical sleuthing skills contributed significantly to the research behind this chapter.

Notes

1 Virginia Woolf, *The Diary of Virginia Woolf, Volume One: 1915–1919*, edited by Anne Olivier Bell (Orlando, FL: Harcourt, 1977), 216.
2 Woolf, *Diary*, 217.
3 Helen Mary Gaskell, 'Hospital Libraries Past and Present', *The Book Trolley* 1, no. 10 (1937): 204.
4 Peter Grant, *Philanthropy and Voluntary Action in the First World War: Mobilizing Charity* (Abingdon: Routledge, 2014), 3.
5 On the War Library, see Sara Haslam, 'Reading, Trauma and Literary Caregiving, 1914–1918: Helen Mary Gaskell and the War Library', *Journal of Medical Humanities* 41, no. 3 (2020): 305–21, and Sara Haslam and Edmund G. C. King, '"Medicinable Literature": Bibliotherapy, Literary Caregiving, and the First World War', *Literature and Medicine* 39, no. 2 (2021): 296–318.
6 'Appendix II: Mrs Gaskell's Story of the War Library 1914–1918', in Maud Warrender, *My First Sixty Years* (London: Cassell, 1933), 294. British Red Cross grants to the War Library amounted to just over £62,983, of which around £27,000 went towards book purchases. See *Voluntary Aid Rendered to the Sick and Wounded at Home and Abroad and to British Prisoners of War, 1914–1919* (London: HMSO, 1919), 272, and 'The War Library', Hospital Library papers, British Red Cross Archives, London, JCO/6/3 (hereafter Hospital Library papers, BRCA).
7 *Voluntary Aid Rendered to the Sick and Wounded*, 270–71.
8 'The War Library', *The Red Cross* (December 1917): 166.
9 *Voluntary Aid Rendered to the Sick and Wounded*, 270–71.
10 Warrender, *My First Sixty Years*, 291–2.
11 Theodore Wesley Koch, *Books in the War: The Romance of Library War Service* (Boston: Houghton Mifflin, 1919), 185.
12 Warrender, *My First Sixty Years*, 292–3.
13 Gaskell, 'Hospital Libraries Past and Present', 204.
14 Gaskell, 'Hospital Libraries Past and Present', 204.
15 Ronald Sturt, 'Hospital Libraries in England and Wales to 1960', in *Hospital Libraries and Work with the Disabled in the Community*, edited by Mona E. Going (London: Library Association, 1981), 39.
16 Cf. Sara Haslam, Jesse Miller, and Laureen Cantwell-Jurkovic, 'The Flow of Comfort: Bibliotherapy, the History of Literary Caregiving, and the Academic Library Today', in *Intersections in Healing: Academic Libraries and the Health Humanities*, edited by Laureen Cantwell-Jurkovic (Lanham, MD: Rowman and Littlefield, 2024), 72.
17 For this wording, see 'Reading in Hospital: Catering for the Patients' Tastes', *Nursing Mirror and Midwives' Journal* (4 October 1930): 10.
18 On wounded veterans in post-war Britain, see Jessica Meyer, 'Wounded in a Mentionable Place: The (In)visibility of the Disabled Ex-Serviceman in Interwar Britain', in *Veterans of the First World War: Ex-Servicemen and Ex-Servicewomen in Post-War Britain and Ireland*, edited by David Swift and Oliver Wilkinson (Abingdon: Routledge, 2019), 158–71.
19 Deborah Cohen, *The War Come Home: Disabled Veterans in Britain and Germany, 1914–1939* (Berkeley and Los Angeles: University of California Press, 2001), 7.
20 See Julien Benda, *Treason of the Intellectuals*, translated by David Broder (1927; London: Eris, 2021), 12–14; and Christopher Lawrence and Anna-K. Mayer, 'Regenerating England: An Introduction', in *Regenerating England: Science, Medicine*

and Culture in Inter-war Britain, edited by Christopher Lawrence and Anna-K. Mayer (Amsterdam: Rodopi, 2000), 2.

21 Margaret Mathieson, *The Preachers of Culture: A Study of English and Its Teachers* (London: Allen and Unwin, 1975), 70–1; Peter Widdowson, *Literature* (London: Routledge, 1999), 46–7.

22 Tomás Irish, *Feeding the Mind: Humanitarianism and the Reconstruction of European Intellectual Life, 1919–1933* (Cambridge: Cambridge University Press, 2023), 93–106; 158–9.

23 Lawrence and Mayer, 'Regenerating England', 10.

24 On the financial state of British libraries after the war, see Alec Ellis, 'English Public Libraries: Years of Crisis, 1914–1919', *Journal of Library History* 22, no. 3 (1987): 277–82. On postwar efforts to 'revitalise' rural areas in Britain by expanding library services, see Alistair Black, *The Public Library in Britain, 1914–2000* (London: British Library, 2000), 22–4.

25 For a wider study of First World War YMCA hut libraries, see Edmund G. C. King, 'E. W. Hornung's Unpublished "Diary," the YMCA, and the Reading Soldier in the First World War', *English Literature in Transition, 1880–1920* 57, no. 3 (2014): 361–87.

26 Basil Yeaxlee, 'Libraries and Adult Education in Rural Areas', *Library Association Record* 23 (April 1921): 89–90; 100.

27 Charles Hagberg Wright, Scheme Submitted to the Red Cross [...] for Providing Hospitals in Great Britain with Literature, January 1919, Hospital Library papers, BRCA.

28 An Appeal to the Red Cross and Order of St. John [1919], Hospital Libraries, 1919–33, King Edward's Hospital Fund for London: Secretariat and Chief Executive Correspondence files, London Metropolitan Archives, A/KE/B/01/04/032 (hereafter King Edward's Hospital Fund papers, LMA).

29 Sturt, 'Hospital Libraries in England and Wales to 1960', 34. Relative value estimations in this chapter are derived from the Measuring Worth calculator: www.measuringworth.com/calculators/ukcompare/ [accessed 15 October 2024].

30 British Red Cross Society and Order of St. John Hospital Library Committee Minute Book, 13 October 1919, Hospital Library sub-committee minutes and meeting papers, British Red Cross Archives, London, JCM/7/1/1/1 (hereafter Minute Book, BRCA).

31 Sturt, 'Hospital Libraries in England and Wales to 1960', 34.

32 Response to application under the War Charities Act, 1916, Local Government Committee, London County Council, case no. 1030, 8 April 1920, British Red Cross Society and Order of St. John Hospital Library papers, Public Control Department: Registration of Charities files, London Metropolitan Archives, PC/CHA/4/46 (hereafter Registration of Charities files, LMA). The multiple handwritten deletions and insertions on this part of the form suggest that it took several iterations to arrive at this final wording.

33 See Martin Gorsky, 'Public, Private and Voluntary Hospitals: Economic Theory and Historical Experience in Britain, c.1800–2010', in *The Political Economy of the Hospital in History: The Construction, Funding and Management of Public and Private Hospital Systems*, edited by Jeronia Pons, Margarita Vilar Rodriguez, and Martin Gorsky (Huddersfield: Huddersfield University Press, 2020), 181–2.

34 'Soldier Critics: Mr. Birrell on Their Need of Books', *The Times* (17 August 1918): 8. The book in question may have been a copy of *The Scottish Reciter*, edited by Ernest Guy Pertwee (London: George Routledge and Sons, 1915).

35 'Soldier Critics', 8.

36 British Red Cross Society and Order of St. John Hospital Library, *Second Annual Report of the Library Committee with Statement of Accounts* (October 1920–October 1921), 22.

A full run of annual reports can be found in the British Red Cross Society and Order of St. John Hospital Library papers, Registration of Charities files, LMA.

37 British Red Cross Society and Order of St. John Hospital Library, *Seventh Annual Report of the Library Committee with Statement of Accounts* (1 October 1925–30 September 1926), 50.

38 British Red Cross Society and Order of St. John Hospital Library, *Third Annual Report of the Library Committee with Statement of Accounts* (October 1921–October 1922), 23.

39 British Red Cross Society and Order of St. John Hospital Library, *Ninth Annual Report of the Library Committee with Statement of Accounts* (1 October 1927–30 September 1928), 36.

40 Gaskell, 'Hospital Libraries Past and Present', 207; British Red Cross Society and Order of St. John Hospital Library, *Fourth Annual Report of the Library Committee with Statement of Accounts* (October 1922–October 1923), 28.

41 See Mary Mahoney's chapter in this volume for an account of the anecdote as a form of evidence in interwar American bibliotherapeutic rhetoric.

42 See Ron Dudai, '"Can You Describe This?" Human Rights Reports and What They Tell Us About the Human Rights Movement', in *Humanitarianism and Suffering: The Mobilization of Empathy*, edited by Richard Ashby Wilson and Richard D. Brown (Cambridge: Cambridge University Press, 2009), 252.

43 British Red Cross Society and Order of St. John Hospital Library, appeal for funds, 18 October 1933, British Red Cross and St John Hospital Library papers, Records of the Pilgrim Trust, London Metropolitan Archives, LMA/4450/C/01/0019 (hereafter Pilgrim Trust papers, LMA).

44 British Red Cross Society and Order of St. John Hospital Library, appeal for funds, August 1933, Pilgrim Trust papers, LMA.

45 David Lindsay, Lord Balniel, to T. Jones, 19 July 1933, Pilgrim Trust papers, LMA.

46 Sturt, 'Hospital Libraries in England and Wales to 1960', 39; Minute Book, BRCA, 25 May 1933.

47 Lord Balniel to Pilgrim Trust, October 1933, Pilgrim Trust papers, LMA.

48 Minute Book, BRCA, 3 May 1934. Toc H was another charity with its origins in a First World War voluntary service initiative – it had originally provided rest and recreation for British soldiers behind the lines. Continued after the war as 'a living war memorial', it became a social service charity whose members conducted hospital visits and generally sought to 'fight for a fair and just society'. See Linda Parker, 'A Living Memorial – The Toc H Movement and Talbot House', in *War and Memorials: The Age of Nationalism and the Great War*, edited by Frank Jacob and Kenneth Pearl (Leiden: Brill, 2019), 209–10.

49 Balniel to Jones, 19 July 1933.

50 Minute Book, BRCA, 3 February 1933.

51 See, for instance, the earlier statement of the new policy in 'Books for the Hospitals: Cooperation with the Libraries', *The Times* (10 March 1931): 17.

52 Minute Book, BRCA, 18 June 1930.

53 In a handwritten marginal note in the Pilgrim Trust papers, Hewetson is described as 'a disgruntled ex-employee of the Red X Library' who 'learnt his job from them and is now getting a good deal of support'. See British Red Cross Society and Order of St. John Hospital Library, appeal for funds, 18 October 1933, Pilgrim Trust papers, LMA.

54 'Hospital Collections: A Warning and Useful Advice', *Bognor Regis Observer* (2 February 1938): 6. On an earlier incident involving fraudulent collections for the charity, see 'National Hospital Library Society', *Truth* (5 February 1936): 206. Serious concerns

about the National Hospital Library Society had been raised as early as 1933 by the British Charities Association; its representatives worked behind the scenes with the *Truth* to expose the NHLS's irregularities. See Minute Book, BRCA, 28 November 1933.

55 See Marjorie Emmeline Cohen, digitised record card, British Red Cross Volunteers during WWI database, https://vad.redcross.org.uk/record?rowKey=44914 [accessed 10 September 2024].

56 For the award of Roberts's MBE, see *Supplement to the London Gazette* (30 March 1920): 3822.

57 Sturt, 'Hospital Libraries in England and Wales to 1960', 41.

58 Gaskell, 'Hospital Libraries Past and Present', 206.

59 Sturt, 'Hospital Libraries in England and Wales to 1960', 37.

60 Sir Bruce Bruce-Porter, 'The Need for Libraries in Hospitals as Part of the Scheme of Curative Medicine', *Journal of State Medicine* 38, no. 12 (1930): 710.

61 Bruce-Porter, 'The Need for Libraries in Hospitals', 711; 710; 713.

62 British Red Cross Society and Order of St. John Hospital Library, *Eleventh Annual Report of the Library Committee with Statement of Accounts* (1 October 1929–30 September 1930), 4.

63 'The Red Cross in Peace', *The Times* (21 May 1930): 21.

64 British Red Cross Society and Order of St. John Hospital Library, *Twelfth Annual Report of the Library Committee with Statement of Accounts* (1 October 1930–30 September 1931), 3.

65 'Fifty-Third Annual Conference', *Library Association Record Supplement* (December 1930): xx.

66 Jennifer J. Connor, 'Prescribed Reading: Patients' Libraries in North American Tuberculosis Institutions', *Libraries & Culture* 27, no. 3 (1992): 260–2.

67 Connor, 'Prescribed Reading', 260.

68 See 'Guild of Hospital Librarians', *Bulletin of the American Library Association* 29, no. 1 (1935): 48–9. On presentations by American hospital librarians at the 1930 British Library Association conference in Cambridge, see 'Reading in Hospital', 10.

69 See Virginia Berridge, 'Health and Medicine', in *The Cambridge Social History of Britain, 1750–1950*, edited by F. M. L. Thompson (Cambridge: Cambridge University Press, 1990), 202; 207.

70 Cf. Suman Gupta, *Political Catchphrases and Contemporary History: A Critique of New Normals* (Oxford: Oxford University Press, 2022), 171.

71 Marjorie E. Roberts to H. R. Maynard, 10 July 1931, King Edward's Hospital Fund papers, LMA.

72 Bruce-Porter, 'The Need for Libraries in Hospitals', 713; 'Reading in Hospital', 10.

73 Haslam and King, 'Medicinable Literature', 299.

74 Quoted in Haslam and King, 'Medicinable Literature', 305.

75 On the gendered nature of this discourse, see Haslam and King, 'Medicinable Literature', 305.

76 Eve Colpus, *Female Philanthropy in the Interwar World: Between Self and Other* (London: Bloomsbury, 2018), 33.

77 [Marjorie E. Roberts], *The British Red Cross Society and Order of St. John Hospital Library: Its Origin, Aim and Development* (London, [1930]), 3–4.

78 Marjorie E. Roberts, 'The Hospital Library', *Nursing Mirror and Midwives' Journal* (27 September 1930): 526.

79 Roberts, 'The Hospital Library', 526.

80 Roberts, 'The Hospital Library', 526.

81 Marjorie E. Roberts, 'The Hospital Library Movement: Origin and Development', *Bulletin of the World Association for Adult Education*, 2nd ser., 8 (February 1937): 26.
82 Marjorie E. Roberts, 'Hospital Libraries', *Nursing Mirror and Midwives' Journal* (31 January 1931): 371.
83 Jean M. Clarke and M. Joy Lewis, 'Obituary: Mona E. Going, 1910–2003', *Health Information and Libraries Journal* 20 (2003): 125.
84 Mona E. Going, interview with Michele Abendstern, 18 January 2002, Health Libraries Group Oral History Project, British Library, London, C1108/02/10–02.
85 Clarke and Lewis, 'Obituary', 125.
86 Going, interview, 18 January 2002.
87 Going, interview, 18 January 2002.
88 L. Stanley Jast, *The Library and the Community* (London: Thomas Nelson, 1939), 189.
89 Quoted in Paul Sturges, 'British Librarianship and the First World War: A Commentary', *Journal of Library History* 22, no. 3 (1987): 286.
90 Haslam, Miller, and Cantwell-Jurkovic, 'The Flow of Comfort', 70.
91 'Hospital Libraries Abroad', *The Lancet* 231, no. 5972 (1938): 414.
92 Marjorie E. Roberts, 'Hospital Libraries Abroad', *The Lancet* 231, no. 5978 (1938): 751.
93 For more detail about professionalisation in interwar American hospital libraries, see Mary Mahoney's chapter in this volume.
94 Marjorie E. Roberts, 'Hospital Library Activities in England', *Special Libraries* 37, no. 3 (1946): 89.
95 Roberts, 'Hospital Library Activities in England', 90.
96 Roberts, 'The Hospital Library', 526. For the triadic model in interactive bibliotherapy, see Arleen McCarty Hynes and Mary Hynes-Berry, *Biblio/Poetry Therapy – The Interactive Process: A Handbook*, 3rd ed. (St. Cloud, MN: North Star Press, 2012), 4–5.
97 [Norah] Mackenzie, 'Psychology', in *Manual for Hospital Librarians*, edited by C. E. A. Bedwell (London: Library Association, 1947), 32.
98 [Barbara] Paget-Cooke, 'The Approach to the Patient', in *Manual for Hospital Librarians*, 34.
99 Paget-Cooke, 'The Approach to the Patient', 36.
100 Paget-Cooke, 'The Approach to the Patient', 36.
101 Paget-Cooke, 'The Approach to the Patient', 37.
102 Andrew Abbott, *The System of Professions: An Essay on the Division of Expert Labour* (Chicago: University of Chicago Press, 1988), 323–4; 88–90; 184.
103 Cf. Colpus, *Female Philanthropy in the Interwar World*, 33.
104 Roberts, *The British Red Cross Society and Order of St. John Hospital Library*, 3.

References

Abbott, Andrew. *The System of Professions: An Essay on the Division of Expert Labour*. Chicago: University of Chicago Press, 1988.

Benda, Julien. *Treason of the Intellectuals*, translated by David Broder. 1927; London: Eris, 2021.

Berridge, Virginia. 'Health and Medicine'. In *The Cambridge Social History of Britain, 1750–1950*, edited by F. M. L. Thompson, 171–242. Cambridge: Cambridge University Press, 1990.

Black, Alistair. *The Public Library in Britain, 1914–2000*. London: British Library, 2000.

'Books for the Hospitals: Cooperation with the Libraries', *The Times* (10 March 1931): 17.

British Red Cross Society and Order of St. John Hospital Library. *Annual Reports of the Library Committee with Statement of Accounts*, 1919–1939. Public Control Department: Registration of Charities files, London Metropolitan Archives, PC/CHA/4/46.

Bruce-Porter, Bruce. 'The Need for Libraries in Hospitals as Part of the Scheme of Curative Medicine', *Journal of State Medicine* 38, no. 12 (1930): 710–15.

Clarke, Jean M., and M. Joy Lewis, 'Obituary: Mona E. Going, 1910–2003', *Health Information and Libraries Journal* 20 (2003): 125–6.

Cohen, Deborah. *The War Come Home: Disabled Veterans in Britain and Germany, 1914–1939*. Berkeley and Los Angeles: University of California Press, 2001.

Colpus, Eve. *Female Philanthropy in the Interwar World: Between Self and Other*. London: Bloomsbury, 2018.

Connor, Jennifer J. 'Prescribed Reading: Patients' Libraries in North American Tuberculosis Institutions', *Libraries & Culture* 27, no. 3 (1992): 252–78.

Dudai, Ron. '"Can You Describe This?" Human Rights Reports and What They Tell Us About the Human Rights Movement'. In *Humanitarianism and Suffering: The Mobilization of Empathy*, edited by Richard Ashby Wilson and Richard D. Brown, 245–64. Cambridge: Cambridge University Press, 2009.

Ellis, Alec. 'English Public Libraries: Years of Crisis, 1914–1919', *Journal of Library History* 22, no. 3 (1987): 272–84.

'Fifty-Third Annual Conference', *Library Association Record Supplement* (December 1930).

Gaskell, Helen Mary. 'Hospital Libraries Past and Present', *The Book Trolley* 1, no. 10 (1937): 203–7.

Going, Mona E. Interview with Michele Abendstern, 18 January 2002, Health Libraries Group Oral History Project, British Library, London, C1108/02/10–02.

Gorsky, Martin. 'Public, Private and Voluntary Hospitals: Economic Theory and Historical Experience in Britain, c.1800–2010'. In *The Political Economy of the Hospital in History: The Construction, Funding and Management of Public and Private Hospital Systems*, edited by Jeronia Pons, Margarita Vilar Rodriguez, and Martin Gorsky, 181–220. Huddersfield: Huddersfield University Press, 2020.

Grant, Peter. *Philanthropy and Voluntary Action in the First World War: Mobilizing Charity*. Abingdon: Routledge, 2014.

'Guild of Hospital Librarians', *Bulletin of the American Library Association* 29, no. 1 (1935): 48–9.

Gupta, Suman. *Political Catchphrases and Contemporary History: A Critique of New Normals*. Oxford: Oxford University Press, 2022.

Haslam, Sara. 'Reading, Trauma and Literary Caregiving 1914–1918: Helen Mary Gaskell and the War Library', *Journal of Medical Humanities* 41, no. 3 (2020): 305–21.

Haslam, Sara, and Edmund G. C. King. '"Medicinable Literature": Bibliotherapy, Literary Caregiving, and the First World War', *Literature and Medicine* 39, no. 2 (2021): 296–318.

Haslam, Sara, Jesse Miller, and Laureen Cantwell-Jurkovic. 'The Flow of Comfort: Bibliotherapy, the History of Literary Caregiving, and the Academic Library Today'. In *Intersections in Healing: Academic Libraries and the Health Humanities*, edited by Laureen Cantwell-Jurkovic, 63–83. Lanham, MD: Rowman and Littlefield, 2024.

'Hospital Collections: A Warning and Useful Advice', *Bognor Regis Observer* (2 February 1938): 6.

'Hospital Libraries Abroad', *The Lancet* 231, no. 5972 (1938): 414–15.

Hospital Library papers, British Red Cross Archives, London, JCO/6/3.

Hospital Library sub-committee minutes and meeting papers, British Red Cross Archives, London, JCM/7/1/1/1.

Hynes, Arleen McCarty, and Mary Hynes-Berry. *Biblio/Poetry Therapy—The Interactive Process: A Handbook*, 3rd ed. St. Cloud, MN: North Star Press, 2012.

Irish, Tomás. *Feeding the Mind: Humanitarianism and the Reconstruction of European Intellectual Life, 1919–1933*. Cambridge: Cambridge University Press, 2023.

Jast, L. Stanley. *The Library and the Community*. London: Thomas Nelson, 1939.

King, Edmund G. C. 'E. W. Hornung's Unpublished "Diary," the YMCA, and the Reading Soldier in the First World War', *English Literature in Transition, 1880–1920* 57, no. 3 (2014): 361–87.

King Edward's Hospital Fund for London: Secretariat and Chief Executive Correspondence files, London Metropolitan Archives, A/KE/B/01/04/032.

Koch, Theodore Wesley. *Books in the War: The Romance of Library War Service*. Boston: Houghton Mifflin, 1919.

Lawrence, Christopher, and Anna-K. Mayer. 'Regenerating England: An Introduction'. In *Regenerating England: Science, Medicine and Culture in Inter-war Britain*, edited by Christopher Lawrence and Anna-K. Mayer, 1–23. Amsterdam: Rodopi, 2000.

Mackenzie, Norah. 'Psychology'. In *Manual for Hospital Librarians*, edited by C. E. A. Bedwell, 23–33. London: Library Association, 1947.

Mathieson, Margaret. *The Preachers of Culture: A Study of English and Its Teachers*. London: Allen and Unwin, 1975.

Meyer, Jessica. 'Wounded in a Mentionable Place: The (In)visibility of the Disabled Ex-Serviceman in Interwar Britain'. In *Veterans of the First World War: Ex-Servicemen and Ex-Servicewomen in Post-War Britain and Ireland*, edited by David Swift and Oliver Wilkinson, 158–71. Abingdon: Routledge, 2019.

'National Hospital Library Society', *Truth* (5 February 1936): 206.

Paget-Cooke, Barbara. 'The Approach to the Patient'. In *Manual for Hospital Librarians*, edited by C. E. A. Bedwell, 34–7. London: Library Association, 1947.

Parker, Linda. 'A Living Memorial—The Toc H Movement and Talbot House'. In *War and Memorials: The Age of Nationalism and the Great War*, edited by Frank Jacob and Kenneth Pearl, 209–28. Leiden: Brill, 2019.

Public Control Department: Registration of Charities files, London Metropolitan Archives, PC/CHA/4/46.

'Reading in Hospital: Catering for the Patients' Tastes', *Nursing Mirror and Midwives' Journal* (4 October 1930): 10.

Records of the Pilgrim Trust, London Metropolitan Archives, LMA/4450/C/01/0019.

'The Red Cross in Peace', *The Times* (21 May 1930): 21.

Roberts, Marjorie E. *The British Red Cross Society and Order of St. John Hospital Library: Its Origin, Aim and Development*. London, [1930].

Roberts, Marjorie E. 'Hospital Libraries', *Nursing Mirror and Midwives' Journal* (31 January 1931): 371.

Roberts, Marjorie E. 'Hospital Libraries Abroad', *The Lancet* 231, no. 5978 (1938): 751.

Roberts, Marjorie E. 'The Hospital Library', *Nursing Mirror and Midwives' Journal* (27 September 1930): 526.

Roberts, Marjorie E. 'Hospital Library Activities in England', *Special Libraries* 37, no. 3 (1946): 87–91.

Roberts, Marjorie E. 'The Hospital Library Movement: Origin and Development', *Bulletin of the World Association for Adult Education*, 2nd ser., 8 (February 1937): 26–31.

'Soldier Critics: Mr. Birrell on Their Need of Books', *The Times* (17 August 1918): 8.

Sturges, Paul. 'British Librarianship and the First World War: A Commentary', *Journal of Library History* 22, no. 3 (1987): 285–93.

Sturt, Ronald. 'Hospital Libraries in England and Wales to 1960'. In *Hospital Libraries and Work with the Disabled in the Community*, edited by Mona E. Going, 27–67. London: Library Association, 1981.

Supplement to the London Gazette (30 March 1920): 3822.

Voluntary Aid Rendered to the Sick and Wounded at Home and Abroad and to British Prisoners of War, 1914–1919. London: HMSO, 1919.

'The War Library', *The Red Cross* (December 1917): 166.

Warrender, Maud. *My First Sixty Years*. London: Cassell, 1933.

Widdowson, Peter. *Literature*. London: Routledge, 1999.

Woolf, Virginia. *The Diary of Virginia Woolf, Volume One: 1915–1919*, edited by Anne Olivier Bell. Orlando, FL: Harcourt, 1977.

Yeaxlee, Basil. 'Libraries and Adult Education in Rural Areas', *Library Association Record* 23 (April 1921): 89–101.

Part III

Contemporary Critical Interventions

9 The Bibliotherapy Novel

Representations of Literary Caregiving and the Crisis of Print Culture, 1919–2019

Jesse Miller

In *Bring on the Books for Everybody: How Literary Culture Became Popular Culture*, Jim Collins argues that the rise of digital media in the twenty-first century has not signaled the end of literary culture, as defenders of print have often worried, but rather has enabled its transformation into a new form of popular culture.[1] Rather than replacing literature, new technologies and infrastructures (like e-readers, online social book reviewing platforms, and big box bookstores) have changed how and where people read literary fiction. These material changes have been accompanied by a redefinition of why people read. Against the backdrop of anxious assessments about the crisis of print and the shrinking number of serious readers, we find a growing community of twenty-first-century book devotees who, contra longstanding academic pronunciations against passionate, affective, identificatory reading, turn to literature for an emotionally transformative, therapeutic experience.[2] Readers are encouraged and validated in such therapeutically motivated reading by articles with titles like 'Why Reading Books Makes You a Better Person, According to Science,' which speaks of 'readers report[ing] being less stressed and less depressed, and having higher levels of self-esteem and a greater ability to cope with challenges,'[3] and 'Dickens Better for Mental Health than Self-Help Books,' which suggests that 'classic works of literature by William Shakespeare, Charles Dickens and other great writers can boost your brain and relieve depression, chronic pain and dementia.'[4] To select their next read, they might browse through *The Novel Cure: An A to Z of Literary Remedies*, a literary reference guide organized around literary cures for serious as well as playful ailments such as 'abandonment,' 'coffee, can't find a decent cup of,' and 'zestlessness.'[5] Or they might book a virtual appointment for a bibliotherapy consultation through the London-based The School of Life for a custom book prescription. Or they might pay a visit to Oh Hello Again bookshop in Seattle, Washington, which 'specializes in bibliotherapy, or using books to help with life's various problems,' and whose shelves are organized by malady.[6] Even the books they select might self-consciously advocate these very literary values. As Collins writes, 'The use value of reading quality fiction – what we read it *for* – has become a central issue in novels that insist on their ability to perform a vitally important function.'[7] In a growing number of popular novels that feature characters who see themselves – like the audience

DOI: 10.4324/9781003471561-13

to whom such books are marketed – as self-consciously literary, 'we find literary fiction insisting on its therapeutic value.'[8]

While Collins notes a range of contemporary fiction that exhibits these values, nowhere is this trend more apparent than in the international spate of recent novels that feature bibliotherapists as characters helping their customers become more healthy by crafting identities as literary selves, including the *New York Times* Bestseller *The Little Paris Bookshop* (2015) (originally published as *Das lavendelzimmer* in 2013) by German novelist Nina George[9] and the Vince Corso series (including *La lettrice scomparsa* [*The Missing Reader*] (2016), *Ogni coincidenza ha un'anima* [*Every Coincidence Has a Soul*] (2018), and *Uccido chi voglio* [*I Kill Who I Want*] (2020)) by Italian novelist Fabio Stassi.[10] These bibliotherapy novels are set in worlds where the value of literature has been put into question and that place literary caregiving at their thematic center. Haslam and King describe 'literary caregiving' to be the empathetic provision of literature as a palliative for readers' mental and emotional needs.[11] With plots shaped around ills in need of a cure, these novels represent such practices of literary caregiving, drawing on the language of medicine to describe individual and social problems, and self-reflexively exploring the usefulness of reading literature as a therapy particularly well suited to addressing such problems. In offering up these representations of literary caregiving, bibliotherapy novels participate in the refunctioning of literature at a time when print culture is seen to be in crisis, elevating it to the status of medicine, insisting on its power to change readers, and sanctioning personal, passionate, therapeutic reading.

The reasons for the growth in these contemporary discourses and practices of bibliotherapeutic reading are many. They include the waning influence of the academy on matters of taste, the convergence of print and digital media, the impact of neoliberalism and its free market policies on culture, and the growth and global circulation of a wellness discourse that insists upon the individual's responsibility towards maximizing their wellbeing.[12] But its roots are in the early twentieth-century United States, in which we find transformations to which our current moment forms an echo: a waning influence of religious institutions and values and the search for new social norms and definitions of the good life, the confluence of print with film and radio, and the concomitant rise of mass forms of media, the specialization of literary studies as it distinguished itself from unprofessional modes of reading, the emergence of consumer capitalism, and developments in the science of mind including therapeutic practices aimed at promoting mental health. These changes came together to form what the sociologist Philip Rieff termed 'therapeutic culture.'[13] It makes sense, then, that the term bibliotherapy was first coined in print in 1916.[14] Medicalized language about literature's potentially harmful effect on readers has long accompanied transformations in print culture, reflecting anxieties about the impact of media on the bodies and minds of its audience.[15] From the beginning of the twentieth century, the discourse of bibliotherapy has responded to this tendency, insisting that if we read in the right way, literature can offer a therapeutic respite from the contemporary, media-saturated, mental pathology-producing world.

Rather than simply engaging in a critique of this trend and its reduction of literature to a therapeutic tool and of social problems to individual pathologies, here I explore the therapeutic culture within and through which literary caregiving holds such meaning today. In describing books as medicine, how do bibliotherapy novels rearticulate the drama of life: its characters, its trials, its equipment, its aims, and its ends?[16] What forms of life do they make imaginable and unimaginable? Studying literature is an important part of the project of understanding literary caregiving and therapeutic culture more generally, both because literature is transformed within this culture (including what one reads, how one reads, and why one reads) and because literature is one of the modes through which this set of beliefs and values is articulated, transmitted, solicited, and challenged. In this chapter, I examine the representation of literary caregiving in fiction, arguing that in drawing on medical metaphors to stage debates about the value of literature, fiction about therapeutic reading actively participates in the refunctioning of literary value, offering a vision of literary care against the backdrop of a perceived crisis of print culture. The chapter shows how these bibliotherapy narratives make a case for the continued importance of print literature, drawing on the popular genre of the detective tale to link aesthetic experience to the diagnosis, care for, and cure of individual and collective ills. Concurrently, in emphasizing the relationship between reading and wellbeing, they participate in the construction of a therapeutic subject, for whom discovering a deep, 'authentic', desiring self, and maintaining and maximizing the mental and emotional health of that self, is at the centre of the project of achieving the good life.[17]

I begin by tracing the bibliotherapy novel back to the early twentieth century, to American writer Christopher Morley's *The Haunted Bookshop* (1919). Not only is this seldom-studied novel the first to feature a bibliotherapist as a character, but it also exemplifies the way the discourse of literary care offered a narrative response to social, political, and economic problems. I follow this by analyzing Nina George's *The Little Paris Bookshop* and Fabio Stassi's short story 'The Shape of an Island,' part of his larger Vince Corso novel series, demonstrating how they transpose many of the same thematic concerns and formal features from Morley's work to insist upon the value of literature in the digital age. This chapter thus supplements growing recent work on the history of therapeutic reading by insisting upon literature as an important site for examining the way metaphors and narratives motivate, shape, script, and comment upon material sites and practices of reading as they circulate through time and across Western cultures.

Detecting the beginnings of the bibliotherapy novel

Book historian Roger Darnton argues that looking to representations of reading can provide information about the 'ideals and assumptions underlying reading in the past,' which led people to invest themselves in literature and shaped the ways that they did so.[18] An important part of such representations is the metaphors through which reading is described. These imply certain attitudes towards the act of reading and a set of beliefs about how and why one should read. These in turn shape lived practices of reading. As Lakoff and Johnson write in *Metaphors We Live By*,

> Metaphors may create realities for us, especially social realities. A metaphor may thus be a future action. Such actions will, of course, fit the metaphor. This will in turn reinforce the power of the metaphor to make experience coherent. In this sense, metaphors can be self-fulfilling prophecies.[19]

As Darnton points out, in eighteenth century Germany, commentators used metaphors of health and illness, diet and digestion, to describe reading, thus indicating a belief in reading's physical effects on the reader, and in the morally important work of regulating such effects.[20] The metaphor of books as medicine implies a whole worldview regarding literature in which readers are patients afflicted by some kind of illness; reading is an improving, therapeutic practice by which the reader can move towards their goal of health; and the authorities who guide readers in proper, therapeutic reading are doctors or bibliotherapists. These tropes of literary care set certain constraints on the kinds of narratives through which we talk about and enact reading. What kinds of phenomenon are considered ills treatable by literature, what kinds of literature can treat those ills, and what is considered health will vary from one instance to another, shaped by a range of cultural and historical factors. But the story that literature's value inheres in its capacity to transform a reader from a negative state to a positive one (when the right thing is read properly), is always implied when a book is described as medicine. Analyzing works of fiction that dramatize these tropes of literary care thus offers insight into this particular vision of literature's value.

The history of the novel features many different kinds of plots about readers. Often, as in the case of Cervantes' *Don Quixote,* Austen's *Northanger Abbey,* and Flaubert's *Madame Bovary*, these novels about novel readers highlight the dangers of improper reading. They tell stories of characters who, in reading too passionately, lose a sense of distinction between themselves and the characters they love, and thus between fantasy and reality. As Karen Littau points out, such narratives exhibit the fear that

> if novel reading is processed sensually, through the body, the danger is that readers might switch off their minds, allow themselves to be absorbed so utterly in the fiction, and identify so closely with what they read that they might well succumb, animally, to its pleasures.[21]

And so in featuring such readers as characters, these novels offer their actual readers guidance in how they should and should not read. Novels about bibliotherapists similarly offer their readers guidance. But their plots focus not on the dangers of reading too passionately, but rather on the healthful benefits of passionate reading, when properly carried out. This is demonstrated in American writer Christopher Morley's *The Haunted Bookshop*.[22] The novel is set in the wake of the First World War and tells the story of the unlikely friendship between

Roger Mifflin, a genteel, anti-modern seller of second-hand books, and a self-styled bibliotherapist, and Aubrey Gilbert, a young modern adman. Together with the beautiful, wealthy young shop assistant Titania Chapman, they stumble upon and ultimately thwart a pro-German plot to assassinate President Wilson, who is bound for the Peace Conference at Versailles. They believe that through the provision of good books, they are inoculating the world against another bout of violent madness.[23] Along the way, they find ample time to debate the value of literature in modern America.

Christopher Morley was himself interested in the place of literature in early twentieth-century life. Cultural historian Joan Shelley Rubin describes him as a middlebrow cultural mediator.[24] He was a highly educated man of letters who sought to uphold the literary values of the Genteel Tradition against the rising tide of modern mass culture while making those values accessible to a broadening public of middle-class readers anxious to distinguish themselves from the masses by becoming cultured, but unsure of how.[25] As Rubin describes Morley's middlebrow blend of genteel and modern sensibilities, Morley embodied 'an animus toward modernism and commerce coupled with a facility for advertising and a personal and literary style that represented departures from Arnoldian understandings of culture and criticism.'[26] Born in 1890 in Haverford, Pennsylvania, he enrolled in Haverford College in 1906 and after graduating traveled to the UK where he attended Oxford as a Rhodes Scholar from 1910 to 1913. At that time, he returned to the US and began working as an entry-level editor for the publisher Doubleday. During these years, he became acquainted with the business side of literary creation, a knowledge of which he was later to integrate into his representations of book culture in his successful early novels. Over the course of his career, he was a columnist for the *New York Evening Post*, an editor of *Ladies' Home Journal*, a founder of the *Saturday Review of Books*, and an original member of the Book-of-the-Month-Club selection committee. He was also a prolific writer of novels, essay collections, and poetry, and a gregarious figure in the scene of artists and intellectuals based around Greenwich Village, especially in the 1920s and 1930s when he frequented the famous Gotham Book Mart and organized social groups such as the Three Hours for Lunch Club and later the Baker Street Irregulars. The latter, founded in 1934, was a group of passionate readers of Arthur Conan Doyle's Sherlock Holmes stories who, led by Morley, engaged in the pretense that the famous detective was a real historical figure. They held parties and conferences in honor of their role model and wrote books and essays mock-seriously celebrating and studying Holmes' life.[27] Their playful emulation of the detective, the mingling of high and low culture, and the blurring of the distinctions between fantasy and reality are all found first in *The Haunted Bookshop,* Morley's novel exploring the healing power of books.

The metaphor of literature as medicine is at the core of this novel. Morley's protagonist Roger Mifflin is a 'practitioner of bibliotherapy.'[28] At the entrance of his bookshop, a sign reads, 'malnutrition of the reading faculty is a serious thing. Let us prescribe for you.'[29] Roger sees books as a form of medicine, and the role of the bookseller as that of a kind of medical specialist, prescribing books in response to the particular mental and emotional illnesses of his customers, just as a doctor prescribes medicine for physical illnesses. As literary scholar Jaime Harker has argued, in his role of literary doctor of the mind and emotions, Roger is representative of the aspirations of the middlebrow cultural mediator, with his faith in the power of books to 'educate, ennoble, and transform.'[30] But if, for Roger, books can improve their readers, this is understood not only in cultural and moral terms, but psychological and medical ones as well. That people are suffering grave psychological ills is evident to Roger as he reflects on the Great War. The social, economic, and technological conditions of modern life have made people ill. Roger believes the war itself was caused by a kind of widespread mental illness, in which violent instinct overpowered the healthy human restraint that undergirds civilization:

> The terrific catastrophe of the war has made [people] realize that their minds are ill. The world was suffering from all sorts of mental fevers and aches and disorders, and we never knew it. Now our mental pangs are only too manifest. We are all reading, hungrily, hastily, trying to find out – after the trouble is over – what was the matter with our minds.[31]

By housing the ghosts of the past, 'the hopes and gentlenesses and dreams of men and women,' he believes literature can provide readers with the imaginative equipment they need to better themselves, to overcome their base impulses, and survive in the modern world.[32] Thus, he proclaims, 'I think the bookseller can play as useful a part as any man in rebuilding the world's sanity.'[33] But in the wake of the war, he wonders whether humans possess such a capacity for sanity any longer.

In the novel's opening chapters, the focus of the drama is on Roger's attempts to convince others of the therapeutic value of literature. He wants to offer literary cures to his customers, and also to cure his own crisis of faith in the virtues of humanity. In framing bookselling as a medical practice, he stakes a claim against his fellow booksellers, who treat literature as a mere commodity. When one jokes that Roger is 'confusing merchandise with metaphysics,'[34] he insists, 'my mind would blow out its fuses if I had to abide by the dirty little considerations of supply and demand.'[35] He also insists on the value of books against the newly popular medium of cinema. Speaking of the effects that engaging with cultural products can have on the health of the audience, Roger warns his young female assistant Titania about the false cures that cinema offers to its spectators. Like following a dietary regimen, at its most successful – that is, when it is with 'real grain'[36] or real art – the act of consuming media enables one to transform one's life for the better. But Roger explains that these consumers are let down when they turn to mass forms of entertainment, such as the cinema, to achieve sustenance. Although the masses seldom realize it, far from nutritious, mass culture consists only of 'paltry husks':

> They think they're amused because they don't know what real amusement is! Laughter and prayer are the two noblest habits of man; they mark us off from the brutes. To laugh at cheap jests is as base as to pray to cheap gods. To laugh at Fatty Arbuckle is to degrade the human spirit.[37]

According to Roger, what motivates the cinema-goer is the legitimate desire to satisfy a longing for 'the things that comfort and console and make life seem worth while.'[38] But, reflecting his middlebrow perspective, it is only through reading quality, literary books, he believes, that people's psychological needs can be truly satisfied.

Roger, then, would likely not be a fan of *The Haunted Bookshop*, which, as a detective thriller, itself takes the form of a mass cultural genre.[39] As the story progresses, it takes on more and more qualities of an action film as the characters discover that, despite the war's conclusion, the health of the world is still uncertain. Two German spies, masquerading as a pharmacist and a chef, plan to assassinate President Wilson by planting a bomb disguised as a book on the ship that is meant to take him to the Peace Conference at Versailles. The German pharmacist, Dr. Weintraub, is the dark foil to Roger. Where Roger has transformed his bookstore into a pharmacy, prescribing books to fulfill the needs of his patients' battered souls, and to treat those illnesses that led to the civilization-destroying war, Dr. Weintraub represents those violent symptoms of modernity as he transforms his pharmacy into a laboratory in which books are literally hollowed out and turned into bombs. As the narrative demonstrates, the necessary literary cure is not to escape from modernity through the genteel, spiritualizing pleasures of literature. Instead, what is necessary is to play the part of the detective, diving full-bodied into the dangerously enervating modern world of cars and trains, movies and machines, telephones and electric lights, advertising and adventure. This is what happens when Roger and Aubrey get caught up in the plot. Middle-class Aubrey, driven by his desire for Titania, the daughter of a rich businessman, follows what he's learned from movies and advertising to trace the German plot and thwart their destructive plans. In the end, the health of his beloved Titania and of the country secured, he becomes 'the hero of this film.'[40]

As a result of his participation in this adventure, Roger comes to a new appreciation of the culture and technology of modernity, as Titania's father agrees to support his dream of owning a fleet of bookmobiles to bring bookselling to the people. Cleaning up his shop, he proclaims, 'This is just what I needed. I was getting into a rut […] I'm thinking seriously of putting in a vacuum cleaner and a cash register. Titania was quite right, the place was too dirty.'[41] Modern technology, in this conclusion, is found to be a support of literary culture, not its enemy. He also comes to a new understanding of the relationship between health and literature. If illness, in this novel, is associated with the violent impulses of war, sanity is associated with peace. Contra Woodrow Wilson's nationalist, isolationist 'America First' policy, Roger embraces the slogan 'America Last' as a necessary part of the return of world peace and sanity, and prays for 'some new conception of national neighbourhood' one which requires 'some new realization of the sanctity of life – all life, animal as well as human.'[42] Such a realization, he believes, will spring from an awareness that the vitality of all living things is, paradoxically, rooted in the universal dis-ease of desire, whose motive power impels all beings from insects to humans:

> What is it that we find in every form of life? Desire of some sort – some unexplained motive power that impels even the smallest insect on its queer travels.

> You must have watched some infinitesimal red spider on a fence rail, bustling along – why and whither? Who knows? And when you come to man, what a chaos of hungers and impulses keep thrusting him through his cycle of quaint tasks.[43]

While he confesses that the attempt to alleviate 'mental fevers and aches and disorders' is a valid, and perhaps even universal one, 'that the mind should actually be satisfied would prove that it exists only as idiocy!'[44] This new account of human sanity, of the human as a member of a larger collectivity of vital beings all fundamentally disabled by their ineradicable desire, rejects the distinction between noble, spiritually enlightened human, and violent, instinctual, brute, to which he had clung earlier in the novel. Such distinctions, he realizes, led to the war, 'the brute mass-impulse, the pride and national spirit, the instinctive simplicity of men that make them worship what is their own above everything else.'[45] What is necessary is not the genteel repression of embodied desire, but rather a therapeutic channeling and sublimation of it towards healthy ends – something he comes to believe that reading can facilitate.

What is Morley's purpose in placing his bibliotherapist into such a plot? In part, this is a commentary by Morley about literary taste, an insistence on the value of popular genres like detective fiction, despite the lack of respect they receive from highbrow professional readers like academics and book reviewers. This is the same impulse behind his founding of the Baker Street Irregulars. But the form of the detective genre is itself significant. By framing anti-social actions as pathological impulses, the plot melds the typical trajectory of a detective tale, which proceeds from mystery to enlightenment and crime to justice, with a therapeutic trajectory, a transformation from illness to health. The reader is invited into this process, the carefully designed detective plot stimulating the motive force of their desire to reach the conclusion while empowering that reader with a sense of authorship over those desires as they attempt to solve the case along with the book's characters, albeit from a safe vantage point. When they put down the book and plunge back into the modern world of consumer culture, it is as literary selves, leading characters of their own lives.[46] In making this claim I am suggesting, by contrast to Joan Shelley Rubin's account of *The Haunted Bookshop*, that more than just 'us[ing] a mystery plot as a framework for literary allusions, recommendations, and remarks on the function of reading,' we might see this novel's engagement with popular genre fiction as central to Morley's populist vision of therapeutic reading.[47]

The bibliotherapy novel in translation

If, for a long time, Morley's Roger Mifflin was the only self-consciously styled bibliotherapist to appear within the pages of a novel, in recent years he has been joined by an international cast of fictional, therapeutic booksellers, responding, despite the century that separates them, with surprisingly similar tools to similar anxieties about the future of print culture. Where Roger worried over the degenerating effects of cinema, billboards, and rising consumerism, today it is global neoliberalism and the alienating, over-connecting, hyper-distracting internet against which a new generation of fictional literary caregivers sets to work with their pharmaceutical libraries. I will discuss two contrasting examples here. My argument is not that these characters, and the contemporary texts they inhabit, are direct translations or derivations of Morley's novel, though it is possible that it was an influence. Instead, I want to suggest that by featuring bibliotherapist protagonists and using the book-as-medicine metaphor as a guiding trope in their stories, contemporary authors express a certain common attitude towards the power of literature in response to a media environment in flux. This is dramatized through a somewhat constrained range of narrative possibilities, their plots driven by efforts to induce therapeutic transformations from illness to health. And yet, as Morley's novel makes clear, there is more than one way for books to be medicinal. The tropes and narratives of literary caregiving, while supplying a framework of possibility, are in these two examples enacted as different kinds of narratives, with distinct models of care and visions of literature's therapeutic value in the technologically-mediated, globalized present.

Nina George's *The Little Paris Bookshop* highlights the persistence of many of the tropes of literary care featured in Christopher Morley's novel. First published in German in 2013 and translated into English in 2015, it tells the story of Jean Perdu, a bibliotherapist who has largely cut himself off from personal attachments in the twenty years since his lover died. Like Roger in *The Haunted Bookshop,* Jean is suspicious of modern technology, rejecting e-book readers and cellular phones as harmful distractions. And like Roger at the end of *The Haunted Bookshop*, Jean owns a mobile bookstore, *The Literary Apothecary.* It's a barge loaded with books and other literary trinkets, moored on the Seine in Paris at the novel's beginning. But the novel's plot mainly follows Jean's travels on the book barge down south and into Provence. The ideas about literature espoused by Jean draw on the metaphor of books as medicine to articulate the idea that reading literature can positively impact readers, fulfilling their emotional needs and transforming their lives. As he puts it, 'A book is both medic and medicine at once. It makes a diagnosis as well as offering therapy. Putting the right novels to the appropriate ailments: that's how I sell books.'[48] Thus, far more than just offering his customers information or entertainment, the bookseller's lofty aim is 'to treat feelings that are not recognized as afflictions and are never diagnosed by doctors.'[49] Books, according to Jean, do not just replace conventional therapy, they are 'the only remedy for countless, undefined afflictions of the soul.'[50] And so he 'sell[s] books like medicine,' recommending particular titles to customers according to their individual needs.[51] In this way, his approach to bookselling emphasizes a distinction between literature and other commodities. While Jean sells all sorts of literary knick-knacks on his book barge, from mystery novel-themed toilet paper to salt and pepper shakers shaped like author busts, he is regretful of this commodification of literature. 'Using [books] as currency didn't come easily to him,' the narrator explains, 'for he knew their true worth.'[52]

Though not a detective novel like *The Haunted Bookshop*, *The Little Paris Bookshop* is structured around a locked room, a dead body, and a mystery. The body is that of Jean's lover, Manon, who died of cancer twenty years before the start of the novel. Unable to process his grief, Jean has locked the room in his apartment where he and Manon had spent much of their time together and has cut himself off from emotional attachments and any sensual pleasures that might remind him of her. The only thing that has helped him is reading a book called *Southern Lights.* And here is the mystery: though he would like to thank the author for this book which has been for him 'a homeopathic dose of happiness [...] the only balm that could ease Jean's pain,' it was published under a mysterious pseudonym.[53] So he sets off from Paris on *The Literary Apothecary* to the south of France finally to visit Manon's grave, and to discover the true identity of *Southern Lights'* author. From here on, the book takes on the form of a quest, in which the protagonist seeks out a significant object, with a variety of challengers and helpers he meets along the way. This journey enacts a conceptual crossing from the urban, technology-filled world of Paris, characterized by the mind, habit, and numbness, to the rural world of Provence, characterized by freedom and the pleasures of the body. This crossing is dramatized through Jean's therapeutic transformation, his processing of grief, and his coming to acknowledge fresh desires and appreciate embodied existence, from physical exertion to eating to sex.

The novel traces a transformation not only of Jean but of his understanding of literature. Early in the novel, he expresses his belief in 'The boundless possibilities offered by books. They would always be enough. They would never stop loving their readers. They were a fixed point in an otherwise unpredictable world.' But over the course of his journey, he realizes that he had come to rely on books too much, valuing them more than his relationships with other people. Thus, he concludes, 'Books can do many things, but not everything. We have to live the important things, not read them. I have to ... experience my book.'[54] While reading is an important part of his therapeutic transformation, he realizes he ultimately must move beyond books to experience, becoming the protagonist of his own life.

The generic conventions of the mystery and quest that George writes through do not only shape this narrative. They model a particular way of relating to the world, of shaping one's life as narrative: to live as a protagonist oriented by the pull of desire, plunging into the world to seek the solution for puzzles, the object of quests. As George explains in an interview, she imagines her novel as a kind of medicine:

> [*The Little Paris Bookshop*] is both a kind of cleansing and a literary form of solace. It penetrates areas of the soul where old and grand emotions are hidden. Grief, melancholy, regrets that we are not sixteen anymore, compassion, the desire to be loved by our parents, finding the place where we feel whole, and understanding the fears in our dreams. The book cleanses these wounds – and above all, it provides solace.[55]

It is significant, then, that the novel contains as paratexts both 'Jean Perdu's Emergency Literary Pharmacy,' a list of books mentioned within the novel, framed as 'fast-acting medicines for minds and hearts affected by minor or moderate emotional turmoil,'[56] and a list of recipes for dishes typical of Provence, to where Jean travels in the novel. Here we have both medic and medicine, the labelling and privileging of mundane discontents as illnesses and the offering of books and food as their cure. The reader is in this way invited to take part in the experiences depicted within the novel, to plunge both into books and other sensuous experiences in the world. Reading and eating share not only a common descriptive vocabulary of taste and consumption but are placed on an even footing as meaningful, sensuous, curative experiences.

Like Christopher Morley and Nina George, Italian writer Fabio Stassi has also created a fictional universe around the practice of bibliotherapy. His dramatization of bibliotherapy over the course of a series of novels shares many similarities with that of the other two authors. Like them, he draws on the language of medicine to describe books, and his dramas are driven by plots about cases in need of cure mingled with mysteries in need of solving. But Stassi, and his bibliotherapist protagonist, are more ambivalent about the power of literature to bring happiness. That protagonist is Vince Corso, a middle-aged man living in Rome who, after losing his job as a teacher of Italian and literature, invents a new career for himself: bibliotherapy. In the course of meeting patients, listening to their stories, and prescribing them stories, Corso is often thrust into the role of detective solving mysteries. There is indeed something of the hardboiled private eye about him: the simple direct style of his narration, his pessimism about the world and the possibility of enacting meaningful change within it.

Vince is a witness to the suffering and sadness his patients endure, himself a victim of these same pains, this same sense of inadequacy, the result of living in a highly imperfect world. In response to his patients' cry '*Help me, Mr. Corso,*'[57] he offers care in the form of literature. 'Don't worry' he tells one patient 'whatever your distress may be, at some point in time a writer has written about it. All you need to do is go to a bookstore.'[58] But Vince is ambivalent about the whole practice. While he might be passionate about reading, he also 'know[s] in advance that [he] wouldn't be able to fix their problems.'[59] Worse, he realizes from experience that reading literature might give rise to new problems, offering readers unrealizable fantasies and taking them away from, rather than closer to, vibrant, lived experience in the world. This has been the case for Vince, who, like the other fictional bibliotherapists, is haunted by ghosts of the past captured in the pages of books:

> I've been living in a universe overrun with ghosts for a long time now. My memory is flooded with indices, title pages, and back covers. It has lost the shape and borders of its tangible experience. Every book that I read takes me farther away.[60]

But while this may lead Vince to see himself as something of an imposter, parading under the title of professional while peddling imperfect cures, he is not entirely cynical about his aims. 'I continue to love literature recklessly,' he insists.

> I continue to welcome my patients and explain – for whatever it might be worth – that no act is more human than reading and that even unintentional

> reading can be medicinal. But the words of others can't save you if they don't become your own.[61]

So, if reading literature isn't able to fix readers' problems and make them happy, why does Vince continue to prescribe books to patients? What is Stassi's vision of literary care? This comes across clearly in his story 'The Shape of an Island.'[62] In this story, Vince is visited by a lawyer, Orlando, who is seeking help with a family problem. He is distraught over discovering that his son is deeply depressed and has barely left his room in two years. He seeks insight from the bibliotherapist. Can Vince help him understand how this disaster came to be? Can Vince tell him what went wrong, and whether he is to blame? By turning to literature, he can. The story follows Vince's bibliotherapy session, in which he listens to Orlando's story of his son and their relationship, and, with some careful detective work to deduce the proper literary prescription, offers up literature that provides a new vantage point from which to understand the situation. His suggestions, Japanese novelist Furukawa Hideo's *Belka* and Sicilian essayist Gesualdo Bufalino's 'Light and Mourning,' reveal an unexpected connection between Japanese and Sicilian cultures, and between the Japanese epidemic of *hikikomori* – people stricken by an intense form of social withdrawal – and Orlando's son's own mental ailment. The story concludes with the revelation that Orlando had, just before visiting Vince, murdered his son out of guilt, a sense that he was the cause of his son's failures and that those failures reflect his own. But Vince had deduced this long before. In the end, Vince may not have cured his patient, but he does solve the case.

As the ending highlights, the story is in many ways a classic detective tale. As with Roger, Aubrey, and Titania in *The Haunted Bookshop*, Vince is like a private detective who, presented with a case, uses careful observation of the facts available to him to identify the culprit of the crime that has been committed. In drawing on generic conventions of the detective story, Stassi plays with the relationship between detective and medical cases, as can be seen in the following exchange:

> 'Is it true that you have a solution for every case you encounter?'
> 'My cases are psychological. I don't solve them. I merely offer literary remedies.'
> 'Remedies for what exactly?'
> 'For my patients' unhappiness. I suggest novels, that's all.'

In both detective and medical cases, a professional is faced with an individual who has transgressed norms (of health or of the law), and it is that professional's role to restore order. In a detective tale, that transgression is a crime, and the detective must use careful observation to assign a motive and identify the culprit. These are the terms in which Orlando poses the medical problem to Vince: 'this situation is a puzzle, or as you might prefer to call it, a crime with no apparent motive.' In a medical case, the transgression is a pathology, and the doctor's job is to bring the patient back to normal health. The bibliotherapist accomplishes this by diagnosing the malady and prescribing 'literary remedies.' In this story, Vince attempts to do both.

But Stassi thwarts genre conventions. While a classic detective tale is resolved when the detective identifies the culprit, fixing blame and criminality on an individual criminal, Vince insists instead on social causes for the transgressions at the heart of this case. His interest is in understanding the social causes that have led Orlando's son to socially withdraw, and Orlando to commit an act of murder. 'It seems to me that it would be a dangerous mistake to connect everything back to the family or to a single individual, in this case, to the father,' Vince says.

> To explain your son's voluntary exile, I would say that today's mental breakdowns are, for the most part, caused by social ills, rather than individual or family ones [… .] The stability of the system rests on the emotional instability of the people who live within it, and especially on young people.

Orlando resists this reframing of his narrative, which removes him from the center of the story. He insists on the importance of 'individual responsibility.' But, just as Roger had discovered in reflecting on the nationalist ideology that led to the violence of the First World War in *The Haunted Bookshop*, Vince posits that it is precisely Orlando's self-centeredness that makes him heir to the impulses behind the Second World War, and that led him to murder:

> What you couldn't accept was your sense of guilt. Your son was the incarnation of that guilt. He was the reflection of your own sick need to be the start and finish of every single thing. He was a heroic reply to your idiotic presumption of believing you were God.

Noting Vince's emphasis on the social forces driving individual behavior (criminal and pathological) is important for understanding the model of literary care put forward by Stassi. In this story, literature is more diagnostic than directly therapeutic. It offers insight not just into unnamed feelings, but into the culture from which those feelings and the literature that describes them emerge, by mapping the relationship between a society and the tendencies of its inhabitants. Reading literature thus offers new frames through which to see the world and to act within it. Stassi, then, does not celebrate the curative power of literature in the same way that George does. Where George's novel describes books as offering readers pleasurable, sensuous experiences akin to eating, Stassi's stories treat literature much more cognitively. Words, and the stories that they form, have an effect, an impact that is intensely personal. But this is less about sensual pleasure than it is about meaning. Readers transform works of literature by bringing their own meaning to it, and they are shaped by these meanings in turn. The illness to be cured in Stassi's bibliotherapy is not emotional numbness, but narcissism. Thus, he states, 'Reading, for me, has always been a way of taking stock of my own limitations.'[63] In this account, literature helps the reader see beyond the individual perspective, offering insight into culture, the shared, symbolic worlds of meaning that shape how and why people act. Through literary care, Stassi proposes, readers can follow writers in transforming that culture, rewriting one's personal narrative by challenging the rules and conventions that govern them. When Orlando asks him 'Do you really believe that books can help?' He replies, 'I'm certain of it. Everything can be rewritten in literature.'

Conclusion: A world of healthy book people

Placing these three bibliotherapy narratives side-by-side reveals the persistence of tropes of literary care across time and space. Despite their differences, these stories insist upon literature's transformative power through the language of medicine, of doctors and patients, and of health and illness. They draw on a popular genre, the detective story, to plot the movement from illness to health, maximize their reach, and articulate their understanding of the relationship between literature, reader, and the world. The circulation of these tropes not only across time, but geographically, offers evidence of the international spread of bibliotherapeutic accounts of literary value and, more broadly, of a specifically American, therapeutic culture, including a form of therapeutic subjectivity in which identity is rooted not in nationality, but in deep, individual desires.[64] Indeed, the stories themselves emphasize literature's power in promoting connections and relationships across national borders based upon shared, essential forms of psychological need. While they tell stories that are grounded in place and culture, they promote universalizing notions of desire and healing that offer the possibility of reaching across national divides. Nina George articulates this worldview in an interview, explaining:

> There is a dedicated community of people in the world who will always be able to connect with each other across all languages, boundaries, and religions. It is the 'Readers' Club.' People who read a lot, starting at a very young age, are people who were raised by books. They have learned about forms of love and hate, kindness, respect, and ideas that are different from their own. They experience the world as something infinitely larger than before. They enjoy the indescribable feeling of having found their true selves. We readers are book people.[65]

Analyzing these bibliotherapy novels has offered insight into just this worldview, which relies on a particular set of metaphors and narratives by which to articulate, validate, and promote the values and practices of such book people. This vision of literary care includes the belief that literature is a uniquely valuable kind of commodity, that its future is threatened by newer forms of inferior media, that mental and emotional issues are a significant problem in need of novel solutions, that one can and should read for pleasure, that when the correct books are read in the right way that pleasure can transform one's thoughts and feelings for the better, that what is considered good to read is dependent on these therapeutic effects, that those effects are specific to the individual reader and their needs, and that readers can be guided in selecting the right books by knowledgeable, empathetic authorities. While sensitive to the social and technological conditions giving rise to readers' discontent, analysis of the bibliotherapy novel shows how this worldview of literary care displaces structural inequality and global power struggles to contemporary media and their intimate effects, its horizon of cure ending at the fantasy life of the individual. More than just mapping this bibliotherapeutic worldview, though, I want to suggest that by attending to creative writers' working in language, we gain insight into the language that constitutes our world, such as the language of the therapeutic – a language that not only describes the world but also frames it in particular ways, soliciting identification and offering an orientation on the world and the problems it poses, the characters we might play, the motives we might be guided by, and the plots we might enact.

Notes

1 Jim Collins, *Bring on the Books for Everybody: How Literary Culture Became Popular Culture* (Durham: Duke University Press, 2010).

2 See, for example, Sven Birkerts, *Changing the Subject: Art and Attention in the Internet Age* (Minneapolis, MN: Graywolf Press, 2015); Ted Striphas, *The Late Age of Print: Everyday Book Culture from Consumerism to Control* (New York: Columbia University Press, 2009).

3 Christina Desmarais,"Why Reading Books Makes You a Better Person, According to Science," *Inc.*, July 3, 2018, www.inc.com/christina-desmarais/why-reading-books-makes-you-a-better-person-according-to-science.html.

4 Andrew Gregory, "The Pick-me-up Papers: Dickens better for mental health than self-help books," *The Times*, March 1, 2020, www.thetimes.co.uk/article/the-pick-me-up-papers-dickens-better-for-mental-health-than-self-help-books-bn9xd88j2.

5 Ella Berthoud and Susan Elderkin, *The Novel Cure From Abandonment to Zestlessness: 751 Books to Cure What Ails You* (New York: Penguin Books, 2014).

6 'FAQs', Oh Hello Again Bookshop, accessed February 19, 2021, https://web.archive.org/web/20220523053656/https://ohhelloagain.com/pages/faqs

7 Collins, *Bring on the Books*, 4.

8 Collins, *Bring on the Books*, 5.

9 Nina George, *The Little Paris Bookshop*, trans. Simon Pare (New York: Broadway Books, 2015).

10 Fabio Stassi, *La lettrice scomparsa* [*The Missing Reader*] (Palermo: Sellerio editore, 2016). Fabio Stassi, *Every Coincidence Has a Soul,* Unpublished Manuscript, trans. Oonagh Stransky 2021. *Ogni coincidenza ha un'anima* (Palermo: Sellerio editore, 2018). Fabio Stassi, *Uccido chi voglio* [*I Kill Who I Want*] (Palermo: Sellerio editore, 2020). Other examples of contemporary bibliotherapy novels featuring representations of literary caregiving include Ellery Adams, *The Secret, Book & Scone Society* (New York: Kensington Books, 2017); Jenny Colgan, *The Bookshop on the Corner* (New York: William Morrow, 2016); Laurence Cossé, *A Novel Bookstore*, trans. Alison Anderson (New York: Europa Editions, 2010); Veronica Henry, *How to Find Love in a Bookshop* (New York: Pamela Dorman Books, 2017); Matthew Sullivan, *Midnight at the Bright Ideas Bookstore* (New York: Scribner, 2017); and Michaël Uras, *Aux petits mots, les grands remèdes* [*Take Two Chapters and Call Me in the Morning]* (Paris: Préludes, 2020).

11 Sara Haslam and Edmund G. C. King, '"Medicinable Literature": Bibliotherapy, Literary Caregiving, and the First World War', *Literature and Medicine* 39, no. 2 (2021), 296–318.

12 On the rise of therapeutic modes of reading, see Timothy Aubry, *Reading as Therapy: What Contemporary Fiction Does for Middle-Class Americans* (Iowa City: University of Iowa Press, 2011); Beth Blum, *The Self-Help Compulsion: Searching for Advice in Modern Literature* (New York: Columbia University Press, 2020); Leah Price, *What We Talk About When We Talk About Books* (New York: Basic Books, 2019). On the emergence of wellness discourse see Carl Cederström, and André Spicer, *The Wellness Syndrome* (Cambridge: Polity Press, 2015).

13 Philip Rieff, *The Triumph of the Therapeutic: Uses of Faith after Freud* (Chicago: University of Chicago Press, 1966). Though its terminology may be indebted to the writings of Freud, the way that these therapeutic ideas were taken up in the US to produce its own culture and ethos, is unique. As Rieff writes, 'Psychological man is, I suggest, more native to American culture than the Puritan sources of that culture would indicate' (58).

14 The term was used in the 1916 essay 'A Literary Clinic' by writer and Unitarian minister Samuel McChord Crothers. In 1914 and 1915, Crothers was already speaking on this theme in lectures to librarians. On the publication and meaning of this essay, see Jesse Miller, 'Medicines of the Soul: Reparative Reading and the History of Bibliotherapy', *Mosaic* 51, no. 2 (2018): 17–34.

15 Karin Littau, *Theories of Reading: Books, Bodies, and Bibliomania* (Cambridge: Polity Press, 2006).

16 Kenneth Burke, *The Philosophy of Literary Form* (1941; reis., Berkeley, CA: University of California Press, 1973). Burke's method of dramatistic analysis informs my project in this chapter.

17 Christopher Lasch, *The Culture of Narcissism: American Life in an Age of Diminishing Expectations* (New York: W.W. Norton, 1979).

18 Robert Darnton, "First Steps Toward a History of Reading," *Australian Journal of French Studies* 23, no. 1 (1986), 16.

19 George Lakoff and Mark Johnson, *Metaphors We Live By* (Chicago: University of Chicago Press, 1980), 56.

20 Darnton, "First Steps," 16.

21 Littau, *Theories of Reading*, 65.

22 Christopher Morley, *The Haunted Bookshop*, (1919; reis., New York: Melville House Publishing, 2013).

23 Michael Neiberg, *The Treaty of Versailles: A Concise History* (New York: Oxford University Press, 2017). Morley's optimism regarding the impact of the Peace Conference was premature. Historians now attribute the strict financial reparations imposed on Germany by the Treaty of Versailles as a significant cause for the rise of the Nazis in Germany and the start of the Second World War.

24 Joan Shelley Rubin, *The Making of Middlebrow Culture* (Chapel Hill: University of North Carolina Press, 1992).

25 George Santayana, "The Genteel Tradition in American Philosophy," *The Genteel Tradition in American Philosophy and Character and Opinion in the United States* (1911; reis., New Haven: Yale University Press, 2009) 3–20. The genteel tradition refers to the nineteenth-century New England cultural elite who attempted through their writings to maintain literary, moral, and social hierarchies.

26 Rubin, *Making of Middlebrow*, 138.

27 Michael Saler, "'Clap if You Believe in Sherlock Holmes': Mass Culture and the Re-Enchantment of Modernity, c. 1890–c. 1940," *The Historical Journal* 46, no. 3 (2003): 599–622.

28 Morley, *Haunted*, 8.
29 Morley, *Haunted*, 14.
30 Jaimie Harker, *America the Middlebrow: Women's Novels, Progressivism, and Middlebrow Authorship between the Wars* (Amherst, MA: University of Massachusetts Press, 2007), 13.
31 Morley, *Haunted*, 17.
32 Morley, *Haunted*, 104.
33 Morley, *Haunted*, 108.
34 Morley, *Haunted*, 42.
35 Morley, *Haunted*, 43.
36 Morley, *Haunted*, 102.
37 Morley, *Haunted*, 102–103.
38 Morley, *Haunted*, 103.
39 John Scaggs, *Crime Fiction* (London: Routledge, 2005).
40 Morley, *Haunted*, 228.
41 Morley, *Haunted*, 220.
42 Morley, *Haunted*, 150.
43 Morley, *Haunted*, 150.
44 Morley, *Haunted*, 151.
45 Morley, *Haunted*, 107.
46 Peter Brooks, *Reading for the Plot: Design and Intention in Narrative* (Cambridge, MA: Harvard University Press, 1984). Brooks discusses the relationship between the design of detective plots and readerly desire (23–36).
47 Rubin, *Making of Middlebrow*, 134.
48 George, *Little Paris,* 28.
49 George, *Little Paris,* 23.
50 George, *Little Paris,* 27.
51 George, *Little Paris,* 27.
52 George, *Little Paris,* 143.
53 George, *Little Paris,* 32.
54 George, *Little Paris,* 316.
55 George, *Little Paris,* 401.
56 George, *Little Paris,* 385.
57 Stassi, *Every Coincidence*, 2.
58 Stassi, *Every Coincidence*, 4.
59 Stassi, *Every Coincidence*, 3.
60 Stassi, *Every Coincidence*, 12.
61 Stassi, *Every Coincidence*, 12.
62 Fabio Stassi, "The Shape of an Island," trans. Oonagh Stransky, *Exchanges: Journal of Literary Translation* (Fall 2019), https://web.archive.org/web/20240723225403/https://exchanges.uiowa.edu/issues/iterations/the-shape-of-an-island/.
63 Stassi, *Every Coincidence*, 5.
64 It is worth noting that in each of the three stories under discussion, that subjectivity is a white masculinity in crisis, and its cure involves a reformulation of that masculinity from one characterized as autonomous and unfeeling, to one which is relational and sensitive, yet still, for all of that, in control.
65 George, *Little Paris,* 401.

References

Adams, Ellery. *The Secret, Book & Scone Society*. New York: Kensington Books, 2017.

Aubry, Timothy. *Reading as Therapy: What Contemporary Fiction Does for Middle-Class Americans*. Iowa City: University of Iowa Press, 2011.

Berthoud, Ella and Susan Elderkin. *The Novel Cure: From Abandonment to Zestlessness: 751 Books to Cure What Ails You*. New York: Penguin Books, 2014.

Birkerts, Sven. *Changing the Subject: Art and Attention in the Internet Age*. Minneapolis, MN: Graywolf Press, 2015.

Blum, Beth. *The Self-Help Compulsion: Searching for Advice in Modern Literature*. New York: Columbia University Press, 2020.

Brooks, Peter. *Reading for the Plot: Design and Intention in Narrative*. Cambridge, MA: Harvard University Press, 1984.

Burke, Kenneth. *The Philosophy of Literary Form*. 1941; Berkeley, CA: University of California Press, 1973.

Cederström, Carl and André Spicer. *The Wellness Syndrome*. Cambridge: Polity Press, 2015.

Colgan, Jenny. *The Bookshop on the Corner*. New York: William Morrow, 2016.

Collins, Jim. *Bring on the Books for Everybody: How Literary Culture Became Popular Culture*. Durham: Duke University Press, 2010.

Cossé, Laurence. *A Novel Bookstore*, trans. Alison Anderson. New York: Europa Editions, 2010.

Crothers, Samuel McChord. "A Literary Clinic." *The Atlantic* 118, no. 3 (September 1916): 291–301.

Darnton, Robert. "First Steps toward a History of Reading." *Australian Journal of French Studies* 23, no. 1 (1986): 5–30.

Desmarais, Christina. "Why Reading Books Makes You a Better Person, According to Science." *Inc.*, July 3, 2018. www.inc.com/christina-desmarais/why-reading-books-makes-you-a-better-person-according-to-science.html.

George, Nina. *The Little Paris Bookshop*. Translated by Simon Pare. New York: Broadway Books, 2015.

Gregory, Andrew. "The Pick-me-up Papers: Dickens Better for Mental Health Than Self-Help Books," *The Times*, March 1, 2020, www.thetimes.co.uk/article/the-pick-me-up-papers-dickens-better-for-mental-health-than-self-help-books-bn9xd88j2.

Harker, Jaime. *America the Middlebrow: Women's Novels, Progressivism, and Middlebrow Authorship between the Wars*. Amherst, MA: University of Massachusetts Press, 2007.

Haslam, Sara and Edmund G.C. King. "'Medicinable Literature': Bibliotherapy, Literary Caregiving, and the First World War," *Literature and Medicine* 39, no. 2 (2021): 296–318.

Henry, Veronica. *How to Find Love in a Bookshop*. New York: Pamela Dorman Books, 2017.

Lakoff, George, and Mark Johnson. *Metaphors We Live By*. Chicago: University of Chicago Press, 1980.

Lasch, Christopher. *The Culture of Narcissism: American Life in an Age of Diminishing Expectations*. New York: W.W. Norton, 1979.

Littau, Karin. *Theories of Reading: Books, Bodies, and Bibliomania*. Cambridge: Polity Press, 2006.

Miller, Jesse. "Medicines of the Soul: Reparative Reading and the History of Bibliotherapy." *Mosaic* 51, no. 2 (2018): 17–34.

Morley, Christopher. *The Haunted Bookshop*. 1919; New York: Melville House Publishing, 2013.

Neiberg, Michael S. *The Treaty of Versailles: A Concise History*. New York: Oxford University Press, 2017.

Oh Hello Again Bookshop. "FAQs.". Accessed February 19, 2021. https://web.archive.org/web/20220523053656/https://ohhelloagain.com/pages/faqs.

Price, Leah. *What We Talk About When We Talk About Books*. New York: Basic Books, 2019.

Rieff, Philip. *The Triumph of the Therapeutic: Uses of Faith after Freud.* Chicago: University of Chicago Press, 1966.

Rubin, Joan Shelley. *The Making of Middlebrow Culture*. Chapel Hill: University of North Carolina Press, 1992.

Saler, Michael. "'Clap if You Believe in Sherlock Holmes': Mass Culture and the Re-Enchantment of Modernity, c. 1890-c. 1940." *The Historical Journal* 46, no. 3 (2003): 599–622.

Santayana, George. "The Genteel Tradition in American Philosophy." *The Genteel Tradition in American Philosophy and Character and Opinion in the United States*. New Haven: Yale University Press, 2009: 3–20. First published 1911.

Scaggs, John. *Crime Fiction*. London: Routledge, 2005.

Stassi, Fabio. *Every Coincidence Has a Soul.* Translated by Oonagh Stransky from *Ogni coincidenza ha un'anima.* Palermo: Sellerio editore, 2018. Unpublished manuscript January 7, 2021.

Stassi, Fabio. *La lettrice scomparsa*. Palermo: Sellerio editore, 2016.

Stassi, Fabio. "The Shape of an Island," Translated by Oonagh Stransky. *Exchanges: Journal of Literary Translation* (Fall 2019),https://web.archive.org/web/20240723225403/https://exchanges.uiowa.edu/issues/iterations/the-shape-of-an-island/.

Stassi, Fabio. *Uccido chi voglio*. Palermo: Sellerio editore, 2020.

Striphas, Ted. *The Late Age of Print: Everyday Book Culture from Consumerism to Control.* New York: Columbia University Press, 2009.

Sullivan, Matthew. *Midnight at the Bright Ideas Bookstore*. New York: Scribner, 2017.

Uras, Michaël. *Aux petits mots, les grands remèdes* [*Take Two Chapters and Call Me in the Morning]*. Paris: Préludes, 2020.

10 'I Liked Them a Lot ... but I Feel Like I Don't Know Them Fully?'

Implications of Recent Research in Immersion and Engagement for Digital Therapeutic Reading

Laura Dietz

In 2020, digital bibliotherapy came into its own. Research on the effects of COVID-19 on reading practices began almost as soon as the crisis did, and with good reason: from the earliest weeks of lockdown, reading increased, and so did expectations regarding the benefits reading would provide. Surveys confirmed an immediate net increase in overall reading (though many read less, due to factors including expanding work and domestic duties, increased news consumption, and worry and stress, these were outnumbered by those who read more).[1] Reasons for reading changed more notably still. Citizens in lockdown were inundated with book recommendations, online literary events, celebrity bedtime stories, and exhortations to read through the crisis.[2] Rationales layered self-improvement and entertainment: books were put forward as a means of putting time to 'good' use, virtuous self-discipline to tame the hours between workouts and online guitar lessons, and in the same breath proffered for passing the time, casting reading as a counterpoint to Zadie Smith's widely shared writing-as-banana-bread metaphor (another illustration of how reasons for pursuing cultural activity were complex and often contradictory).[3] But prominent among rationales for reading were health and wellbeing.[4] News coverage on lockdown reading lingered on the promise of reading for solace, relief, and healing.[5] Explicit comparisons between books and medicine were easy to find: as Taffy Brodesser-Anker put it (appropriately, in a *New York Times* article where authors shared 'books that bring them comfort'): 'beneath all this external crisis our souls are still wretched and needy and require their own antibiotics and Purell and masks and toilet paper'.[6] As a respondent in my own reading survey explained in March 2021, reflecting on a year of confinement, isolation, danger, and fear, 'where previously reading was a nice thing to do, within covid reading e-books has largely been for mental health and escapism. It's to shut out the world'.[7]

This mass turn towards 'the idea that reading can have a beneficial effect on mental health'[8] is rightly identified as a watershed moment for bibliotherapy. But it represented a shift not only in terms of volume – the number of individuals reading for wellbeing or the number of hours spent – but in terms of platform. 2020 is also

DOI: 10.4324/9781003471561-14

the year when school, university, library, and bookshop closures forced readers – many for the first time – to digital[9] books. In the U.S., according to the Association of American Publishers (AAP), e-book sales in 2020 increased by more than 16%, double the increase enjoyed by print, and audiobook revenue increased by more than 17%;[10] an especially startling result given the drastic decline in commuting during lockdown and corresponding reduction in time spent in a popular setting for audiobook and Kindle reading. This was the case for respondents in my 2021 survey who reported reading fewer e-books because they were no longer taking Kindles on trains or the subway. The surge was such that by January 2021, Arts Council England had announced more than £300,000 in grants for libraries expanding their e-book and digital audiobook collections to help respond to the '146% increase in demand for digital stock at libraries during the coronavirus crisis'.[11] In my own 2021 and 2022 surveys, 34% of respondents reported reading e-books more than before the pandemic. The most commonly cited reasons were, predictably, closed (or open but unacceptably high-risk) libraries and bookshops. Only 14% reported less e-book reading; major reasons included the aforementioned on-hold commutes, but also screen fatigue, with print serving as a means to 'counteract all the zoom screen time'.[12] The increase in audiobook listening (particularly from library loans, an increase that would not appear in the AAP's sales statistics) was even more dramatic: 41% reported listening to audiobooks more than they did before the pandemic, compared to only 10% reporting less.

Even before the pandemic, digital had emerged as a critical component in the delivery of bibliotherapy in community settings. Despite its short history as a mainstream means of reading,[13] digital widens access in a number of crucial ways. Most prominently, the lower cost and vastly greater range of human-read audiobook options extend the reach of charity schemes such as the Royal National Institute of Blind People (RNIB)'s venerable Talking Books, as well as library collections and commercial options, and e-books can typically be rendered into computer-generated synthetic speech by an e-reading app or (where Digital Rights Management does not disrupt this) other smartphone and tablet apps.[14] Readers with impaired vision can benefit from e-books' adjustable text size, but also the higher contrast of backlit screens.[15] Customisable line length and line spacing can reduce fatigue for some readers with dyslexia, though for these readers backlit screens have been found in some studies to exacerbate fatigue and reduce reading speed.[16] The lighter weight and one-handed reading (or for audiobooks, no-handed reading) are exceptionally important for readers with arthritis.[17] But most critically for the COVID-19 era, digital books allowed instant, round-the-clock access for multiple users regardless of mobility or geographical location.[18] Doctors Emmanuel Stip, Linda Östlundh, and Karim Abdel Aziz explored therapeutic reading for healthcare workers in their 2020 paper 'Bibliotherapy: Reading OVID during COVID'. Delving into personal experiences of coping under intolerable conditions, they found reading invaluable at the very moment when print was often inaccessible; but for them, e-books came to the rescue. 'Sometimes, in our exile, we are not lucky to have taken a library in our suitcases with the chosen books and in a familiar language. Fortunately, there are electronic libraries and e-books'.[19]

Notably, Stip, Östlundh, and Abdel Aziz don't frame this cherished reading as lesser in any way because of being on screen. On-screen Ovid is described as providing the reader with an authentic and beneficial encounter with literature, without qualifiers. There is no mention of disappointment with format, or frustration with a second-choice delivery option (even if second-choice status may be implied when they describe 'chosen books' as items one would pack in a suitcase rather than download to a smartphone). Rather, they foreground relief that any access is possible, and report that the reading has been the 'therapy' they sought, that e-books have served as 'talismans' they needed; the 'window on a world' that only a book could offer at a dark time.[20] Embedded in that relief is the most pressing question regarding digital bibliotherapy: though their confidence that therapeutic reading is platform-agnostic is based on authentic personal experience, is that confidence warranted? The 2020s are the time to examine digital bibliotherapy and consider how emerging evidence on reader experiences of e-reading reveals aspects that may affect the bibliotherapeutic process.

The expansion of empirical research on how e-reading may affect aspects of 'literary reading' (as opposed to more utilitarian reading for information purposes, generally studied separately)[21] can potentially deepen our understanding of how, or whether, digital platforms may affect other aspects of the therapeutic reading experience. Many dimensions of e-book and digital audiobook reading are ripe for investigation: for example, how audiobook listening can promote wellbeing by developing literary skills in a different, and complementary, manner than print reading,[22] or how layered multiplatform access, the now-commonplace practice of reading a given text on paper, on screen, or via audio depending on location, affects reading frequency and sense of intimacy and ownership.[23] But one particularly urgent dimension is narrative immersion. 'The unique nature of cognitive and emotional immersion that unfolds when individuals make sense of, and respond to, narrative content is a central focus of researchers interested in the persuasive effects of narrative' and 'research is now more sensitive to the medium-specific nature of immersion'.[24] This chapter will consider the role of immersion in giving readers a sense of engagement *with*, authentic experience *of*, and lasting emotional connection *to* a digital book. It will contrast the medium materiality model with the cognitive map model, and consider the role of interactivity in bibliotherapy using digital fiction.[25] In its conclusion, the chapter will discuss how strategies to remove potential barriers to immersion can inform therapeutic reading using digital books.

Getting Lost in a Digital Book

The study of immersion and transportation in digital therapeutic reading is starved of data. One reason is the emphasis of bibliotherapy research to date on non-fiction texts, particularly self-help books, rather than literary works such as novels, plays, and poetry.[26] As Troiscanko puts it, 'bibliotherapy with fiction or poetry is often practiced but rarely researched' (a split recognizable in the experiences of the Ovid-reading medics) and 'assumptions about the inevitably edifying nature of art are frequent, and realistic acknowledgements of the complexity of both literature and human beings are oddly rare'.[27] Another reason is that 'much work on bibliotherapy to date has centred on texts in print' and 'qualitative and statistical evaluations of the value of reading in a digital format remain in their infancy'.[28] This lacuna is important because the aspects of digital reading yet to be fully investigated are not peripheral, but central to bibliotherapy. If the bibliotherapeutic process begins, as many models specify, with identification or involvement,[29] any digital barrier to identification or involvement could be potentially devastating to the process. There is, unfortunately, a shortage of empirical research on any aspect of digital reading, though key studies on immersion and digital reading, immersion and digital fiction, and some studies on bibliotherapy and digital fiction, discussed below, offer a path ahead.[30]

Bibliotherapists know all too well the challenges of synthesising research findings when reading research is carried out in so many fields, with such a range of methodologies. The experience of being 'lost in a book' is widely examined,[31] but there are competing terms for describing it as well as competing methods for measuring it. Being lost in a book involves (temporary) forfeiture of other things, including forms of attention that would in other contexts be desirable: it is a state where readers 'lose track of time, fail to observe events going on around them' in a literary reverie akin to Csikszentmihalyi's concept of 'flow' as 'a complete focus on an activity accompanied by a loss of conscious awareness of oneself and one's surroundings'.[32] Hence, terms to describe it highlight departure as much as arrival; surrender of one mode for the sake of a more complete presence in another. Researchers custom-build their terminology, finessing what forms of focus are of interest and what forms of forfeiture are under consideration, to redefine for the purposes of a specific study or sub-field terms such as transportation, absorption, or engagement. This populates a taxonomy of immersion that differentiates forms including narrative, psychological, emotional, spatio-temporal, social, ludic, and even a separate sub-category for 'literary'.[33] Popular metrics for measurement of attention include Green and Brock's transportation scale (2000), Busselle and Bilandzic's narrative engagement scale (2009), and Kuijpers, Hakemulder, Tan, and Doicaru's story world absorption scale (2014).[34] Each has its own grouping of narrative experiences studied together, not all of which relate to reading: Busselle and Bilandzic's experiments, for example, use film and television, but their theories are applied by other researchers to 'sustained attention to and open reflection on the world of story' as encountered in novels and stories as well.[35] Most metrics rely heavily on questionnaires to capture participant's impressions of a given narrative encounter. But some studies, particularly more recent ones, also attempt to quantify responses to a literary text via measurement of pupil dilation, eye tracking (measuring how long a participant's gaze rests on a given word or line, how often a participant rescans a given passage, etc.), blink rate, and other observable physiological responses.[36] As revealing as such experiments can be in, for example, Eekhof, Kuijpers, Faber, Gao, Mak, van den Hoven, and Willems's 2021 paper 'Lost in a Story, Detached from the Words', the fact that many experimental setups require participants to read in a lab, listening to an audiobook while gazing into a camera or reading on a desktop computer with a camera mounted on top, make it easier to compare two different texts read on the same platform (say, a novel deemed 'literary' and a novel deemed 'commercial') than the same text in different formats.[37] Experiments that do compare formats, like those described below, are rare but revealing, and particularly ingenious in design. Most importantly to bibliotherapists, their theories on mechanism offer some early insights into how barriers to immersion for digital reading might be overcome.

Leaving the World Behind: Departure from the Physical Interface

At the moment of reading immersion, the physical world left behind includes one's physical interface with the text, be it Codex or Kindle or smartphone. It is the moment when there is no effective barrier between the reader and the story or 'world of stories you can dive into', or as one study participant put it, 'reading on a Kindle I forget I'm reading on a Kindle … apart from the fact that it's not as heavy'.[38] The idea of a forgettable interface echoes – for some respondents consciously, for others perhaps unconsciously – Amazon marketing. Amazon's stated goal has long been for a Kindle not to dazzle or delight, but rather 'disappear': to, in Jeff Bezos's words in a 2007 letter to Amazon shareholders, 'get out of the way, *just like a physical book*, so readers could become engrossed in the words' [emphasis mine].[39] But that moment of disappearance is delayed, potentially indefinitely, for the subset of readers who 'find it very difficult to engage with a text that is on screen'.[40]

Across existing studies of engagement with digital texts, and indeed across studies of digital reading more generally, participants most often frame the challenge for digital as closing the gap with print, not outperforming print. Many are confident that digital is 'as good': that for them platform is irrelevant and the reading experience is the same: 'I have no particular favourite medium', 'I don't really have a preference', or 'I really don't care if it's print or electronic most of the time' (the latter also confirming that some of the time, they most certainly do care).[41] E-books are, for these readers, one format among many, neither sought after nor preferred: 'I read in all formats: hard copy, paperback/hardback, audiobook, e-audiobook, ebook, mp3, manuscript, advanced readers, flipster … the format is unimportant'.[42] Gathering qualitative data from a group of university employees using Kindles for a full year, just after its 2007 U.S. product release, Clark, Goodwin, Samuelson, and Coker found participants 'united in their opinion that … the print book functions as an inconspicuous container once the participant began reading'.[43] It is possible that transportation via digital reading is a skill developed via practice; if so, this points to ever-easier immersion as experience with e-reading (and exposure to a greater range of e-reading platforms, each with their own advantages) ushers a larger proportion of readers into a coveted 'inconspicuous container' category. Clark, Goodwin, Samuelson, and Coker determined that experience with the interface was not by itself enough to make the device 'get out of the way' as Bezos hoped. Roughly half 'did become accustomed to the Kindle as a reading device' and 'it did eventually fade into the background' – some within moments – but for the other half, the Kindle remained a stubbornly 'noticeable, obtrusive device'.[44] This obtrusiveness was more than a nuisance: as 'they were not fully engaged with the text as they would be if reading a traditional book'[45] their entire reading experience was affected.

For some respondents in my own surveys, the 'physicality' of a print book is described as important, as where print is cited 'better for remembering / more of a physical memory aspect'.[46] This potentially supports Mangen and Kuiken's medium materiality model, discussed further below. However, one draws attention to the fact that the physical object only really matters when 'the content is not all that engaging'.[47] To bibliotherapists, this reminder that books are not interchangeable – just as readers are not – is unsurprising, to say the least.

For those who do experience barriers to immersion, this interference can be consequential. The barrier may not be impenetrable, as they can still read the book, but some respondents describe what is to them a profound difference in their connection to the book and to the author. They explain that 'when you're reading on a Kindle, or whatever [the reading device] … they're not as attached to the author or something?'[48] A relationship, in multiple senses, is depleted. As a result, there is a level of comprehension or apprehension placed out of reach: 'some of the ones I've read on Kindle only so far, I really enjoyed them, I liked them a lot … but I feel like I don't know them fully?'[49] *Feel* may suggest that the subjectivity of these experiences renders effects of any such depletion unquantifiable. However, recent studies on emotion and reading, such as Lei, Willems, and Eekhof's on how measuring reading speed of emotional vs neutral words reveasl individual differences in need for affect and narrative absorption, demonstrate how techniques such as eye tracking open up possibilities for quantitative and mixed methods studies – and with them, new avenues for bibliotherapy research.[50]

In 2008, Clark, Goodwin, Samuelson, and Coker's participants were limited to texts that could be read on a first-generation Kindle. In the 2020s, readers enjoy a vastly expanded menu of device options; in my own studies, a large majority of participants had used more than one e-reading device in the past 12 months (for example, reading on a phone, on a laptop, and on a tablet at different times). But most of the e-books they read were still of the kind one could read on a Kindle: non-enhanced, what McCracken calls 'transitional', and Phillips 'vanilla', e-books.[51] Such texts ('vanilla' remaining the most popular form of e-book, representing the great majority of loans, free downloads, and sales) do not take advantage of potential enhancements such as multimedia content or internal or external links (other than those standard for a given app or device, such as search functions or Kindle X-ray and popular highlights), the sorts of enhancements that would prevent a text being presented on paper. For what Bell, Ensslin, Ciccoricco, Rustad, Laccetti, and Pressman define as digital fiction, works that must remain on screen or they will lose functionality and/or meaning, the immersion situation is even more complex.[52]

This issue of interactivity is central in Ensslin, Skains, Riley, Haran, Mackiewicz, and Halliwell's 2016 paper 'Exploring Digital Fiction as a Tool for Teenage Body Image Bibliotherapy', with immersion one-dimension under study.[53] Digital interactive fiction is believed to have huge potential for immersive reading experiences.

Green and Jenkins' earlier empirical studies of paper-based interactive fiction, where readers are guided through numbered short chapters in different branching paths based on their in-story choices (for example, to open a door or follow a character, as in *Choose Your Own Adventure* books) had found interaction generally conducive to transportation and identification.[54] Ensslin, Skains, Riley, Haran, Mackiewicz, and Halliwell hypothesised that 'certain conventions of DF [digital fiction] give it a high *potential* as bibliotherapy: non-visible protagonists and conventional use of the second person perspective permitting the reader/player to personify the role and its relevant choices; multiple communication modes combining text, image and sound; and interactivity that further engages the reader/player in the narrative choices' [emphasis theirs], making investigation of its clinical applications a priority.[55] However, early 'empirical hypertext reading studies (e.g. Gardner 2003, Pope 2006, Miall and Dobson 2001)' from the very end of the 20th century documented the 'perceived alienating effects of hypertext as a basis for storytelling'.[56] This needed to be tested again with 21st-century readers. For their body image study, Ensslin and her co-authors used existing texts, not stories specially designed. The chosen texts were a variety of interactive digital fictions that ranged from purely hypertext to more elaborate forms making greater use of animations and game-like interfaces. Their main finding was that for their participants, using their set of texts, digital fiction was not an effective tool. The problem was not the technology, which was familiar,[57] but the stories. There were other barriers to do with subject matter and 'weirdness', but a primary issue was structure.[58] 'Obfuscated, subtle, or absent narrative structures' are 'conventional' for DF but 'unfamiliar' for general readers, and 'largely confused participants'.[59] 'In most cases, participants found it difficult to relate to the female protagonists', in part because of the 'multilinearity and perceived lack of [traditional narrative] closure of the text'.[60] In sum, despite its potential, 'purpose-built DFs' are needed, and such purpose-built texts will probably need to be more linear, offer more closure, and generally be considerably more conventional: in other words, more like the kind of books one can purchase from Amazon for reading on a Kindle, in terms of content as well as form.[61]

Bell, Ensslin, van der Bom, and Smith later looked specifically at immersion in a single and even more complex work: a 2015 digital fiction installation by Andy Campbell and Judi Alston called WALLPAPER. An artwork that combined text with sound, visuals, and gamified interactivity in a gallery space, it unsurprisingly presented a hugely intricate immersion situation. The researchers found evidence that immersion in this setting was not a 'completely absorbing experience', something binary where one is in or out, but an 'intermittent process', a 'less totalising experience than previously assumed' where different forms of immersion, such as ludic or spatial or social, were more or less prominent at different stages.[62] The metaphor of a switchboard (in the 'sense of a mixing desk') captured both the array of potential experiences available to the same person in the same installation and the agency of that person in adjusting the levels, as it were, on competing forms of immersion.[63] Further, different forms could be antagonistic, as where focus on ludic aspects could compete with other forms of immersion, such as narrative or emotional (as when focus on in-game goals pushed out attention to plot or character). The researchers proposed a hierarchy of immersion where spatio-temporal immersion must come first: without transportation to a story world, narrative and ludic immersion never have the chance to begin. Interactivity introduced an additional level of engagement, yet had the potential to interrupt immersion at any point.[64] To use game studies terminology, WALLPAPER's interaction elements were just as likely to 'pop' readers out of the experience as to 'push' them in.[65]

Creating Models for Screen Immersion

Complementing the rich data on individual experiences of reading immersion found in qualitative studies, quantitative studies offer some insight into possible mechanisms. Two competing models, the medium materiality model and the cognitive map model, suggest entirely different strategies to address immersion issues.

In 'Lost in an iPad: Narrative Engagement on Paper and Tablet' (2014), Mangen and Kuiken present a medium materiality model in which haptics of turning the page, holding completed pages in the left hand, and other physical elements of handling a print book are indispensable to grasping one's place in the text, which in turn is indispensable to remembering, understanding, and engaging with a text.[66] In this model, the dislocation felt by some readers when reading a reflowable e-book (exemplified by respondents in my own surveys who reported that they 'don't like not having a physical eye-view of where [they are] in the book' and miss turning pages when 'turning pages tells you where you are in the story – part of the reading experience – knowing that the climax is coming etc.') presents an insoluble problem.[67] In a 2x2 study giving participants the same text on an iPad and as a stapled booklet (with the researchers acknowledging that this was an atypical print format, which may have affected results), Mangen and Kuiken found a small but statistically significant reduction of narrative engagement when the material was presented as non-fiction, though not when the same text was presented as fiction.[68] Despite this intriguing possibility that some genres are more affected by format than others, the researchers concluded that without 'physical, tactile, and spatiotemporally fixed cues' giving readers additional information on their progress towards completing a text, 'overview of the text's organization and structure … may be diminished'.[69] To further test their hypothesis and examine e-ink instead of a backlit screen, Mangen (this time with Olivier and Velay) designed a follow-up experiment comparing the print condition with a Kindle. There, print demonstrated more consistent advantage: 'on most tests subjects performed identically whatever the reading medium … on measures related to chronology and temporality, those who had read in the print pocket book, performed better than those who had read on a Kindle'.[70] Drawing on both sets of results, the new conclusion was that knowing one's place in the text was critical, and that screen reading environments were irreparably impoverished when it came to the kind of cues available when reading in print.

Hou, Rashid, and Lee, however, hypothesised that digital reading platforms are too diverse to generalise, and that proposed examining not just reading on different devices, but reading using different presentations on the same device. Their experiment compared readers' engagement with a Marvel Comics graphic novel in print form, fixed-layout PDF form on iPad, and in a dynamic panel-by-panel presentation on iPad, and their findings indicated reduced engagement for only the dynamic presentation: the non-reflowable PDF proved just as engaging as print.[71] Their conclusion is that difficulty in forming a cognitive map of the text stems from reflow, not a loss of tactile or spatiotemporally fixed cues. If true, the solution to the problem would then be straightforward: reading comics in PDF rather than panel-by-panel presentations, and by extension 'vanilla' novels in PDF rather than reflowable .AZW or .EPUB form. Such a shift would carry heavy costs, given that abandoning reflowable formats would mean surrendering adjustable text size, line length, line spacing, and colour and contrast, some of the very affordances that make digital more accessible to some readers with visual impairments and/or dyslexia. But for readers facing immersion barriers, such trade-off could be, at least some of the time, worthwhile.

Another solution, of course, would be to abandon digital bibliotherapy altogether: to respond to the complexity of and controversy surrounding digital immersion by relegating e-reading to 'emergency book' status, suitable for Ovid-hungry medics sheltering in place but the format of last resort for anyone with choice. A flight to paper is romantic as well as simple, catering to readers still frayed by format wars that attempted to pit print reading (and print readers) against digital, framing e-books in particular as enemies of literature.[72] The seductiveness of the reflexively anti-digital stance is illustrated by an anecdote from the reviewer and critic Laura Miller. Miller reviewed Maryanne Wolf's *Reader, Come Home* (2018), an indictment of e-reading that extends the pro-print argument of her influential *Proust and the Squid* (2000).[73] As Miller reported:

> Reading about Wolf's experiment reminded me of the weekend last year when I sunk into the velvet folds of Jennifer Egan's Manhattan Beach, a novel that is not at all slow but rather slowing. It demonstrated an uncanny power to still my jittering mind and return me to the long, trancelike reading bouts of my early 20s, when I devoured fat Henry James novels for fun. How much more satisfying this was than the facile and addictive consumption of social media that takes up way too much of my time!
>
> I went looking on my shelves for a copy of Egan's novel, wondering if I could find on a randomly accessed page some trace of that magic. Finally **I remembered that I'd read Manhattan Beach in PDF form**, on my iPad.
>
> The screen didn't lessen the potency of the novel's spell. It would be nice if Wolf caught up with the times and stopped fretting about e-books and the notion that they inhibit this kind of immersion.[74]

Conclusion

What, then, are the implications for bibliotherapists today? Until further research is available, results like those discussed here offer some practical options.

It is premature to turn away from digital bibliotherapy, or to assume that print is always best, or even typically best. The profound advantages of quick, easy access, of frequently lower costs (to readers and to institutions) and of accessibility (for individuals and for locked down societies) are too great to discard. Respondents in my surveys who explained that COVID made them converts to e-reading (as with 'love them now! Was sceptical about the reading experience before but turns out it's great') spoke for many: the number of people at least open to e-reading has permanently increased.[75] Further, the barriers noted above are not universally or even consistently experienced: all evidence is that this impact is felt by some readers, at some times, with specifics as to 'the "who", the "what", the "where" and the "when" questions, which can be of great help in attacking the more difficult "whys" and "hows" ', remaining extremely limited.[76] It is also, however, premature to adopt interactive fiction for bibliotherapy. For all its potential, and for all the theoretical interest, experiments to date have revealed a complex and extremely difficult to standardise immersion situation, and unpromising results. The digital texts that represent the best-understood, and safest choices, for bibliotherapy at this time are 'vanilla': the texts that do not take advantage of the affordances of the digital to add features and functionality. These texts, those that could be translated back to print form with minimal adjustment, also allow for the closest head-to-head comparison for readers or bibliotherapists seeking to compare a given reader's experiences across platforms. For the time being, bibliotherapists may wish to recommend a free edition of *Alice in Wonderland* on Kindle rather than *Alice or iPad* or one of its many imitator apps.

For bibliotherapists working today, a first step would be making awareness of format standard. Therapists could make readers' record-keeping regarding mode of reading as commonplace as record-keeping on titles read (keeping in mind that many readers swap between platforms and devices, reading an e-book on Kindle during a lunch hour, listening to the same book via Audible narration while driving home, and then continuing the story with a print copy while reading in a favourite chair at home in the evening).[77] This would require tracking the specifics of interface, particularly reflowable vs non-reflowable, as well as print vs e-book vs audio.

A second step would be continuous consideration of format in addressing issues with immersion. Therapists could, where such issues arise, propose experimenting with non-reflowable formats or with print alternatives (much as they would propose experimenting with digital if cost, access, or difficulty in reading small and non-adjustable type were barriers to reading print books). Crucially, therapists would wish to consider such a fix as the right one in context, not a permanent prescription: existing evidence does not support locking readers forever into categories of 'digital' or 'print'. Sensitivity and flexibility are better watchwords; in the face of evidence that context matters, and the knowledge that digital reading platforms advance and digital readers gain experience and confidence, consistency would be foolish indeed.

Research on immersive reading, digital reading, and bibliotherapy continues apace, and all will yield a greater understanding of encounters with digital texts and how they affect (when they do affect) bibliotherapeutic processes. But there is a strong case for targeted research on digital bibliotherapy. Such studies could underpin targeted examination of the mechanisms of digital reading immersion, emotional connection, and ultimately positive outcomes; data that will be relevant to all bibliotherapeutic research. The COVID-19 pandemic has shone a spotlight on the value, relevance, and importance of therapeutic reading, and at the same time on the fragility of circulation systems: we can no longer ignore how a sudden change of circumstances, be they societal or personal, can force us to revise our strategies for obtaining and reading books. The need for Ovid during COVID will, we all pray, be time-limited. But the need for Ovid-on-demand, and for open options as to format and platform for our therapeutic reading, is only beginning.

Notes

1 'World Book Night: One in Three Reading More during Lockdown', *BBC News*, 23 April 2020, sec. Entertainment & Arts, www.bbc.com/news/entertainment-arts-52379327; Porter Anderson, 'Coronavirus Impact: A New Survey by Italian Publishers Sees "Abandonment of Reading"', *Publishing Perspectives*, 16 July 2020, https://publishingperspectives.com/2020/07/coronavirus-impact-a-new-survey-by-italian-publishers-sees-reading-dropping/; Porter Anderson, 'Coronavirus Impact: Nielsen Book India on Readers in the Pandemic', *Publishing Perspectives*, 15 July 2020, https://publishingperspectives.com/2020/07/coronavirus-impact-india-publishing-industry-nielsen-book-impact-study-pandemic-covid19/; Laura Dietz, 'Projection or Reflection? The Pandemic Bookshelf as a Mirror for Self-Image and Personal Identity', *English Studies* 103, no. 5 (4 July 2022): 675–89, https://doi.org/10.1080/0013838X.2022.2087034.

2 Dietz, 'Projection or Reflection?'; Laura Dietz and Leah Henrickson, 'Introduction: Books on Screen', *Participations* 19, no. 3 (2023): 259-271.

3 Zadie Smith, *Intimations*, 2020, www.penguin.co.uk/books/321775/intimations-by-smith-zadie/9780241492383; Tessa Hadley, 'Intimations by Zadie Smith Review – a Wonderful Essayist on the Lockdown', *The Guardian*, 1 August 2020, sec. Books, www.theguardian.com/books/2020/aug/01/intimations-by-zadie-smith-review-a-wonderful-essayist-on-the-lockdown.

4 Much of the advice was class-specific; see Sally Blackburn-Daniels and Edmund G. C. King, 'Bookshelves, Social Media and Gaming', *English Studies* 103, no. 5 (2022): 653–59.

5 Corinna Norrick-Rühl and Shafquat Towheed, 'Introduction', in *Bookshelves in the Age of the COVID-19 Pandemic*, ed. Corinna Norrick-Rühl and Shafquat Towheed (London: Palgrave Macmillan, 2022), 1–27.

6 Elisabeth Egan and Tina Jordan, 'Celeste Ng, Ann Patchett, Min Jin Lee and Others on the Books That Bring Them Comfort', *The New York Times*, 18 March 2020, sec. Books, www.nytimes.com/2020/03/18/books/comfort-books-celeste-ng-ann-patchett-and-others-coronavirus.html.

7 Survey 2021.

8 Edmund G. C. King, Sara Haslam, and Siobhan Campbell, 'Bibliotherapy: How Reading and Writing Have Been Healing Trauma since World War I', *The Conversation*, 15 November 2018, http://theconversation.com/bibliotherapy-how-reading-and-writing-have-been-healing-trauma-since-world-war-i-106626.

9 Digital reading can be used to describe a wide array of formats, though there remain competing definitions, including many that narrow 'digital books' or 'digital fiction' to only

some media, platforms, or styles. 'Digital fiction', for example, has been defined by Alice Bell, Astrid Ensslin, Dave Ciccoricco, Hans Rustad, Jess Laccetti, and Jessica Pressman as 'fiction written for and read on a computer screen that pursues its verbal, discursive and/or conceptual complexity through the digital medium, and would lose something of its aesthetic and semiotic function if it were removed from that medium', which makes reading digital fiction different from reading a PDF scan that faithfully reproduces a print original (see Alice Bell et al., 'A [S]Creed for Digital Fiction', *Electronic Book Review*, 7 March 2010, https://electronicbookreview.com/essay/a-screed-for-digital-fiction/.) As Matthew Rubery has observed, it remains commonplace to deny that audiobooks count as reading, despite the fact that this treats blind and partially sighted people as non-readers or inferior readers; see Matthew Rubery, *The Untold Story of the Talking Book* (Cambridge, MA: Harvard University Press, 2016). This chapter will take an inclusive view, and embrace e-books, audiobooks, interactive fiction, hybrid forms, etc.

10 Elizabeth A. Harris, 'Surprise Ending for Publishers: In 2020, Business Was Good', *The New York Times*, 29 December 2020, sec. Books, www.nytimes.com/2020/12/29/books/book-publishing-2020.html. As AAP membership does not include Amazon, a major publisher as well as distributor of e-books, 16% is likely to underestimate the true scale of the increase.

11 Mark Chandler, 'ACE Makes £152,000 Grant for Library e-Books and Audio', *The Bookseller*, 21 January 2021, www.thebookseller.com/news/ace-awards-152000-grant-library-e-books-and-audio-1233873.

12 Survey 2021.

13 Laura Dietz, 'The Short Story and Digital Media', in *The Edinburgh Companion to the Short Story in English* (Edinburgh University Press, 2018), 125–44, https://doi.org/10.1515/9781474400664-011.

14 RNIB, 'Talking Books', RNIB, accessed 28 February 2024, www.rnib.org.uk/living-with-sight-loss/independent-living/reading-and-books/talking-books/; RNIB, 'Text-to-Speech in eBooks', RNIB, accessed 28 February 2024, www.rnib.org.uk/living-with-sight-loss/independent-living/reading-and-books/text-to-speech-in-ebooks/.

15 Angus Phillips, *Turning the Page: The Evolution of the Book* (Abingdon: Routledge, 2014), 37–38.

16 Matthew H. Schneps et al., 'E-Readers Are More Effective than Paper for Some with Dyslexia', *PLOS ONE* 8, no. 9 (18 September 2013): e75634, https://doi.org/10.1371/journal.pone.0075634; Luz Rello and Ricardo Baeza-Yates, 'How to Present More Readable Text for People with Dyslexia', *Universal Access in the Information Society* 16, no. 1 (1 March 2017): 29–49, https://doi.org/10.1007/s10209-015-0438-8; British Dyslexia Association, 'Visual Difficulties', British Dyslexia Association, accessed 18 December 2023, www.bdadyslexia.org.uk/dyslexia/neurodiversity-and-co-occurring-differences/visual-difficulties.

17 Laura Dietz, 'Credible Texts: Legitimacy and Reputation of E-Books and E-Novels' (PhD diss., University College London, 2019), 220–221.

18 Steffen Moritz et al., 'New Wine in an Old Bottle? Evaluation of myMCT as an Integrative Bibliotherapy for Obsessive-Compulsive Disorder', *Journal of Obsessive-Compulsive and Related Disorders* 16 (2018): 2, https://doi.org/10.1016/j.jocrd.2017.12.009.

19 Emmanuel Stip, Linda Östlundh, and Karim Abdel Aziz, 'Bibliotherapy: Reading OVID During COVID', *Frontiers in Psychiatry* 11 (2020), www.frontiersin.org/articles/10.3389/fpsyt.2020.567539.

20 Stip, Östlundh, and Abdel Aziz, 'Bibliotherapy'.

21 Anne Mangen, 'The Digitization of Literary Reading', *Orbis Litterarum* 71, no. 3 (2016): 243–44, https://doi.org/10.1111/oli.12095.

22 Emily Best, 'Audiobooks and Literacy: A Rapid Review of the Literature' (National Literary Trust, 2020), https://cdn.literacytrust.org.uk/media/documents/Audiobooks_and_literacy_2020.pdf.

23 Laura Dietz, *E-Books and 'Real Books': Digital Reading and the Experience of Bookness* (Cambridge: Cambridge University Press, 2024).

24 Freya Sukalla et al., 'Embodiment of Narrative Engagement: Connecting Self-Reported Narrative Engagement to Psychophysiological Measures', *Journal of Media Psychology: Theories, Methods, and Applications* 28, no. 4 (2016): 175, https://doi.org/10.1027/1864-1105/a000153; Alice Bell et al., 'Immersion in Digital Fiction', *International Journal of Literary Linguistics* 7, no. 1 (29 January 2018): 2, https://doi.org/10.15462/ijll.v7i1.105.

25 Anne Mangen and Don Kuiken, 'Lost in an iPad: Narrative Engagement on Paper and Tablet', *Scientific Study of Literature* 4, no. 2 (1 January 2014): 150–77, https://doi.org/10.1075/ssol.4.2.02man; Jinghui Hou, Justin Rashid, and Kwan Min Lee, 'Cognitive Map or Medium Materiality? Reading on Paper and Screen', *Computers in Human Behavior* 67, no. C (1 February 2017): 84–94, https://doi.org/10.1016/j.chb.2016.10.014; Astrid Ensslin et al., 'Exploring Digital Fiction as a Tool for Teenage Body Image Bibliotherapy', *Digital Creativity* 27, no. 3 (2 July 2016): 177–95, https://doi.org/10.1080/14626268.2016.1210646.

26 Stip, Östlundh, and Abdel Aziz, 'Bibliotherapy'; Moniek M. Kuijpers, 'Bibliotherapy in the Age of Digitization', *First Monday*, 30 September 2018, https://doi.org/10.5210/fm.v23i10.9429; Emily T. Troscianko, 'Fiction-Reading for Good or Ill: Eating Disorders, Interpretation and the Case for Creative Bibliotherapy Research', *Medical Humanities* 44, no. 3 (1 September 2018): 201–11, https://doi.org/10.1136/medhum-2017-011375.

27 Troscianko, 'Fiction-Reading for Good or Ill', 207.

28 Nick Canty, 'Bibliotherapy: Its Processes and Benefits and Application in Clinical and Developmental Settings', *Logos* 28, no. 3 (30 November 2017): 39, https://doi.org/10.1163/1878-4712-11112133.

29 Canty, 'Bibliotherapy', 35.

30 Matt Hayler, *Challenging the Phenomenology of Technology: Embodiment, Expertise and Evolved Knowledge* (Basingstoke: Palgrave Macmillan, 2015); Mangen and Kuiken, 'Lost in an iPad'; Hou, Rashid, and Lee, 'Cognitive Map or Medium Materiality?'; Bell et al., 'Immersion in Digital Fiction'; Astrid Ensslin, Alice Bell, and Jen Smith, 'Immersion, Digital Fiction, and the Switchboard Metaphor' *Participations* 16, no. 1 (2019); Ensslin et al., 'Exploring Digital Fiction as a Tool for Teenage Body Image Bibliotherapy'.

31 Victor Nell, *Lost in a Book: The Psychology of Reading for Pleasure* (New Haven: Yale University Press, 1998).

32 Rick Busselle and Helena Bilandzic, 'Measuring Narrative Engagement', *Media Psychology* 12, no. 4 (23 November 2009): 324, https://doi.org/10.1080/15213260903287259.

33 Ensslin, Bell, and Smith, 'Immersion, Digital Fiction, and the Switchboard Metaphor'.

34 Melanie C. Green, Timothy C. Brock, and Geoff F. Kaufman, 'Understanding Media Enjoyment: The Role of Transportation Into Narrative Worlds', *Communication Theory* 14, no. 4 (2004): 311–27, https://doi.org/10.1111/j.1468-2885.2004.tb00317.x; Busselle and Bilandzic, 'Measuring Narrative Engagement'; Moniek M. Kuijpers et al., 'Exploring Absorbing Reading Experiences: Developing and Validating a Self-Report Scale to

Measure Story World Absorption', *Scientific Study of Literature* 4, no. 1 (2014): 89–122, https://doi.org/10.1075/ssol.4.1.05kui.

35 Kuijpers, 'Bibliotherapy in the Age of Digitization'.

36 Often drawing on methodologies pioneered by Human-Computer Interaction researchers and others studying immersion in games: another instance, like that of the WALLPAPER interactive story installation discussed later, of the dovetailing of reading and gaming immersion research.

37 Lynn S. Eekhof et al., 'Lost in a Story, Detached from the Words', *Discourse Processes* 58, no. 7 (9 August 2021): 595–616, https://doi.org/10.1080/0163853X.2020.1857619.

38 Focus group 1 participants 3, 1.

39 Amazon, '2007 Letter to Shareholders', 2008, 1, www.sec.gov/Archives/edgar/data/1018724/000119312508084145/dex991.htm.

40 Survey 2015.

41 Survey 2014, 2016, 2015.

42 Survey 2015.

43 Dennis T. Clark et al., 'A Qualitative Assessment of the Kindle E-book Reader: Results from Initial Focus Groups', *Performance Measurement and Metrics* 9, no. 2 (1 January 2008): 125, https://doi.org/10.1108/14678040810906826.

44 Clark et al., 'A Qualitative Assessment of the Kindle E-book Reader', 125.

45 Clark et al., 'A Qualitative Assessment of the Kindle E-book Reader', 125. For more obtrusiveness as a fundamental stage in technology adoption, marking a boundary (which can be crossed more than once, with obtrusiveness intensifying as well as fading at different stages) between non-integrated device and full integrated technology, see Hayler, *Challenging the Phenomenology of Technology: Embodiment, Expertise and Evolved Knowledge*.

46 Survey 2016.

47 Survey 2016.

48 Focus group 1 participant 5.

49 Focus group 1 participant 3.

50 Anqi Lei, Roel M. Willems, and Lynn S. Eekhof, 'Emotions, Fast and Slow: Processing of Emotion Words Is Affected by Individual Differences in Need for Affect and Narrative Absorption', *Cognition and Emotion* 37, no. 5 (4 July 2023): 997–1005, https://doi.org/10.1080/02699931.2023.2216445.

51 Ellen McCracken, 'Expanding Genette's Epitext/Peritext Model for Transitional Electronic Literature: Centrifugal and Centripetal Vectors on Kindles and iPads', *Narrative* 21, no. 1 (2013): 105–124; Phillips, *Turning the Page: The Evolution of the Book*.

52 Bell et al., 'A [S]Creed for Digital Fiction'.

53 Ensslin et al., 'Exploring Digital Fiction as a Tool for Teenage Body Image Bibliotherapy'.

54 Melanie C. Green and Keenan M. Jenkins, 'Interactive Narratives: Processes and Outcomes in User-Directed Stories', *Journal of Communication* 64, no. 3 (1 June 2014): 483–486, https://doi.org/10.1111/jcom.12093.

55 Ensslin et al., 'Exploring Digital Fiction as a Tool for Teenage Body Image Bibliotherapy', 19.

56 Ensslin et al., 'Exploring Digital Fiction as a Tool for Teenage Body Image Bibliotherapy', 12, 5.

57 Alice Bell, Astrid Ensslin, and Hans Kristian Rustad, eds., *Analyzing Digital Fiction*, Routledge Studies in Rhetoric and Stylistics 5 (New York: Routledge, 2014), 17.

58 Bell, Ensslin, and Rustad, *Analyzing Digital Fiction*, 185.

59 Ensslin et al., 'Exploring Digital Fiction as a Tool for Teenage Body Image Bibliotherapy', 17.
60 Ensslin et al., 'Exploring Digital Fiction as a Tool for Teenage Body Image Bibliotherapy', 12.
61 Ensslin et al., 'Exploring Digital Fiction as a Tool for Teenage Body Image Bibliotherapy', 19.
62 Bell et al., 'Immersion in Digital Fiction', 1, 19, 18.
63 Ensslin, Bell, and Smith, 'Immersion, Digital Fiction, and the Switchboard Metaphor', 19.
64 Ensslin, Bell, and Smith, 'Immersion, Digital Fiction, and the Switchboard Metaphor'.
65 Bell et al., 'Immersion in Digital Fiction', 17.
66 Mangen and Kuiken, 'Lost in an iPad'.
67 Survey 2015, 2016.
68 Mangen and Kuiken, 'Lost in an iPad', 162, 167.
69 Mangen and Kuiken, 'Lost in an iPad', 152.
70 Anne Mangen, Gérard Olivier, and Jean-Luc Velay, 'Comparing Comprehension of a Long Text Read in Print Book and on Kindle: Where in the Text and When in the Story?', *Frontiers in Psychology* 10 (2019): 1, www.frontiersin.org/articles/10.3389/fpsyg.2019.00038.
71 Hou, Rashid, and Lee, 'Cognitive Map or Medium Materiality?' It's essential to underscore that the researchers did not compare fiction with non-fiction, or work with purely textual material. Before generalising their findings across all-text novels, or non-fiction of any kind, additional experiments would be needed.
72 Simone Murray, *The Digital Literary Sphere: Reading, Writing, and Selling Books in the Internet Era* (Baltimore: Johns Hopkins University Press, 2018); Leah Price, *What We Talk About When We Talk About Books* (New York: Basic Books, 2019); Jessica Pressman, *Bookishness: Loving Books in a Digital Age* (New York: Columbia University Press, 2020).
73 Laura Miller, 'Just Read the Book Already', *Slate*, 16 August 2018, https://slate.com/culture/2018/08/reader-come-home-by-maryanne-wolf-reviewed.html.
74 Miller, 'Just Read the Book Already'.
75 Survey 2022.
76 Robert Darnton, 'First Steps Toward a History of Reading', *Australian Journal of French Studies* 51, no. 2/3 (2014): 155.
77 Dietz, *E-Books and 'Real Books': Digital Reading and the Experience of Bookness*.

References

Amazon. '2007 Letter to Shareholders', 2008. www.sec.gov/Archives/edgar/data/1018724/000119312508084145/dex991.htm.

Anderson, Porter. 'Coronavirus Impact: A New Survey by Italian Publishers Sees "Abandonment of Reading"'. *Publishing Perspectives*, 16 July 2020. https://publishingperspectives.com/2020/07/coronavirus-impact-a-new-survey-by-italian-publishers-sees-reading-dropping/.

———. 'Coronavirus Impact: Nielsen Book India on Readers in the Pandemic'. *Publishing Perspectives*, 15 July 2020. https://publishingperspectives.com/2020/07/coronavirus-impact-india-publishing-industry-nielsen-book-impact-study-pandemic-covid19/.

BBC News. 'World Book Night: One in Three Reading More during Lockdown'. 23 April 2020, sec. Entertainment & Arts. www.bbc.com/news/entertainment-arts-52379327.

Bell, Alice, Astrid Ensslin, David Ciccoricco, Hans Rustad, and Jess Laccetti and Jessica Pressman. 'A [S]Creed for Digital Fiction'. *Electronic Book Review*, 7 March 2010. https://electronicbookreview.com/essay/a-screed-for-digital-fiction/.

Bell, Alice, Astrid Ensslin, and Hans Kristian Rustad, eds. *Analyzing Digital Fiction*. New York: Routledge, 2014.

Bell, Alice, Astrid Ensslin, Isabelle van der Bom, and Jen Smith. 'Immersion in Digital Fiction'. *International Journal of Literary Linguistics* 7, no. 1 (29 January 2018). https://doi.org/10.15462/ijll.v7i1.105.

Best, Emily. 'Audiobooks and Literacy: A Rapid Review of the Literature'. National Literary Trust, 2020. https://cdn.literacytrust.org.uk/media/documents/Audiobooks_and_literacy_2020.pdf.

Blackburn-Daniels, Sally, and Edmund G. C. King. 'Bookshelves, Social Media and Gaming'. *English Studies* 103, no. 5 (2022): 653–659. https://doi.org/10.1080/0013838X.2022.2094575.

British Dyslexia Association. 'Visual Difficulties'. British Dyslexia Association. Accessed 18 December 2023. www.bdadyslexia.org.uk/dyslexia/neurodiversity-and-co-occurring-differences/visual-difficulties.

Busselle, Rick, and Helena Bilandzic. 'Measuring Narrative Engagement'. *Media Psychology* 12, no. 4 (23 November 2009): 321–347. https://doi.org/10.1080/15213260903287259.

Canty, Nick. 'Bibliotherapy: Its Processes and Benefits and Application in Clinical and Developmental Settings'. *Logos* 28, no. 3 (30 November 2017): 32–40. https://doi.org/10.1163/1878-4712-11112133.

Chandler, Mark. 'ACE Makes £152,000 Grant for Library e-Books and Audio'. *The Bookseller*, 21 January 2021. www.thebookseller.com/news/ace-awards-152000-grant-library-e-books-and-audio-1233873.

Clark, Dennis T., Susan P. Goodwin, Todd Samuelson, and Catherine Coker. 'A Qualitative Assessment of the Kindle E-book Reader: Results from Initial Focus Groups'. *Performance Measurement and Metrics* 9, no. 2 (1 January 2008): 118–129. https://doi.org/10.1108/14678040810906826.

Darnton, Robert. 'First Steps Toward a History of Reading'. *Australian Journal of French Studies* 51, no. 2/3 (2014): 152–177.

Dietz, Laura. 'Credible Texts: Legitimacy and Reputation of E-Books and E-Novels'. PhD diss., University College London, 2019.

———. *E-Books and 'Real Books': Digital Reading and the Experience of Bookness*. Cambridge: Cambridge University Press, 2025.

———. 'Projection or Reflection? The Pandemic Bookshelf as a Mirror for Self-Image and Personal Identity'. *English Studies* 103, no. 5 (4 July 2022): 675–689. https://doi.org/10.1080/0013838X.2022.2087034.

———. 'The Short Story and Digital Media'. In *The Edinburgh Companion to the Short Story in English*, edited by Paul Delaney and Adrian Hunter, 125–44. Edinburgh University Press, 2018. https://doi.org/10.1515/9781474400664-011.

Dietz, Laura, and Leah Henrickson. 'Introduction: Books on Screen'. *Participations* 19, no. 3 (2023): 259–271.

Eekhof, Lynn S., Moniek M. Kuijpers, Myrthe Faber, Xin Gao, Marloes Mak, Emiel van den Hoven, and Roel M. Willems. 'Lost in a Story, Detached from the Words'. *Discourse Processes* 58, no. 7 (9 August 2021): 595–616. https://doi.org/10.1080/0163853X.2020.1857619.

Egan, Elisabeth, and Tina Jordan. 'Celeste Ng, Ann Patchett, Min Jin Lee and Others on the Books That Bring Them Comfort'. *The New York Times*, 18 March 2020, sec. Books.

www.nytimes.com/2020/03/18/books/comfort-books-celeste-ng-ann-patchett-and-others-coronavirus.html.

Ensslin, Astrid, Alice Bell, and Jen Smith. 'Immersion, Digital Fiction, and the Switchboard Metaphor' 16, no. 1 (2019).

Ensslin, Astrid, Lyle Skains, Sarah Riley, Joan Haran, Alison Mackiewicz, and Emma Halliwell. 'Exploring Digital Fiction as a Tool for Teenage Body Image Bibliotherapy'. *Digital Creativity* 27, no. 3 (2 July 2016): 177–195. https://doi.org/10.1080/14626268.2016.1210646.

Green, Melanie C., Timothy C. Brock, and Geoff F. Kaufman. 'Understanding Media Enjoyment: The Role of Transportation into Narrative Worlds'. *Communication Theory* 14, no. 4 (2004): 311–327. https://doi.org/10.1111/j.1468-2885.2004.tb00317.x.

Green, Melanie C., and Keenan M. Jenkins. 'Interactive Narratives: Processes and Outcomes in User-Directed Stories'. *Journal of Communication* 64, no. 3 (1 June 2014): 479–500. https://doi.org/10.1111/jcom.12093.

Hadley, Tessa. 'Intimations by Zadie Smith Review – a Wonderful Essayist on the Lockdown'. *The Guardian*, 1 August 2020, sec. Books. www.theguardian.com/books/2020/aug/01/intimations-by-zadie-smith-review-a-wonderful-essayist-on-the-lockdown.

Harris, Elizabeth A. 'Surprise Ending for Publishers: In 2020, Business Was Good'. *The New York Times*, 29 December 2020, sec. Books. www.nytimes.com/2020/12/29/books/book-publishing-2020.html.

Hayler, Matt. *Challenging the Phenomenology of Technology: Embodiment, Expertise and Evolved Knowledge*. Basingstoke: Palgrave Macmillan, 2015.

Hou, Jinghui, Justin Rashid, and Kwan Min Lee. 'Cognitive Map or Medium Materiality? Reading on Paper and Screen'. *Computers in Human Behavior* 67, no. C (1 February 2017): 84–94. https://doi.org/10.1016/j.chb.2016.10.014.

King, Edmund G. C., Sara Haslam, and Siobhan Campbell. 'Bibliotherapy: How Reading and Writing Have Been Healing Trauma since World War I'. *The Conversation*, 15 November 2018. http://theconversation.com/bibliotherapy-how-reading-and-writing-have-been-healing-trauma-since-world-war-i-106626.

Kuijpers, Moniek M. 'Bibliotherapy in the Age of Digitization'. *First Monday*, 30 September 2018. https://doi.org/10.5210/fm.v23i10.9429.

Kuijpers, Moniek M., Frank Hakemulder, Ed S. Tan, and Miruna M. Doicaru. 'Exploring Absorbing Reading Experiences: Developing and Validating a Self-Report Scale to Measure Story World Absorption'. *Scientific Study of Literature* 4, no. 1 (2014): 89–122. https://doi.org/10.1075/ssol.4.1.05kui.

Lei, Anqi, Roel M. Willems, and Lynn S. Eekhof. 'Emotions, Fast and Slow: Processing of Emotion Words Is Affected by Individual Differences in Need for Affect and Narrative Absorption'. *Cognition and Emotion* 37, no. 5 (4 July 2023): 997–1005. https://doi.org/10.1080/02699931.2023.2216445.

Mangen, Anne. 'The Digitization of Literary Reading'. *Orbis Litterarum* 71, no. 3 (2016): 240–62. https://doi.org/10.1111/oli.12095.

Mangen, Anne, and Don Kuiken. 'Lost in an iPad: Narrative Engagement on Paper and Tablet'. *Scientific Study of Literature* 4, no. 2 (1 January 2014): 150–177. https://doi.org/10.1075/ssol.4.2.02man.

Mangen, Anne, Gérard Olivier, and Jean-Luc Velay. 'Comparing Comprehension of a Long Text Read in Print Book and on Kindle: Where in the Text and When in the Story?' *Frontiers in Psychology* 10 (2019). www.frontiersin.org/articles/10.3389/fpsyg.2019.00038.

McCracken, Ellen. 'Expanding Genette's Epitext/Peritext Model for Transitional Electronic Literature: Centrifugal and Centripetal Vectors on Kindles and iPads'. *Narrative* 21, no. 1 (2013): 105–124.

Miller, Laura. 'Just Read the Book Already'. *Slate*, 16 August 2018. https://slate.com/culture/2018/08/reader-come-home-by-maryanne-wolf-reviewed.html.

Moritz, Steffen, Marit Hauschildt, Sarah Catherine Murray, Anya Pedersen, Michael Krausz, and Lena Jelinek. 'New Wine in an Old Bottle? Evaluation of my MCT as an Integrative Bibliotherapy for Obsessive-Compulsive Disorder'. *Journal of Obsessive-Compulsive and Related Disorders* 16 (2018): 88–97. https://doi.org/10.1016/j.jocrd.2017.12.009.

Murray, Simone. *The Digital Literary Sphere: Reading, Writing, and Selling Books in the Internet Era*. Baltimore: Johns Hopkins University Press, 2018.

Nell, Victor. *Lost in a Book: The Psychology of Reading for Pleasure*. New Haven: Yale University Press, 1998.

Norrick-Rühl, Corinna, and Shafquat Towheed. 'Introduction'. In *Bookshelves in the Age of the COVID-19 Pandemic*, edited by Corinna Norrick-Rühl and Shafquat Towheed, 1–27. London: Palgrave Macmillan, 2022.

Phillips, Angus. *Turning the Page: The Evolution of the Book*. Abingdon: Routledge, 2014.

Pressman, Jessica. *Bookishness: Loving Books in a Digital Age*. New York: Columbia University Press, 2020.

Price, Leah. *What We Talk About When We Talk About Books*. New York: Basic Books, 2019.

Rello, Luz, and Ricardo Baeza-Yates. 'How to Present More Readable Text for People with Dyslexia'. *Universal Access in the Information Society* 16, no. 1 (1 March 2017): 29–49. https://doi.org/10.1007/s10209-015-0438-8.

RNIB. 'Talking Books'. RNIB. Accessed 28 February 2024. www.rnib.org.uk/living-with-sight-loss/independent-living/reading-and-books/talking-books/.

———. 'Text-to-Speech in eBooks'. RNIB. Accessed 28 February 2024. www.rnib.org.uk/living-with-sight-loss/independent-living/reading-and-books/text-to-speech-in-ebooks/.

Rubery, Matthew. *The Untold Story of the Talking Book*. Cambridge, MA: Harvard University Press, 2016.

Schneps, Matthew H., Jenny M. Thomson, Chen Chen, Gerhard Sonnert, and Marc Pomplun. 'E-Readers Are More Effective than Paper for Some with Dyslexia'. *PLOS ONE* 8, no. 9 (18 September 2013): e75634. https://doi.org/10.1371/journal.pone.0075634.

Smith, Zadie. *Intimations*, 2020. www.penguin.co.uk/books/321775/intimations-by-smith-zadie/9780241492383.

Stip, Emmanuel, Linda Östlundh, and Karim Abdel Aziz. 'Bibliotherapy: Reading OVID during COVID'. *Frontiers in Psychiatry* 11 (2020). www.frontiersin.org/articles/10.3389/fpsyt.2020.567539.

Sukalla, Freya, Helena Bilandzic, Paul D. Bolls, and Rick W. Busselle. 'Embodiment of Narrative Engagement: Connecting Self-Reported Narrative Engagement to Psychophysiological Measures'. *Journal of Media Psychology: Theories, Methods, and Applications* 28, no. 4 (2016): 175–186. https://doi.org/10.1027/1864-1105/a000153.

Troscianko, Emily T. 'Fiction-Reading for Good or Ill: Eating Disorders, Interpretation and the Case for Creative Bibliotherapy Research'. *Medical Humanities* 44, no. 3 (2018): 201–11. https://doi.org/10.1136/medhum-2017-011375.

11 Trauma and Literature

Current Bibliotherapeutic Practices and Literary Trauma Studies in Sweden

Katarina Båth

Songs are sown by those who mourn
But from singing joy is born.[1]

The quote above is from the Finland-Swedish romantic-idealist poet Zacharias Topelius (1818–1898) and is one of many examples of how authors throughout history have portrayed the cathartic effect of literature; it is from the wound, from sorrow that literature often arises, and it is by working through the painful memories literarily that one can hope to achieve reconciliation and liberation from sorrow. Another, more modern perspective on how literature accesses numbed, painful feelings within us is Kafka's famous statement about literature as an axe for the frozen sea within: 'I think we ought to read only the kind of books that wound or stab us. If the book we're reading doesn't wake us up with a blow to the head, what are we reading for? [...] A book must be the axe for the frozen sea within us.'[2] Kafka wants literature to tear open wounds. From a modern, psychoanalytic perspective, the image might be applied to accessing traumatized, frozen feelings within.

Both quotations can be related to a long tradition of seeing both trauma and the healing of trauma as intimately connected with literary fiction.[3] In tracing the historical trajectory of literary engagement with wounds, pivotal examples such as Aristotle's notion of *catharsis*, Apollo as the 'dual god of medicine and poetry', Christianity's veneration of Jesus' wounds, and Freud's trauma theory illustrate the centrality of the wound in poetic expression and its potential role in literary fiction as a means to heal mental wounds in Western cultural history.[4] Today, interest in the ability of literature to process painful emotions and assist with mental healing is cultivated in the field of literary trauma studies and in the practices known as bibliotherapy, or poetry therapy.[5]

Exploring different ideas about how literature (fiction and poetry) and the reading and/or writing of fiction or poetry can have healing effects, is a particular interest for me. The purpose of this chapter is twofold: first I will give a short overview of the current bibliotherapy and *Shared reading* practices that are expanding at this time in Sweden. (In Finland, bibliotherapy has a longer tradition, but in

DOI: 10.4324/9781003471561-15

Sweden, it is not until the last decade that a rising interest has evolved.[6]) This part of the chapter also builds upon interviews with three Swedish practitioners: two bibliotherapy educators and one *Shared Reading* Group Leader.[7]

Secondly, and as one outcome of my review of current practice in this specific time and place, I want to initiate a dialogue between the contemporary practice of creative bibliotherapy and the field of literary trauma studies, in order to explore the different ways in which reading can have healing effects. I will critically reflect upon the diverse ways in which fiction and poetry can help us cope with grief and process mental traumas, if we acknowledge that reading is an event that blurs and often reverses the relationship between subject and object – in ways that help us heal through the text.[8]

Much of the bibliotherapeutic research being done is focused on 'demonstrating the effectiveness of bibliotherapy' and finding evidence that it works – or perhaps does not.[9] My contribution combines an overview of the Nordic practice, with a reflection on what the reading of literature does to our vulnerable subjects. Hopefully, this can serve as a starting point for further dialogue between the fields of bibliotherapy and literary trauma studies, which – although they share an interest in questions regarding trauma, literature, and recovery – are two different fields with little overlap that have developed out of different contexts. Where literary trauma studies are more theoretically focused on ways literary texts can depict traumatic experiences, bibliotherapy is a more human-oriented practice with a focus on healing as a result. As Mazza puts it: 'in poetry therapy the focus is on the person, not the poem' – '[c]lients are not asked to identify the "true" meaning of a poem, but rather the personal meaning'.[10] Despite or because of these differences I hope that the dialogue initiated here might generate new thoughts both on the healing effects of reading as well as on how traumas and vulnerability can help us interpret literature.

Current Bibliotherapy and *Shared Reading* Practices in Sweden and Finland

The concept of bibliotherapy has developed into a broad umbrella term, covering a wide range of aims, methods, and orientations all over the world. As Liz Brewster points out in her chapter 'Bibliotherapy: A Critical History', 'there have been many interpretations of what constitutes bibliotherapy, who should deliver it and how it should be delivered'.[11] As a form of therapeutic treatment, it has its roots mainly in the US and UK, but projects where literature and art are used for therapeutic purposes can be found all over the world.[12]

The broad definition of bibliotherapy is 'the use of literature to promote mental health', but depending on the setting, target group, working method, and the material, the procedures vary. For instance, institutional bibliotherapy takes place at a hospital or a prison; clinical bibliotherapy is supervised by a doctor or psychologist and has the explicit aim 'to encourage insight and behavioural change'; and developmental bibliotherapy is more about general self-development and maintenance of mental health for people 'who did not have any diagnosis of mental health problems'.[13] McCarthy Hynes and Hynes-Berry differentiated 'reading bibliotherapy' (prescriptive reading) from 'interactive bibliotherapy' where the social interaction in a reading group and 'the triad of participant-literature-facilitator' becomes important.[14] Against this background, one could describe the bibliotherapeutic practice that is currently on the rise in Sweden and has a longer tradition in Finland, as mainly developmental, interactive/creative bibliotherapy.

In the Nordic countries, *kirjallisuusterapia* [literature therapy] has its longest tradition in Finland. One of the central figures of Finnish bibliotherapy is the cultural psychologist Juhani Ihanus. He describes how the Finnish interest in bibliotherapy started to grow in the 1940s. In the 1950s, reading groups at hospital libraries were developed.[15] The first regular literature therapy groups were initiated in Finland in the late 1970s and the first European organization for bibliotherapy was established in Finland in 1981.[16] The Finnish Association for Literature Therapy has a scientific journal, *Kirjallisuusterapia* [Literature Therapy], and a website.[17]

The 'Finnish model' of bibliotherapy has a focus on expressive and creative writing. The patient/participant is to be aided to find, and use, healing words. Ihanus has published five anthologies on bibliotherapy, and in the above-mentioned anthology he describes how he views literature therapy as a kind of 'word art therapy'. It is supposed to be a 'word adventure', a process where finding 'the healing words' is key.[18] Several of the other contributions in Ihanus' anthology also have a focus on expressive/creative writing, such as therapeutical diaries, therapy writing, and life writing.[19] Finnish bibliotherapist Päivi Kosonen describes, in a series of articles, bibliotherapy as a form of 'identity work', where the literature serves as a 'reflective other' aiding participants in articulating and addressing painful memories. Fiction and poetry are thus viewed as expressive mediums, artistic forms capable of unlocking deeper layers of memory, thus providing participants with the opportunity to verbalize painful experiences.[20]

The Finnish bibliotherapy tradition has some similarities with the process Mazza depicted in *Poetry Therapy*, where using poetry in personal ways is central. Ihanus' description of the healing effect of words also has points of contact with how Philip Davis (who works in close collaboration with *The Reader Organization* and is married to Jane Davis, the initiator of *Shared Reading*) describes his view of literature and reading. In *Reading and the Reader: The Literary Agenda* (2013), Philip Davis stresses how literature and lyrical words have a different effect on us from everyday language's way of describing: He talks about 'meaning intuited' and how the right poem can help you articulate your emotions; the poem 'gives the word, but you feel its meaning'.[21]

In Sweden, interactive bibliotherapy (the collective reading of fiction or poetry to improve mental health) has become increasingly widespread and popular only in the last decades. Before the early 2000s, the term was rarely used in cultural discussions, and the activities described as bibliotherapeutic were very few. However, since around 2010, creative, interactive bibliotherapy has become increasingly common.[22] The typical form of bibliotherapy in Sweden is open reading groups at libraries or targeted groups at local health centres aimed at people with relatively mild mental health problems; the interest in this form of 'reading treatment' is growing.[23] Parallel to this, the British concept of *Shared Reading*[24] has also been imported to Sweden, and there are now many educated *Shared Reading* group leaders in several places in Sweden, and a few bigger research projects founded on *Shared Reading*-practices have also been conducted.[25]

Since 2017, Ersta Sköndal University College has offered the course 'The Bibliotherapeutic Work Procedure', targeted towards librarians, social workers, and other professionals, and the number of applicants has been high.[26] When they advertised the new course in spring 2017, over 200 people expressed interest, and they have been able to offer approximately 22–24 places each year since then.[27] The university course is the first of its kind in the country, and since bibliotherapy is a fairly new form of activity in Sweden, but one that has attracted a lot of attention and interest, Swedish libraries have called for more information about how bibliotherapy works and its benefits and risks.[28]

As bibliotherapy becomes more common in Sweden, it is mainly the Finnish model that is being imported, but the reading process seems to be given a more central function in the Swedish bibliotherapy groups, compared with the word focus and creative writing in Finland.[29] The new university course at Ersta Sköndal was initiated by Pia Bergström, a social worker and teacher of Finnish origin, who has a bibliotherapy degree from Finland. The course at Ersta Sköndal is directed towards professionals and shorter than the Finnish more formal education, but what is taught at the Ersta Sköndal course is inspired by the Finnish literature therapy model.[30] Theoretically, the course at Ersta Sköndal goes beyond Ihanus' views and the Finnish tradition, being anchored additionally in central Anglo-Saxon (UK/US) theories of bibliotherapy: Hynes & Hynes-Berry, Shrodes, Brewster & McNicol feature on the reading list.

In *Bibliotherapy* (2018), Sarah McNicol outlines the theoretical ground for fiction or poetry-based bibliotherapy. She describes the theories for this type of bibliotherapy as 'associated with reader development and the reading experience' and writes about the potential impact of reading in terms of 'absorption', 'escapism', and 'involvement'.[31] McNicol presents the central theories of the bibliotherapeutic reading process, beginning with Caroline Shrodes' (1949) model: (1) identification and projection, (2) abreaction and catharsis, and (3) insight and integration. She then adds Hynes & Hynes-Berry's development of the model into a four-step bibliotherapeutic process: recognition – examination – juxtaposition (where 'a deeper level of understanding is reached'), and finally – self-application, which occurs when the reader evaluates and integrates her impressions from the literary work of art and 'filters it for their own life situation' in order to create 'a new, deeply personal meaning'.[32]

To these established theories McNicol and Brewster also add a reasoning on the 'interaction of text and reader' and the fact that 'bibliotherapy may not work in the same way [...] for all readers'.[33] 'Reader attributes' such as the will to participate, need for emotional support, demographic characteristics (age, gender), and self-perception will impact the bibliotherapeutic process. And just as readers differ, so do texts: 'not all texts are written to produce the same type of response'.[34]

In the Nordic context attempts to refine this established theory have also been made by Swedish bibliotherapy researcher Cecilia Pettersson, who in a number of studies has examined, and advocated for a user-centered perspective: women on sick leave were interviewed about how reading affected their psychological well-being, self-confidence, and social capacity.[35] A group of people suffering from long-term anxiety and depression partaking in an interactive bibliotherapy group were studied.[36] In her book *Biblioterapi* (2020), Pettersson draws conclusions from her earlier, empirical, participant-oriented studies, and develops concrete, practical advice, including the importance of a literature selection sensitive to the group's needs, carefully planned discussion structures, and openness to modifying approaches throughout the process.[37] So even though one can notice the trend in bibliotherapy studies to establish broad, universal, and somewhat simplistic and undifferentiated models for what a healing reading process should be about, there also exist practical and perhaps nationally or otherwise-inflected attempts to nuance these models.

The bibliotherapy being taught at Ersta Sköndal and the *Shared Reading* initiatives that are spreading in Sweden have the social, interactive aspect of the reading group in common – the shared experience is an important part of both activities. Above-mentioned Pettersson also emphasizes the social, interactive aspects of the reading practice in her study of people suffering from long-term anxiety and depression partaking in an interactive bibliotherapy group. The study shows how the particular combination of reading, and the social gathering of the group, was valued by many participants.[38] Besides Pettersson's research, there are also other earlier Swedish studies on bibliotherapy where the social, interactive aspect of reading together is emphasized in different ways: Inger Eriksson's (2006) dissertation on poetry reading groups for people in the final stages of life is an older example; Eva Selin and Karin Graube's study 'Reading aloud to children in hospital. Bibliotherapy as a community builder' (2017) and Eva Selin's *Läsklubb pågår! En metodbok om högläsning som biblioterapi* (2019) are two more recent examples where a bibliotherapeutic practice (reading aloud for hospitalized children) has generated a methodological description.[39]

Reading about bibliotherapy gives you an approximate idea of what it is and how it works, but, to me, some of the prescriptive models for how reading is supposed to affect a participant appeared somewhat formulaic and unnuanced. Isn't there a contradiction, or paradox, between the chaotically subversive, disruptive force that fiction and poetry can be, and the desire to evoke an expected healing progression with pre-established prescriptions, the type of control needed in healthcare and the medical field?

In order to gain more practical insight into this key question, as understood by central figures in modern Swedish bibliotherapy, I met with two of the teachers at the Ersta Sköndal course, Pia Bergström and Eva Bergstedt and I also participated in a trial bibliotherapy session held by Finnish bibliotherapist Päivi Kosonen.[40]

Eva Bergstedt is a freelance journalist and librarian who has covered the field of bibliotherapy in several articles for the Swedish press.[41] She is one of the current course leaders at Ersta Sköndal. When I asked her why people in

Sweden are drawn to bibliotherapy, she stated three main reasons: (1) you do not have to talk directly about your own problems; (2) you get more words to describe your feelings; and (3) literature and the discussion of literature confirm that you are not alone. The course offered at Ersta Sköndal is to be viewed as an introduction to the bibliotherapeutic work procedure. You do not become a bibliotherapist from participating in it; Eva stresses that such a title should be avoided, out of humility for the limits of one's competence. She is also reluctant to state whether it should always be called bibliotherapy – sometimes 'educative literature discussions' may be a more suitable term for interactive, developmental bibliotherapy.

Many of the bibliotherapy leaders participating in the university course are librarians, and bibliotherapy reading groups are often arranged as a joint venture between a library and a health care center, hospital, or care association so that the group collaborates with an educated therapist. With the right collaboration between librarians and social workers/psychotherapists, it can often be a very rewarding undertaking and positive experience for the participants.[42] Regardless of educational background, the leader of a bibliotherapy reading group needs to be empathetic, and an attentive listener.[43]

Pia Bergström was the initiator of the course offered at Ersta Sköndal. She has a background as a social worker and family therapist with engagement in non-profit associations and volunteer organizations. Her bibliotherapy degree is from Finland, so she is schooled in the 'Finnish model' with its focus on writing, and aiding the participants to expand their experiences and develop personally through the use of literature.[44] When Pia Bergström considers my somewhat theoretical questions on literary views, the healing effects of literature, and if identification or escapism is key for the choice of books, she states her way of thinking and working is different and has other points of departure.

She stresses that the original meaning of the word therapy is *service*.[45] Her work starts with the human, and the needs of the participants. Based on their specific problems, she then searches for useful literature, or word art (for example inspirational cards with proverbs or quotes) that ignites creativity in the participants; stories that make them open up and put words to their own experiences.

One example of how she has worked is the project *Du, Jag, Vi* [*You, Me, We*] which was a group of young people (aged 16–20) having a parent sentenced to jail. She introduced them to books they could relate to, and an important part of the bibliotherapy was talking and writing about passages from the books they were especially moved by. By writing down their thoughts and reactions and reading them aloud to each other, they started over time to transform their views about themselves and their life narratives.[46]

Normally a bibliotherapy group, in Bergtröm's description, consists of 6–8 participants who meet once a week, for a period of around four months, or 15–16 sessions. Each session can be 2 hours long. It always starts by creating a harmonic, calm atmosphere in the room, by doing warm-up exercises, something to make sure everyone in the room feels safe. Then they work with a more specific theme, or text, and each participant writes, maybe two pages. Bergström describes the session as a living process, with a certain rhythm. As a bibliotherapy leader, she must trust the group and their process.

When I participated in the trial bibliotherapy session (we read a passage from the Swedish author Agneta Pleijel's childhood memoirs and then wrote our own texts in response to hers), I found that this was a much more creative, poetic approach to the literary text than what I am used to from regular literature seminars or book circles. It reminded me more of creative writing practices, even though we started out with reading an existing work of literature. The approach, of freely choosing selected parts or sentences from the work at hand which you then develop into your own text, makes the literary text a kind of springboard for the participants' own life stories. For some of those who participated in this trial (predominantly women between 65 and 80 so a group that at least approximately could remember a similar time as the time depicted in Agneta Pleijel's childhood memories) small details in the text made them remember details from their own childhood that had made a strong impact on them. Literary depictions of such trivial things as a window stitch or a certain garment can awaken memories that have been buried for decades.

In February 2021, I interviewed Åsa Sarachu, who works as a *Shared Reading* facilitator and is a member of the *Shared Reading Sweden* network. She begins by emphasizing that *Shared Reading* lacks any therapeutic claims: It is a reading and literature-promoting activity where participants are given space to show vulnerability, but it is not about reading with any explicit aim to solve mental health problems. Instead, this reading community is about the potential of literature to provide support, meaning, and context in our lives. It aims to: (1) spark interest in fiction and poetry, so that the participants discover new literature and become more avid readers, attentive to what the text evokes in them, and (2) promote the social and community aspects of reading: meeting in groups, making new friends, and sharing a moment of togetherness. Even though the explicit therapeutic aim is absent, there are obvious similarities between *Shared Reading* and the activities described above by Bergstedt and Bergström.

Sarachu speaks with warm enthusiasm about how conversations stemming from literature are often rewarding, existential, and deep. The literature read becomes a way to avoid talking directly about oneself, while also evoking memories, leading the discussion between the text and the participants' various life experiences, and childhood memories, that make them see different dimensions of the text.

The *Shared Reading* gatherings are characterized by the lack of pretentiousness and the permissive atmosphere, which is a difference compared to academic literary seminars. The general rule is 'be kind'; you read there and then, and it's the moment of shared reading, of collective, associative conversation, that becomes important. Commonly, short stories which are short enough to be read in their entirety during one session are read – sometimes also poetry, but short stories are more common. The choice of literature is important, it needs to be rich and thought-provoking. The *Shared Reading* network has active circle leaders in several parts of Sweden, including Skåne, Jönköping, Uppsala, and Gävle, and the target groups are very diverse: including within the correctional services and senior associations- or among newly arrived teenagers. *Shared Reading* projects are aimed at specific target groups, but who these groups are varies.[47]

Bibliotherapy and Literary Trauma Theory – The Start of a Conversation

In literary trauma studies – the field I want to critically place in dialogue with bibliotherapy in the remainder of this chapter – the question of literary representation of traumatic experiences is central. Trauma often involves both language – and memory loss, and literary trauma theory studies the ability of fiction to portray and express difficult experiences that need to be worked through but cannot be directly expressed.[48]

Cathy Caruth describes trauma as 'unclaimed experience'.[49] She emphasizes that trauma can hardly be defined by the event that caused it, since different persons react differently to the same events. A traumatic experience is thus often highly individual.[50] How traumatic experiences, loss, and separation, mourning and grief processes, as well as post-traumatic stress syndrome, are portrayed and worked through in fiction and poetry is what literary trauma research is concerned with.

An important part of literary trauma studies is also a special focus on the ethical aspects of reading.[51] These perspectives can perhaps add something to and nuance the bibliotherapeutic models of reading. I mentioned above how identification or recognition is an important part of the bibliotherapeutic process. When I participated in the trial session, several of the participants were quick to confirm how 'they recognized themselves' in the text we had read. The identification paradigm reappears often in bibliotherapy literature and seems to be an important part of the work procedure. Of course, identification can also occur in relation to literary characters with completely different experiences, and this form of identification is also present within bibliotherapeutic practice. But paired with a problem-solving paradigm where you are supposed to mentally heal or develop, one could (possibly generalizing) claim that the formula seems to be: 'you read about what which you want to be cured from'.

In literary trauma studies, what is sometimes called 'over-identification', or 'identification turned into appropriation', is problematized. In *Writing History, Writing Trauma* (2001), Dominick LaCapra distinguishes empathy from identification. He believes that empathy is that double maneuver in which one establishes a bond with the other at the same time as one accepts the other person's 'otherness'. LaCapra discusses 'empathic unsettlement', sensitivity towards the other – towards the text being read – which involves being 'responsive' but resisting 'full identification with, and appropriation of, the experience of the other'. This requires both risking oneself and one's own potential for traumatization, while also recognizing 'that another's loss is not identical to one's own loss'. This is why 'cognition and critical analysis' is an inevitable part of empathy, and why 'it is very important to distinguish empathy from identification'.[52] Empathy 'combines a rapport or bond with the other [...] with an affirmation of otherness', but when you identify with something, you absorb or embody it. The result is that 'the receiver of testimony' – or in this case, the reader, a hypothetical participant in a bibliotherapy group – succumbs to 'projective identification', or secondary trauma.[53] To gain access to, or relive a certain experience of pain, through identifying with a literary work depicting it, doesn't necessarily guarantee that you will be free from it. The literary trauma narrative always balances ambivalently between, on the one hand, a compulsion to repeat that only reinforces the trauma, and *catharsis*, purification.[54]

If identification unproblematized becomes our main way of relating to fiction, you could argue that this creates a kind of narcissistic, appropriative reading that is close to consumerism. In the beginning of this chapter, I quoted Arthur Lerner's statement in the *Journal of Poetry Therapy*: 'in poetry therapy the focus is on the person, not the poem'. But once they've come together, how can he define where one begins and the other ends? This is a critical question. It has to do with where our concern for the person ends and where our understanding of the 'affect' of the poem begins. Isn't an important part of almost all reading processes (at least the ones involving fiction and poetry) that they pull the rug out from under strict definitions where the reader could be considered a separate entity (let's say the subject), and the text is addressed as if not part of the overall interaction (as if the object)? Instead, with literature and poetry, these definitions can readily be seen to be less fixed and less easily distinguishable.[55] Are reading processes just as much power struggles as identificatory or symbiotic mergers? The text we read often takes control and subjectifies – it *does* something to us. The poem may correctively exhort us 'Du muss dein Leben ändern', like the Apollo statue to Rilke's art contemplator, and confront us with parts of ourselves we would rather avoid. Or as Swedish children's literature author Lennart Hellsing put it in a famous, often quoted verse; 'While we read the books, the books read us. / Can books read people? Of course they can! / How else would they know everything about us?'[56] Literature is not just written words on a paper for us to consume or mirror ourselves in; literary texts can also be seen as active agents seeking to transform the passive, depressive reader-object into something more creative.[57]

Fiction and poetry have the capacity both to heal and distress us – to make us feel worse. I quoted Kafka at the beginning of this chapter. His axe metaphor is a famous image of literature's subversive ability to crush us completely. If you read the full quote, Kafka builds his metaphor by stating that we need 'books that affect us like a disaster, that grieve us deeply, like the death of someone we loved more than ourselves, like being banished into forests far from everyone, like a suicide'.[58] I am not saying this shock effect is necessarily a bad thing. But literature's ability to hurt and cause harm isn't much talked about in the bibliotherapy discourse.[59] One exception is the research of Emily Troscianko, who, critical of the identification paradigm, asks: 'If reading about someone the same as yourself is meant to be therapeutic, what makes it different from, say, rereading your own diary entries?'[60] Troscianko did an online survey on the effects of reading fiction among patients recovering from eating disorders. She asked respondents about their reading habits, 'whether they had sought out fiction or nonfiction to help with their disorder and whether any books had been helpful or harmful, and if so how'.[61] The findings showed that reading could be both helpful and harmful. It has the capacity to reinforce negative thought patterns and thus exacerbate the disorder if you are reminded of your illness and for instance zoom in on all depictions of thinness in the story. But reading fiction which gives you the possibility to escape and forget your predicament has reportedly a positive impact.[62] This is also in line with the findings in Cecilia Pettersson's empirical, user-centered research. In Pettersson's study of women's experience of reading fiction during sick leave, she noticed that most chose to read 'lighter', more escapist genre literature that they found relaxing during their sick leave. Identificatory reading was prominent, but more general, in the sense that one could identify with the characters regardless of the kind of life being read about. Pettersson also noted that several of the women spoke about the importance of self-forgetting reading, meaning that they forgot about themselves while reading.[63]

Anne Whitehead writes in *Trauma Fiction* (2004): 'Trauma theory readjusts the relationship between reader and the text, so that reading is restored as an ethical practice'.[64] In bibliotherapy, the ethical considerations concerning the choice of literary texts focus on the users. They come first, and the text is a working tool or a transitional object, chosen with regard to the readers' demands or specific problems. Relational aspects and empathy are crucial in the interactions between participants and between participants and the bibliotherapy leader.

However, within the field of literary trauma studies, it is instead the text that is prioritized and placed in focus. The ethical discussion about reading here concerns how the reader engages with the text, as an 'other' or a witness. As Whitehead states: 'Trauma studies work against medical reductionism by exhorting practitioners to attend to a voice which is not fully known or knowable, and to bear witness'.[65] This voice is found in literature, through poetic and literary expression.

Finally, I want to open up for further thought on how perspectives from the text-focused field of literary trauma studies can enrich and nuance the bibliotherapeutic discourse on how literature heals us. I believe that there are additional perspectives to be added to the debate about identification and escapism within bibliotherapy. A recent publication, *Narrative Medicine: Trauma and Ethics* (2024) eds. Juhl Rasmussen and Sodemann, also attests to the fact that perspectives from trauma theory can rejuvenate the broad field of narrative medicine in ways that invite further contemplation.

The discussion of ethics within the field of literary trauma studies involves raising awareness that literature depicting painful, traumatic experiences necessitates a profoundly ethical response. You cannot simplistically identify with the experiences depicted, nor can you repeat or consume them. Whitehead refers to Shoshana Felman and Dori Laub's influential *Testimony: Crises of Witnessing in Literature, Psychoanalysis, and History* (1992). They argue that 'testimony requires a highly collaborative relationship between speaker and listener', which – transferred into the bibliotherapeutic context I am discussing here – could be understood as book and reader. The listener/reader bears

> a dual responsibility: to receive the testimony but also to avoid appropriating the story as his or her own. A fragile balance is engendered between the

> necessity to witness sympathetically that which testimonial writing cannot fully represent and a simultaneous respect for the otherness of the experience, which resists rendering it too familiar or indulging in too easy an understanding or identification.[66]

Is it not possible to envisage that a form of trauma-informed, empathetic reading could have beneficial therapeutic effects just as identificatory or escapist ones? This is a suggestion to think further upon, but for example, a trauma-informed, empathetic reading could be a combination of self-forgetfulness and care for the pain depicted in the literary work. A reader/participant in bibliotherapy who has experienced something difficult, that he/she suffers from, could, through such trauma-informed reading, re-evaluate their own suffering as something that gives them an empathetic ability to understand and feel compassion for the text, rather than just identifying themselves in it. So to speak, one can 'help' the text to heal, engage with its problems, and in that way, perhaps simultaneously re-evaluate oneself and one's abilities. To some extent, this is probably what many bibliotherapy circles engage in, but thinking of the text as a fellow being, as someone who suffers and needs help, shifts the perspective slightly away from identification and/or escapism.

This may sound like a big step to take, to start talking about the text as a suffering subject. But, influenced by D.W. Winnicott, Ihanus emphasizes the importance of play in bibliotherapy. To him, what distinguishes bibliotherapy from regular psychotherapy is that bibliotherapy has a third – a transitional object – the literary work of art. With the help of the textual transitional object, the reader can depart from the vacuum-sealed existence of monologue and progress to dialogues and polylogues. In the literary-therapeutic situation, numerous alternative realities and interpretations of reality emerge.[67]

This position demonstrates allows for viewing the book as more than a tool, and also as something you have a relationship with, and could care for, like a teddy bear. To stretch it a little further: If the literary text can take part in the reading session as a transitional object, doesn't this open up the possibility of seeing the text as a dialogue partner, someone the reader can care for and try to help?

So instead of limiting our understanding of healing through books to it being about identification and/or self-forgetting escapism, I think maybe we should turn it the other way around. It is you, the reader, who with all your suffering and vulnerability, can help heal the book by listening to it. And in that ability to heal the book, by listening emphatically and creatively to it, lies also a reevaluation of that from which you suffer.

Notes

1 Quote from Zacharias Topelius poem "Sången" ["The Song"] [1842]. Eva Ström and Thomas Sjösvärd helped with the translation to English.

2 Kafka states this in a letter to his friend Oskar Pollak in 1904. See Kafka, Franz, *Briefe 1902–1924* (1958). The English translation of the quote can be found on Goodreads page "Quotable quotes": www.goodreads.com/quotes/237620-i-think-we-ought-to-read-only-the-kind-of.

3 The word *τραῦμα* [trauma] comes from the Greek word for wound. In a modern context (from Freud onwards), the understanding of trauma is rather psychological than physical: it concerns how an overwhelming, psychologically shaking event or experience has left traces so the response comes delayed, afterward. The original wound being repressed, not fully known, creates a compulsion to repeat, leading to prolonged suffering where the trauma affects both memory and identity. See van der Kolk, Bessel, 2015; Caruth, Cathy, 1996.

4 Malmberg, Carl-Johan, *Sår: i myt, kult, bild och dikt*, 2005, 13ff. Mazza, Nicholas, *Poetry Therapy: Theory and Practice*, [2004] 2017, 5f. C.f. Pettersson, Cecilia, 2014, 56–57, Heinö, Agneta, 2004, 4–5.

5 For a recent overview of the field of literary trauma studies, see Davis & Meretoja, 2020; Kurtz, 2018; for an introduction to contemporary bibliotherapy see McNichols & Brewster, 2018; Mazza, *Poetry Therapy: Theory and Practice*, [2004] 2017.

6 Partly, this expansion stems from a number of initiated action driven bibliotherapy and *Shared Reading* research projects, partly from the fact that a Finnish bibliotherapist, Pia Bergström, started a university course in "Bibliotherapy as a working method" in 2017. C.f. Cecilia Pettersson, *Biblioterapi: Hälsofrämjande läsning i teori och praktik* (Stockholm: Appell, 2020), 69–87.

7 Pettersson, *Biblioterapi,* 2020. Those interviewed are bibliotherapy practitioners Pia Bergström and Eva Bergstedt, and the *Shared Reading* Group Leader is Åsa Sarachu.

8 When we read, we immerse ourselves in the experience depicted in the text. We might project our own experiences onto the text, but just as much, the text's subjective experience shapes us and how we perceive. Reading is about opening oneself up and allowing the text to shape oneself. The Swedish children's book author Lennart Hellsing has expressed it as 'while we read the books, the books read us.' The subject/object aspects of reading have been explored by various scholars across multiple disciplines, including hermeneutics, i.e. the work of Hans-Georg Gadamer, and reader-response theory, for example Stanley Fish and Wolfgang Iser. Also, in the field of literary didactics, there are theories such as Louise Rosenblatt's transactional theory of reading, which emphasizes the reciprocal relationship between the reader and the text (cf. Gadamer [1960] 1994; Fish 1980; Iser [1978] 1991; Rosenblatt [1978] 1994).

9 McNicol & Brewster, 2018, 23.

10 Mazza, *Poetry Therapy: Theory and Practice,* [2004] 2017, 4, with reference to Arthur Lerner, "Poetry Therapy Corner", *Journal of Poetry Therapy*, Vol 7, Issue 3, March 1994, 151–154..

11 Brewster, Liz, "Bibliotherapy: A Critical History", in McNicol & Brewster, 2018, 5.

12 Carolyn Shrodes' pioneer dissertation *Bibliotherapy: A Theoretical and Clinical-Experimental Study* (1949) linked bibliotherapy to psychoanalysis. The dynamic interaction between reader and literature was described by Shrodes as a psychoanalytic process with three stages: identification, catharsis, insight. This psychoanalytical understanding of bibliotherapy has continued to be influential.

13 Rubin, Rhea Joyce, 1978; McNicol & Brewster, 2018.

14 McCarthy Hynes, Arleen & Mary Hynes-Berry, *Biblio/Poetry Therapy. The Interactive Process: A Handbook*, [1994] 2012, 4–5.

15 Ihanus, 2004, 20 with reference to Sippola 1985. Ihanus has published several anthologies on bibliotherapy (Ihanus 1985; 1989; 1991; 1995; 2002) and methods involving reading or writing for therapeutic purposes have been applied in rehabilitation as well as in preventative care in hospitals, correctional facilities, and outpatient care.

16 Ihanus, Juhani, "Litteratur och terapi", *Att tiga eller tala. Litteraturterapi – ett sätt att växa*, ed. Anneli Aurela, Juhani Ihanus & Carin Dedijer, transl. Ann-Christine Relander

(Helsingfors: BTJ Kirjastopalvelu, 2004), 13–36. Ihanus work is also translated into English in the volume *Transformative Words. Writing Otherness and Identities* (New York: Nova Publishing, 2019).

17 Finnish Association for Literature Therapy: https://kirjallisuusterapia.net/

18 Ihanus, "Litteratur och terapi", 2004, 13–31.

19 Ihanus et al, 2004; Johansson on therapeutical diaries, 95ff; Enwald on therapy writing, 109ff; Viitaniemi on life writing, 142ff.

20 Kosonen 2018, 25.

21 Davis 2013.

22 Pettersson 2020, 69, 71.

23 Pettersson 2020, 69–87.

24 *Shared Reading* is a concept developed by UK organization *The Reader*. On their website they explain the activity:

> *Shared Reading* groups are open to all and free to attend. A group of people, one of them a trained Reader Leader, reads a great novel, short story or poem aloud. We stop and talk about what we have read. There is no need for group members to read aloud or speak – it's fine to just listen. The idea is to create a space where people feel at ease.
> www.thereader.org.uk/what-we-do/shared-reading/

25 For example, Professor Anders Ohlsson's project, 'Shared Reading and Pain Rehabilitation', The Centre for Languages and Literature, Lund University, and Professor Kerstin Rydbeck's '*Shared Reading* in a Nordic context', a collaboration between several universities, coordinated by Department of Archives – Libraries – Museums, Uppsala University. See Forslid, T., Ohlsson, A., Rydbeck, K., Skjerdingstad, K. I., Steenberg, M. & Tangerås, T. M. (ed.) *Shared Reading i Skandinavia: Teori og praksis* (Oslo: ABM-media AS, 2022), https://skriftserien.oslomet.no/index.php/skriftserien/article/view/796

26 A sixfold of applicants for each spot. C.f. news reports in *Rapport* 12.07.2017: www.svt.se/kultur/biblioterapi-later-manniskor-lasa-sig-friska and in *Kropp och själ*, P1, 'Läsning som läker', 11.07.2017: http://sverigesradio.se/sida/avsnitt/917193?programid=1272.

27 Bergstedt 2018.

28 Pettersson 2014.

29 Kosonen observes that the Swedish interest in bibliotherapy appears to emphasize reading more strongly, contrasting with the Finnish focus on creative writing therapy. This is also evident by Pettersson's review of the Swedish field of bibliotherapy practice, Pettersson 2020, 71–73. Earlier Swedish research on bibliotherapy also has a focus on reading, as seen in the work of Skans Kersti Nilsson & Torsten Pettersson, 2009.

30 Bergström 2018.

31 McNicol and Brewster 2018, 26–27

32 McNicol and Brewster 2018, 30 with reference to Hynes, A. M., and Hynes-Berry, M., *Biblio/Poetry Therapy – The Interactive Process: A Handbook*, North Star Press, 2012, 31.

33 McNicol and Brewster 2018, 31.

34 McNicol and Brewster 2018, 31.

35 Pettersson 2016.

36 Pettersson 2018.

37 Pettersson 2020, 155–193.

38 Cecilia Pettersson, "Psychological well-being, improved self-confidence, and social capacity: Bibliotherapy from a user perspective", *Journal of Poetry Therapy* 31, 2018, 124–134.

39 Inger Eriksson 2006; Eva Selin and Karin Graube 2018. Additional notable studies focusing on bibliotherapy and the potential healing effects of reading conducted in a Nordic context in recent years include: Magnus Persson 2012; Torsten Pettersson, 2008, 2009; Nina Frid 2016; Thor Magnus Tangerås, 2018.

40 I met with Eva Bergstedt 2018.09.28, with Pia Bergström 2018.10.01 and the trial bibliotherapy session with Päivi Kosonen was conducted at the fair Best of Norden, Nordic museum, Stockholm 2018.10.06.

41 Bergstedt 2017a, 2017b, 2017c.

42 Bergström 2018. C.f. Pettersson 2018.

43 Bergström 2018.

44 Cf. Ihanus, "Litteratur och terapi", 2004, p. 20–22. See also Kosonen, who have noticed that "when it comes to the development of therapeutic methods, reading has been overshadowed by writing" in the Finnish model. Kosonen 2018, p. 24. See also Kosonen 2019a, 2019b.

45 From Greek *therapeia* "curing, healing, service done to the sick; a waiting on, service".

46 The project resulted in an anthology: Bergström, P. & Omsén, E. (ed) 2016. *Du jag vi. Om att ha en förälder i fängelse*. Stockholm: Buff Stockholm.

47 Sarachu 2021. For an overview of Shared Reading in Scandinavia, research and practice, see Forslid, T., Ohlsson, A., Rydbeck, K., Skjerdingstad, K. I., Steenberg, M. & Tangerås, T. M. (ed.) *Shared Reading i Skandinavia: Teori og praksis* (Oslo: ABM-media AS, 2022).

48 For an updated introduction to the field of literary trauma theory see Davis and Meretoja 2020, 2–4: "Canonical works of trauma studies by literary critics and theorists Cathy Caruth (1995, 1996) and Shoshana Felman, the psychiatrist Dori Laub (Felman and Laub 1992) and the historian Dominick LaCapra (1994, 2001) laid the foundation for what would become the explosion of trauma studies." Davis and Meretoja, 2020, 3.

49 Caruth 1996.

50 Caruth 1995, p. 3–12.

51 See for instance Martin Modlinger and Philipp Sontag (eds.) anthology *Other People's Pain. Narratives of Trauma and the Question of Ethics* (2011).

52 LaCapra 2001, 41-42, 78-79, 211-213. Cf. Whitehead, *Trauma Fiction*, 2004, 8–9, 35.

53 Whitehead, *Trauma Fiction*, 2004, 8–9; LaCapra 2001, 211-213.

54 Whitehead, *Trauma Fiction,* 2004, 83–84.

55 Gadamer [1960] 1994; Fish 1980; Iser [1978] 1991; Rosenblatt [1978] 1994.

56 Rainer Maria Rilke, "Archaïscher Torso Apollos" and Lennart Hellsing "Böcker ska blänka som solar".

57 C.f. Davis, Philip, *William James* (2022) where he in a similar way argues that James functions as a "human motor force, performing in his readers the equivalent of the work of the spinal cord and the brain's motor cortex, to create movement—mental, emotional, and physical." Davis, *William James*, 2022, 1.

58 Kafka [1904] 1958.

59 I am primarily thinking here of the established bibliotherapy theories that describe various ways in which literature can be healing. However, the shift in bibliotherapy research towards conducting more empirical case studies naturally opens opportunities to also note the ways in which literature can be harmful. C.f. Troscianko 2018b, 201.

60 Troscianko 2018c; https://scroll.in/article/887286/can-reading-a-good-book-help-with-eating-disorders-yes-but-it-can-also-do-harm-says-new-research

61 Troscianko, 2018b, 6.

62 Troscianko, 2018b, 16.

63 Pettersson 2016; c.f. Pettersson, *Biblioterapi*, 2020, 87; 117–120; 122–125.
64 Whitehead, *Trauma Fiction,* 2004, 8.
65 Whitehead, *Trauma Fiction,* 2004, 8.
66 Whitehead, *Trauma Fiction,* 2004, 7–8 with reference to Felman and Laub, *Testimony,* 1992.
67 Ihanus, "Litteratur och terapi", 2004, 27.

References

Bergstedt Eva. 'Alternativ medicin mot livsproblemen', *Svenska Dagbladet* (21 March 2017) www.svd.se/a/vo30l/alternativ-medicin-mot-livsproblemen (retrieved 12 March 2024).

Bergstedt Eva. 'Biblioterapi – ett sätt att hantera barnens självmord', *Svenska Dagbladet* (20 March 2017) www.svd.se/a/j5LAw/biblioterapi-ett-satt-att-hantera-barnens-sjalvmord (retrieved 12 March 2024).

Bergstedt, Eva. Interview with Eva Bergstedt, bibliotherapy leader and journalist, conducted at the Book Fair in Gothenburg, 28 September 2018.

Bergström, Pia. Interview with Pia Bergström, social worker and educationist, bibliotherapy leader, conducted in Stockholm 1 October 2018. Web page to the Association for Bibliotherapy in Sweden: www.biblioterapi.se (retrieved 24 January 2025).

Bergström, Pia, and E. Omsén, eds. *Du jag vi. Om att ha en förälder i fängelse.* Stockholm: Buff Stockholm, 2016.

Caruth, Cathy. 'Introduction'. In *Trauma: Explorations in Memory*, edited by Cathy Caruth, 3–12. Baltimore: Johns Hopkins University Press, 1995.

Caruth, Cathy. *Unclaimed Experience. Trauma, Narrative, and History.* Baltimore: Johns Hopkins University Press, 1996.

Davis, Colin, and Hanna Meretoja, eds. *The Routledge Companion to Literature and Trauma*. London: Routledge, 2020.

Davis, Philip. *Reading and the Reader*. Oxford: Oxford University Press, 2013.

Eriksson, Inger. *Poesiläsning som meningsskapare. En studie om poesigrupper på sjukhem och hospice*. PhD Diss. Lund University, 2006.

Felman, Shoshana, and Dori Laub. *Testimony: Crises of Witnessing in Literature, Psychoanalysis and History*. London: Routledge, 1992.

Fish, Stanley. *Is There a Text in This Class? The Authority of Interpretive Communities.* Cambridge, MA: Harvard University Press, 1980.

Forslid, T., Ohlsson, A., Rydbeck, K., Skjerdingstad, K. I., Steenberg, M. and T. M. Tangerås, eds. *Shared Reading i Skandinavia: Teori og praksis*. Oslo: ABM-media AS, 2022. https://skriftserien.oslomet.no/index.php/skriftserien/article/view/796 (retrieved 12 March 2024).

Frid, Nina. *Läsa, läka, leva! Om läsfrämjande och biblioterapi*. Lund: BTJ Förlag, 2016.

Gadamer, Hans-Georg. *Truth and Method.* 2nd. ed. Translated by Joel Weinsheimer and Donald G. Marshall (1960; New York: Continuum, 1994).

Heinö, Agneta. *'Man behöver inte vara officiellt deprimerad'. Om biblioterapi som biblioteksverksamhet, med Kirklees i England som exempel.* Borås: Högskolan i Borås, Institutionen för Biblioteks- och informationsvetenskap, Bibliotekshögskolan, 2004.

Hellsing, Lennart. 'Böcker ska blänka som solar', www.goodreads.com/quotes/8395428-b-cker-ska-bl-nka-som-solar-och-gnistra-som-tomtebloss-medan (retrieved 12 March 2024).

Hynes, A. M., and M. Hynes-Berry. *Biblio/Poetry Therapy – The Interactive Process: A Handbook*. 3rd. ed. St Cloud, MN: North Star Press, 2012.

Ihanus, Juhani, ed. *Att tiga eller tala. Litteraturterapi – ett sätt att växa*. Translated by Ann-Christine Relander. Helsingfors: BTJ Kirjastopalvelu, 2004.

Ihanus, Juhani. 'Litteratur och terapi'. In *Att tiga eller tala. Litteraturterapi – ett sätt att växa*, edited by Anneli Aurela, Juhani Ihanus and Carin Dedijer. Translated by Ann-Christine Relander, 13–36. Helsingfors: BTJ Kirjastopalvelu, 2004.

Ihanus, Juhani. *Transformative Words. Writing Otherness and Identities*. New York: Nova Publishing, 2019.

Iser, Wolfgang. *The Act of Reading: A Theory of Aesthetic Response*. Baltimore: Johns Hopkins University Press, 1991.

Kafka, Franz. *Briefe 1902–1924*. New York: Schocken Books, 1958. English translation of the quote: www.goodreads.com/quotes/237620-i-think-we-ought-to-read-only-the-kind-of (retrieved 12 March 2024).

Kosonen, Päivi. 'Towards Therapeutic Reading. Part 1: Identity Work. Growth and Development through Reading', *Scriptum: Creative Writing Research Journal* 5, no. 2 (2018): 25–48.

Kosonen, Päivi. 'Towards Therapeutic Reading. Part 2: The Interactive Process of Reading', *Scriptum: Creative Writing Research Journal* 6, no. 1 (2019): 17–39.

Kosonen, Päivi. 'Towards Therapeutic Reading. Part 3: Forms of Shared Reading', *Scriptum: Creative Writing Research Journal* 6, no. 2 (2019): 43–57.

Kropp och själ, P1, 'Läsning som läker', 11 July 2017: http://sverigesradio.se/sida/avsnitt/917193?programid=1272 (retrieved 12 March 2024).

Kurtz, J. Roger, ed. *Trauma and Literature*. Cambridge: Cambridge University Press, 2018.

LaCapra, Dominick. *Writing History, Writing Trauma*. Baltimore: Johns Hopkins University Press, 2001.

Lerner, Arthur. 'Poetry Therapy Corner', *Journal of Poetry Therapy* 7, no. 3 (1994): 151–54.

Malmberg, Carl-Johan. *Sår: i myt, kult, bild och dikt*. Stockholm: Wahlström & Widstrand, 2005.

Mazza, Nicholas. *Poetry Therapy: Theory and Practice*. London: Routledge, 2017.

McNicol, Sarah and Liz Brewster, eds. *Bibliotherapy*. London: Facet, 2018.

Modlinger, Martin, and Philipp Sontag, eds. *Other People's Pain: Narratives of Trauma and the Question of Ethics*. Oxford: Peter Lang, 2011.

Nilsson, Skans Kersti, and Torsten Pettersson. *Litteratur som livskunskap. Tvärvetenskapliga perspektiv på personlighetsutvecklande läsning*. Borås: Högskolan i Borås, 2009.

Ohlsson Anders. 'Shared Reading after Pain Rehabilitation', The Centre for Languages and Literature, Lund University, https://portal.research.lu.se/en/projects/shared-reading-after-pain-rehabilitation (retrieved 12 March 2024).

Persson, Magnus. 'Den friska boken och den sjuka människan. Om litteratur som medicin'. In *Den goda boken. Samtida föreställningar om litteratur och läsning*. Lund: Studentlitteratur, 2012.

Pettersson, Cecilia. *Biblioterapi*. Stockholm: Appell förlag, 2020.

Pettersson, Cecilia. 'Biblioterapi i ett litteraturvetenskapligt perspektiv', *Tidskrift för litteraturvetenskap* 44, no. 1 (2014): 55–65.

Pettersson, Cecilia, 'Psychological Well-being, Improved Self-confidence and Social Capacity: Bibliotherapy from a User Perspective', *Journal of Poetry Therapy* 31, no. 2 (2018): 124–34.

Pettersson, Cecilia. 'Women's Experience of Reading Fiction while on Sick Leave', *LIR Journal*, no. 6 (2016): 48–59.

Pettersson, Torsten. 'Att läsa för att utvecklas'. In *Litteratur som livskunskap. Tvärvetenskapliga perspektiv på personlighetsutvecklande läsning*. Borås: Högskolan i Borås, 2009.

Pettersson, Torsten,. 'Drömmar om verkligheten. Skönlitteraturens potential för existentiell psykoterapi'. In *Bara detta liv. Texter i existentiell psykologi och psykoterapi*, edited by Dan Stiwne. Stockholm: Natur & Kultur, 2008.

Rilke, Rainer Maria. 'Archaïscher Torso Apollos', https://writing.upenn.edu/bernstein/syllabi/readings/Rilke-Archaic.html (retrieved 12 March 2024)

Rosenblatt, Louise. *The Reader, the Text, the Poem: The Transactional Theory of the Literary Work*. New ed. Carbondale: Southern Illinois University Press, 1994.

Rubin, Rhea Joyce. *Using Bibliotherapy. A Guide to Theory and Practice*. Phoenix: Oryx Press, 1978.

Rydbeck, Kerstin. '"Shared Reading" in a Nordic Context', a research project coordinated by Department of Archives – Libraries – Museums, Uppsala University. www.abm.uu.se/forskning/pagaende-forskningsprojekt/shared_reading/ (retrieved 12 March 2024).

Sarachu, Åsa. *Shared Reading*-practitioner, interview over Zoom, 27 February 2021.

Selin, Eva, and Karin Graube. 'Bibliotherapy at Its Best: Reading Aloud in a Swedish Hospital', *Children & Libraries: The journal of the Association for Library Service to Children* 16 no. 2 (2018). https://doi.org/10.5860/cal.16.2.13 (retrieved 12 March 2024).

'*Shared Reading*: How does it work?' The Reader Organization: www.thereader.org.uk/what-we-do/shared-reading/.

Shrodes, Carolyn. *Bibliotherapy. A Theoretical and Clinical-Experimental Study*. PhD Diss: University of California, Berkeley, 1949.

Sippola, Leena. 'Kirjallisuusterapian kehityslinjoja', In *Sanojen liikkeitä. Kirjoituksia kirjallisuus- ja runoterapiasta*, edited by Juhani Ihanus, 11–26. Helsinki: Kirjastopalvelu, 1985.

Sonck, Mikaela. 'Biblioterapi låter människor läsa sig friska', *Rapport* 12 July 2017. www.svt.se/kultur/biblioterapi-later-manniskor-lasa-sig-friska (retrieved 12 March 2024).

Suomen Kirjallisuusterapiayhdistys ry [Finnish Literary Therapy Association] https://kirjallisuusterapia.net/ (retrieved 12 March 2024).

Tangerås, Thor Magnus. *'How Literature Changed My Life'. A Hermeneutically Oriented Narrative Inquiry into Transformative Experiences of Reading Imaginative Literatu*re. PhD Diss., Oslo Metropolitan University, 2018.

Topelius, Zacharias, 'Sången' ['The Song'] (1842). https://topelius.sls.fi/sv/collection/199/text/18285?views=(type:readingtext),(type:comments),(type:facsimiles,nr:13) (retrieved 12 March 2024).

Troscianko, Emily T. 'Can Reading a Good Book Help with Eating Disorders: Yes but It Can also Do Harm Says New Research', *Scroll.in* (23 July 2018): https://scroll.in/article/887286/can-reading-a-good-book-help-with-eating-disorders-yes-but-it-can-also-do-harm-says-new-research (retrieved 26 June 2024).

Troscianko, Emily T. 'Fiction-Reading for Good or Ill: Eating Disorders, Interpretation and the Case for Creative Bibliotherapy Research', *Medical Humanities* 44, no. 3 (2018), 201–11.

Troscianko, Emily T. 'Literary Reading and Eating Disorders: Survey Evidence of Therapeutic Help and Harm', *Journal of Eating Disorders* 6 (2018): 1–17.

Whitehead, Anne. *Trauma Fiction*. Edinburgh: Edinburgh University Press, 2004.

12 Hoping Out Loud

Creative Bibliotherapy and Well-being Strategies

Danni Glover

Introduction

My own work on bibliotherapy has been primarily that of a practitioner. I am interested in its versatility, its ability to be personalised to the communities in which one works, its function as a self-managed therapeutic strategy, and its responsiveness as a practice to the input of those who take part. That is to say, each bibliotherapy experience is unique to the person experiencing it because the outcomes of reading and expressive writing can be considered mainly subjective. My experience as a practitioner of bibliotherapy has had several dimensions: I have worked with shared reading and creative writing; I have worked both prescriptively – according to themes laid out by project funders – and more freely allowing creative conversations with participants to follow any avenue they wished. In general, I can suggest a couple of maxims that have consistently evidenced themselves throughout my work. The first is that bibliotherapy is demonstrably valuable in producing mental well-being outcomes, though it can resist conventional academic rigour by favouring loose, colloquial definitions and not always generating documentation. The second is that bibliotherapy appears to be most successful when allowing people to express emotional states permissively and non-invasively, drawing out experiences which have previously been privately held. Because of its perceived tendency towards the qualitative and even towards the colloquial in practice, and because of its apparently low-impact psychological mandate, there has been much discussion in literature to date about bibliotherapy's legitimacy as a tool for well-being that stands up to academic scrutiny.[1] I would suggest that, rather than presenting obstacles for the academic, this tension presents an opportunity for them to 'lean in' and broaden the collective understanding of how creative therapies can be impactful in subtle but meaningful ways. This chapter is an account of key experiences within my work as a bibliotherapy practitioner (in a post-conflict community situation and working directly with NHS staff during the COVID-19 pandemic), and how bibliotherapy has provided an outlet to people who have struggled to access more established mental health and well-being services, ensuring limited positive outcomes, particularly relating to their experience of hope in challenging circumstances.

DOI: 10.4324/9781003471561-16

Past Perspectives: Shared Reading

My earliest work in this field focused on two main groups: children, particularly looked-after children (i.e., children who are living with foster carers and/or in residential care settings), and older people. In my earliest projects undertaken while working at a Northern Irish arts charity, I worked within a shared reading model, selecting thematically relevant works of (largely public domain) literature which were delivered to referred groups alongside suggestions for the facilitator to open up discussions during and after the reading. The shared reading model developed by the charity involved reading a short story or poem aloud to the group which had been selected with both the audience and pre-defined themes in mind, taking pauses in the text to ask questions which had been developed in collaboration with psychology practitioners and provoke ongoing discussion. In order to mitigate barriers caused by variable literacy skills and confidence with reading, the facilitator read the story aloud to the group, and those who wished were also able to follow along using a paper copy. These stories and the related discussion topics were selected with certain themes in mind, usually themes suggested by the desired outcome measurements of our funders. One major funder, for example, was particularly interested in conversations that raised awareness of resilience in children aged 8–18, which was measured before and after participation in a 12-week block of workshops by way of a low-impact survey developed by the in-house psychology team. This presented a tension between the needs of the funder and the needs of the group; the funder was interested in investigating a psychological concept that, in more rigorously therapeutic contexts, might have been challenging for participants, while the young people who came to the workshops naturally had a more colloquial and personal way of relating to the literature. The work of programming these projects was to resolve that tension and break the concept of 'resilience' into subthemes that were more relatable to children, to identify literature that would open these concepts up for discussion, and to design conversation points that allowed the facilitator to pitch the conversation to the children they were working with at a bespoke level. The groups themselves were referred largely because the young people within them were at risk in some way; many of the young people lived in and around Derry-Londonderry, an area which is notable for being both massively over-represented in local statistics around multiple deprivation and for being a site of significant intergenerational trauma following the decades of sectarian violence there since the 1960s.[2] The experiences of the young people, who were referred to the charity for which I worked, were strongly defined by these factors, and the stories they shared in my workshops often reflected this reality.

It became quickly apparent in these workshops, particularly in groups of young people aged 15+, that their reflections on the literature often did not align neatly with prescribed discussion points suggested by funders. More often than not, discussion was focused on their subjective readings of the stories and how they reflected their own experience. There was often crossover with the discussion points suggested by funders – the stories were, after all, not selected at random – but a process emerged of the young people responding more strongly when they were empowered to direct the conversation themselves, often with surprising and unexpected results. This process was baked into the shared reading model, a technique of bibliotherapy that allows participants to relate to a character and choose to share or retain their reflections based on that relation, rather than the more strenuous effort of relating their experiences wholesale through, for example, writing exercises. One group responded strongly to a reading of Kate Chopin's 'The Story of an Hour' (1894), in which a woman in an unsatisfying marriage receives the ultimately false news that her husband has been killed in an accident and finds that she reacts more with relief than grief. Though this story more closely textually reflects the expression of being freed from a relationship that stopped the main character from achieving her potential – it was selected for this particular group, who had all already engaged with the criminal justice system, to stimulate a conversation about having relationships that foster positive impacts on one's own life – the group unanimously had a more sinister reading. They supposed that the husband acted abusively prior to the events of the story and that the wife drops dead at the end not because of the shock of her complex emotions, but of a kind of suicidal ideation. There is not a hint of this in the text of the story, but over the course of the discussion, they began to open up about experiences in their own lives with abuse and neglect in the home. Though from the perspective of the funder, this session did not make a contribution to their understanding of resilience, from my own point of view (and, I hope, that of the young people who so generously shared their experiences), the session was overwhelmingly positive in providing them with a safe space to share and begin to process traumatic experiences.

Working with older people had a slightly different dimension. In the UK, the Reading Agency partners with organisations across the country to deliver their 'Reading Friends' shared reading programme to older people, among other programmes aimed at various populations.[3] Reading Friends seeks to reduce loneliness through shared reading opportunities facilitated in communities by trained volunteers; unlike much of the work I had undertaken with young people, the only requirement held by the Reading Agency was that the literature we provided be enjoyable and engaging, which gave myself and my team a degree of agency to develop reading lists. Because the work was situated in the community, we also enjoyed the unique advantage of being able to know our participants and their reading preferences quite well. Though older participants had a more diverse and varied taste in terms of the literature enjoyed, the stories which garnered the greatest response in terms of discussion generated were those that served as a prompt for them to discuss the stage of life they were currently at. While our younger participants did well in conversations around skill-building for resilience and processing conflicts that were present in their daily lives, older participants who had already developed those skills over the course of a life well-lived preferred to have conversations that reflected the reality that they had more time behind them than ahead of them and that the time they had ahead was valuable for precisely that reason. The concerns they exhibited were overwhelmingly around maintaining agency as they aged (this was particularly acute for participants with a diagnosis of Alzheimer's disease, or other causes of dementia), preserving a sense of their identity in the face of physical and psychological changes associated with ageing and maintaining an optimistic outlook during this phase of their life. We therefore considered literary selections for this group that had a focus on hope as a thematic anchor, drawing on research by Rick Snyder (among others), who defined hope as 'a positive motivational state that is based on an interactively derived sense of successful (a) agency (goal-directed energy), and (b) pathways (planning to meet goals)'.[4]

By focusing on hope, we could create space for conversations about future planning that were accepting of and empowering to people in a later stage of life; while a younger person might define goal-setting and future planning in terms of education, careers, relationships, or changes to their families, an older person who has already experienced these life events is better supported by social and therapeutic interventions that enable reminiscence about past events as a tool to drive goal setting and future planning that accounts for a person's individual needs. Snyder developed a tool to measure psychological levels of hope, but it also proved a useful concept in a non-academic context, as the language of hope is very widely understood, and therefore it is conceptually very well-suited to form the cornerstone of low-impact exercises to improve well-being. As a concept, hope integrates well into social conversations (i.e., 'I hope that my family and I will have time to get together this week'), but it also has a philosophical or spiritual dimension (i.e., 'I hope I will be able to see my loved ones after I die'). This variety of well-understood meanings, in addition to the defined psychological concept, means that even a question as simple as 'What do you hope for?' can yield a wide variety of answers depending on the mindset of individuals within a group of participants. Subsequent research has also demonstrated that increased levels of hope are correlated with markers of well-being such as life satisfaction, conscientiousness, and optimism. The same research indicates that a high level of hope is associated with lower incidences of ailments such as cancer, chronic pain, and depression and that people with higher levels of hope also tended to binge drink less, perform physical activity more frequently, and sleep better.[5] The outcomes for hope-based bibliotherapy are excellent, both in their objective and subjective markers.

With this understanding of hope and how it can manifest in social, philosophical, and psychological discussions, literature for older audiences was selected to encourage discussions that positively reflected life experiences and found value and hope in the challenge of late-life changes. One such story that was used frequently was James Joyce's classic 'Eveline' (1904; 1914), in which the titular main character decides to leave the father and siblings she cares for in Ireland to go to Argentina with a lover whose sincerity is ambiguous. This story's impact on the groups was unique because it universally elicited strong responses, but these responses were always diverse: some people saw in it the importance of staying loyal to family and some saw in it the value of exploring the world and what it offers. Many discussed times of displacement in their own lives, such as leaving home to get married or being deployed during their armed service. The character of Frank, the lover, was a topic of significant discussion, inspiring people to share stories both of 'the one who got away' and rogues who made them the rue the day they met. Like the Kate Chopin story that was so effective with younger groups, each person brought their own experience to 'Eveline', however unlike the younger groups, the older people tended to respond from a place of reminiscence rather than immediate or recent experience. This reminiscence was particularly supported by Joyce's lush evocation of Eveline's internal plight:

> She stood among the swaying crowd in the station at the North Wall. He held her hand and she knew that he was speaking to her, saying something about the passage over and over again. The station was full of soldiers with brown baggages [*sic*]. Through the wide doors of the sheds she caught a glimpse of the black mass of the boat, lying in beside the quay wall, with illumined portholes. She answered nothing. She felt her cheek pale and cold and, out of a maze of distress, she prayed to God to direct her, to show her what was her duty. The boat blew a long mournful whistle into the mist. If she went, tomorrow she would be on the sea with Frank, steaming towards Buenos Ayres. Their passage had been booked. Could she still draw back after all he had done for her? Her distress awoke a nausea in her body and she kept moving her lips in silent fervent prayer.[6]

Working with these groups informed my subsequent bibliotherapy practice in several ways. The first was to reframe my understanding of bibliotherapy to a real-world practice. My academic background meant that I had some baggage to shake, particularly around a looseness of vocabulary that was anathema to my training, but essential when working directly with members of the public, many of whom were not habitually readers, even as a hobby. I became more comfortable using language such as 'well-being' or 'home' which came up often in discussions with groups but that was academically difficult to define or had plural definitions. The second was to prize highly a person-centred approach to bibliotherapy: not emphasising my own outcomes or readings of texts during bibliotherapy exercises and not trying to sway the discussion at the expense of allowing the room to speak and share freely using the text as a jumping-off point. Finally, I became certain of the potential of bibliotherapy as a tool that created a space for vital conversations that were, if not therapeutic (a term that, in academia at least, resists the colloquial), vital in constructing valuable narratives of self-expression. Rather than creating a new narrative, shared reading experiences appeared to open the valve to what was already true in the minds of people who took part. I have lost count of how often I have heard people say that they were sharing a private experience for the first time in the supportive context of the bibliotherapy workshop. Current trends in bibliotherapy research demonstrate the potential for the practice of bibliotherapy to improve specific health outcomes;[7] in my own practice, I have seen the practice's potential in facilitating well-being in a more general sense. Crucially, it supported a version of well-being that could be self-managed. If a person can read, they can participate in a bibliotherapy practice. There is no requirement for them to consider their emotional problems or adverse life experiences in great depth in order for them to experience the release of expressing themselves and the associated mental health and well-being benefits; these benefits are present even if sharing occurs at what may appear to be a shallow level – that is to say, a person does not need to become very introspective to feel significant affects; they may simply relate the narrative of their experiences.[8] However, I also noted that the expressive section of the workshops – that is, the opportunity for groups to talk about what we had just read together – was more impactful than the reading itself, which provided a useful stimulus for discussion but was less frequently referred back to once the ball was rolling. I began to consider the potential for creative writing exercises which emphasised the act of self-expression as a form of bibliotherapy that could serve as an outlet to express emotional pressures; the release valve was repeatedly alluded to by participants in earlier workshops I facilitated.

Bibliotherapy in the Time of COVID-19: Creative Writing

I was therefore extremely grateful to be invited to join the staff of Dr Siobhan Campbell's 2020 Open University project, 'Creative and Expressive Writing with Frontline Health Care Workers during and after COVID-19'.[9] Dr Campbell and I met in 2018 at a conference she was co-organising chronicling bibliotherapy's origins to the present day, at which I, along with my colleague Aoife Lyons, presented our experience as practitioners among several panels of theorists and researchers. I found these perspectives tremendously enriching, as I hope other presenters found the paper I co-presented, and a theme emerged for the day that bibliotherapy was an artistic and scientific practice that was both understood through practice and enriched practically by research, a truly interdisciplinary undertaking. When Dr Campbell approached me two years later, the idea of mingling at a conference felt so much a thing of the past, as the UK (and much of the rest of the world) was in the throes of a lockdown brought on by a deadly pandemic. These tragic circumstances presented us with an opportunity and an urgency. We knew that expressive and creative writing strategies could be successful tools in aiding the recovery of survivors of violence and trauma, such as veterans and refugees.[10] It was equally true that these exercises can help people cope with impending stressors that they are aware will occur soon.[11] Could it also be the case that these exercises could provide an outlet for health care workers who were dealing with the implications of the pandemic in the most immediate possible way?

The high levels of stress and incidences of mental illness among health care workers globally are well documented.[12] The outbreak of COVID-19 in late 2019 certainly compounded these issues; a study of COVID healthcare workers conducted in China in January and February 2020 reported 'more severe degrees of all measurements of mental health symptoms than other health care workers' including depression, anxiety, insomnia, and distress, with symptoms being most acutely experienced by nurses, women, frontline staff, and staff working in Wuhan hospitals.[13] The United Kingdom's National Health Service is, at the time of writing, the fifth largest employer in the world, and the pandemic highlighted the need for healthcare workers to receive support, compounded by 'the lack of resources needed within the NHS … the risk of burnout … isolation woes and stigmatisation of healthcare staff of being carriers of the virus themselves by some in society'.[14] As our project began, there was no vaccine imminently available for the virus, and therefore it was impossible to infer when healthcare workers might expect this situation to draw to a close, which no doubt was a further factor contributing to their overall distress. If it was possible that creative and expressive writing exercises could have a positive impact on recovering from stressful situations, self-regulating, and independently managing one's emotions, then the staff of the NHS presented us with a uniquely appropriate and accessible case study. The conduit for these workshops came from Mel McEvoy, a Nurse Practitioner in North Tees and Hartlepool NHS Trust, who had experience in staff well-being support and who felt that the potential benefits made the workshops appropriate, along with the adherence to BERA guidelines. The effectiveness of these workshops demonstrated that his instincts were correct.

The team delivered 3 × 90-minute Creative Writing workshops over three months via MS Teams to clinical staff at North Tees and Hartlepool. Campbell's workshop design had up to four writing exercises for each session, some with an extension which could be pursued in the weeks in between. Initially these exercises were not shared in advance, which was highlighted in survey feedback by participants who indicated they would prefer to have advance notice, which was implemented by the third session. These exercises were escalating in their demand for writing acuity and emotional intensity of content shared. In session one, we began with two shared reading exercises followed by some free writing. Participants were read the Mary Oliver poem 'Wild Geese' (2002) and were asked to highlight words and phrases that were particularly resonant for them, then to free-write for a couple of minutes in any style or form they chose about whatever those lines they selected brought up. Two themes emerged in this exercise. The first is that without prompting, the participants used this exercise as a way of comparing and contrasting their lives at home and work and the emotional processes involved in moving between those spheres. One participant lifted a line directly from the poem and wrote on, suggesting that the line itself evoked experiences that were familiar to her:

> *Tell me about despair, yours, and I will not tell you mine to you*
> Meanwhile the world goes on
> I will listen to you cry
> Then I will leave this pod of despair this cloud of despair and masks
> Then I will go home to my evening
> Until together we enter that pod again.

Responses such as this demonstrate that when faced with a piece of literature that asks participants to think about ways in which they are restricted, one reaction was immediately to relate that experience to that of moving between the danger of work and the safety of home. These responses called to mind recent research that suggests frontline health care workers are experiencing stigma, their work being framed both as lifesaving and essential and also as a danger to public health when they move through public spaces.[15]

The second theme suggested by this exercise was identified through participants' understanding and appreciation of the poem. Poetry appreciation carries a stigma of its own, as many people have not encountered poetry since their English lessons at school (if then), and there is a perception that they will read poetry incorrectly or miss the point. This anxiety was reflected in the feedback of participants, who recorded, in spite of workshop facilitators' assurances to the contrary, that they feared taking the wrong message from the poem and therefore doing the free writing exercise incorrectly. This response may suggest a limitation of bibliotherapy; though in theory the exercises are low-impact enough to be practiced independently and at home, in the initial stages people may benefit from the reassurance of practicing with a trained and knowledgeable facilitator who can act as a gateway to forms of literature that do not necessarily inspire comfort and familiarity in the typical reader. 'Wild Geese' is a commonly drawn-on resource for bibliotherapy exercises, not only because it deals quite explicitly with processing emotions and experiencing emotional honesty but also because the poem itself is ambiguously hopeful; it compares the freedom of migrating geese to the pressures of modern human life and suggests that happiness can be found by '[letting] the soft animal of your body love what it loves',[16] but it also acknowledges that the human experience is fraught with distress which can both create pressure to resist reacting authentically to pain and be compounded by that same pressure. In this exercise, the participants universally read the poem as expressing negative emotions, drawing on lines such as 'Tell me about despair, yours, and I will tell you mine', and 'Whoever you are, no matter how lonely'. There was a sense that the poem was speaking directly to their difficulties rather than the things in their life which are uplifting. This reaction to the poem may indicate the immediacy of stress and anxiety in their lives. Several participants took part in these workshops literally during breaks in their working day, while still wearing hospital attire and on hospital premises.

What was also interesting about their responses to 'Wild Geese' was that, despite their expressed anxieties about reading and responding to poetry, their written exercises carried a degree of sophistication that indicated a fairly high comfort level with expressive writing. Metaphor in particular came quite naturally, and most participants included elements of metaphor in their written responses to the poem:

- 'The geese made me think about where I'm from, they're so noisy all day and night and it's like their noise is the same as the noise inside the house, it's where I'm meant to be … it feels free and alive'.
- 'The wild geese know something in me has wildness flying'.
- 'The darkest nights always come with the promise of daylight'.
- 'This is still a beautiful world, but it's night-time now'.
- 'Then I will leave this cloud of despair and masks …'

Metaphor forms a key component of poetry therapy advanced by Nicholas Mazza's R.E.S. (receptive/expressive/symbolic) model, which he suggests '[has] the potential to address the cognitive, affective, behavioural, and spiritual domains of human experience'.[17] Rafael Campo has suggested that poetic language such as metaphor is particularly important for clinical staff to become comfortable with, because

> the work of doctors will always necessarily take place at the intersection of science and art. Physicians who lack a passion for language or who fail to see beauty will be at a loss to translate these wonders [of new technologies and therapies] in the most meaningful terms for their lay patients and into the larger society around us.[18]

Jeanne Sorrell and Vicki Holmes have both separately argued that poetry is a useful skill for nurses in particular to develop.[19] Holmes points out that poetry is an expressive space for reflecting on an experience that is entirely unique to the poet, and that it is 'a way of releasing the mysteries of nursing practice'.[20] The literature both on teaching creative writing (for therapy or for its own merits) and appreciating the value of creative writing practices in healthcare settings, however, misses this observation suggested by our Open University project, that even participants who had not practiced or learned in creative writing techniques were able to use metaphor intuitively and appropriately in a supported setting. The workshop was delivered entirely in English, and this was true for both participants for whom English was their primary language and those for whom it was a secondary language. Metaphor being a key component of the kind of expressive writing that facilitates positive conversations about well-being and health, as well as its function as a natural and intuitive component of language, means that expressive forms of language are especially well-suited to self-managed forms of stress management and emotional release. This observation also echoes my earlier work, in which participants of shared reading workshops expressed that they were discussing aspects of their lives that were always familiar to them but that they had never had an opportunity to express. The use of metaphor to convey the aspects of one's inner life appears to be deeply ingrained in the expression of language in this mode, almost as if it were innate.

Subsequent sessions also began with a lower-impact exercise such as the one prompted by 'Wild Geese' before opening up to exercises that were potentially more challenging both in terms of the work being asked of participants and the scope for them to discuss more sensitive issues in the group. In the second session, an exercise called 'Window on the World' invited participants to imagine a window they were familiar with from their past – both the scene from inside the window and what was being observed outside of it – and to say whatever they wished to the younger self they imagined as the observer. Proponents of 'inner child' therapies suggest that the practice can help patients to uncover and express unmet needs that in their usual life they are in some ways restricted from expressing, a concept that is again evocative of bibliotherapy's ability to draw out unspoken stories from a person participating: not the discovery of something new, but the expression of something deeply known.[21] The setting of the 'window' was a neutral situation designed to anchor the writing in a place and begin a discussion about resilience in the face of vulnerability (suggested in the exercise by Childhood). Inner child therapies have the potential to draw out expressions of deeply held vulnerabilities, as well as trauma, so the exercise was purposefully presented to participants in a positive light, with the suggestion that they offer their child self some positive words about the future. Responses to this exercise were very successful, with participants already offering richly descriptive passages that demonstrated introspection and vulnerability, and, encouragingly, were able to express optimism despite their present-day circumstances, a feature which is commonly associated with strong levels of resilience.[22]

> Rows of terraced roof tops, slate-coloured tiles covered in moss and dirt. Rows of chimneys, some crumbling, some billowing smoke from their large stack. Standing in my attic bedroom, as a small child leaning on tip toes out the old attic windows. Gazing out to the evening sky, rain pouring, dripping down the drain pipes washing into the street. Down below holds the busy street, main road through my estate, always noisy. Glowing yellow light soothing in the night, a constant presence through the night. Black and white strips splash over the road, guiding people to cross safely during the night. lots of people who appear busy always rushing and always pushing. Sudden flash of blue appears across the road, looking closer can see an ambulance, this one is all black. Unknown to me at that time delivering those people to their final resting place in the large house across the street, a funeral home. As a small child the world appears so big and so busy. If there was one message, I would give to that small girl is that you will not always feel this small or so overwhelmed.

Another participant contacted project staff after the workshop to offer a poetic response to the exercise. This was an exciting development for a couple of reasons. Firstly, it indicated that the process of creative writing was becoming enjoyable and accessible enough that participants were writing independently, though no mandatory 'homework' had ever been issued. Secondly, the content of the poem they sent was apropos of their current situation.

> The attic window is dark and scary,
> Its glass cracked and its paintwork faded.
> It's ugly.
> Look at the window they told me laughing
> They wanted to scare me I think.
> But I looked beyond the window and beyond the dark.
> Look beyond the dark and see the light.
> Look beyond the dark and see the blue sky and green grass.
> Look beyond the dark and see that life is going on.
> Look beyond the dark and don't be scared
> Look beyond the dark and don't cry.
> Look beyond the mask

See their faces, see their smiles.
Look beyond the mask and hear their laughter.
Look beyond the mask and see their tears of happiness.
Look out of the window
Look beyond the dark
Look behind the mask
See a normal world.

This was a remarkably sophisticated response. Not only did this participant offer to read aloud with spontaneity, indicating a quickly growing level of comfort with independent creative responses, particularly in a challenging form; but she also created something that spoke to her original, spontaneous piece's themes of childhood vulnerability (in the original exercise, she had written about her sibling claiming they could see Dracula from the window of their bedroom and the fear that inspired) while also relating to her current situation. Here, the mask is both a Halloween mask of terror and a clinical N-95 mask, as well as the emotional mask that is compelled by fear in difficult situations. Had I the opportunity to work more intensively with this participant, I might have asked her who was wearing the mask; her patient in the COVID ward, putting on a brave face in spite of their pain and fear? Or the participant herself, a nurse whose job it was to offer comforting smiles though her own fear was overwhelming? Yes, behind the mask is a normal world, but the mere expression that the participant believed this was true indicated an important development in our understanding of how creative responses to stress and mental well-being lined up: hope was an essential component. She was moved to write in order to give voice to her hope. This is equally true of the scene quoted above written during the workshop. If that participant could give her younger self one message, it would be that she would not always be overwhelmed; a hopeful message that, I think, she needed to hear as an adult as well. Creative writing can give even the least practiced writers the creative space to speak directly to their own emotional needs.

In the final week, the tenor of the exercises escalated slightly in that participants were asked in a more direct way than previously to explicitly engage with their emotions – through writing. They began by writing lists of things they disliked in the world around them. Their suggestions ranged from very mundane (horror films, particular brands of beer) to existential (dogmatism, their perception that the world was less connected and loving than it was in the past). Very few mentions were made of COVID-specific annoyances or disturbances, though the exercise was left open to these elements if they came up. In the subsequent discussion, the group unanimously agreed that they felt there were things that they were 'allowed' to be annoyed about but others that they were not, seemingly associating the emotion of annoyance with the act of complaining, which was particularly acutely expressed when it came to annoyances around either work or the pandemic in general. For example, they 'allowed' themselves to be annoyed about the weather and train schedules, but they did not feel able to freely express their negative feelings about their jobs. Repeatedly they apologised for 'venting' in a space that had been created specifically so they could talk about things they disliked. This apology may be in some way tied to a perception that they have in some ways 'volunteered' to do this extremely dangerous work and amplified by the stigma attached to working with infectious patients in the pandemic context. This stigma was uneasily balanced against the 'clap for our carers' phenomenon; NHS staff were recognised in the public perception both as heroes for putting their lives on the line and as dangerous for the same reason. This also highlighted the disparity between public displays of appreciation for the work of NHS staff and political support for the NHS as an organisation. As Helen Wood and Beveley Skeggs have asked,

> This is the landscape of care that preceded Covid-19 and is seldom made apparent in the nationalised public displays of affection. Recognition and gratitude for care must now turn into care justice. How then do we put the humanity back into care? How do we restore some commitment to alleviating human suffering, and *value* time and emotion to support our basic human love for each other?[23]

Indeed, feminist economic research has long argued for a re-evaluation of the value of care labour, which disproportionately affects women both at home and in the workplace. The COVID-19 pandemic gave this argument a renewed impetus.[24]

One participant specifically highlighted her perspective on this phenomenon as a staff member who supported clinical staff and who had worked in that capacity previously but was now primarily based in an office:

> Most people in this room are patient facing, on the front line. I've struggled with that. As I work operationally, yes I have to work with the angst and the sickness and how am I going to provide a service, and I remember when everyone was clapping for the NHS and I thought 'don't be clapping for me, I've not done anything'. Of all the things I've written [in these workshops] I can't write about COVID without humour – I can't relate to patients. Some of my nurses said to me today 'If you could just see them begging to die, some of them' and I think to myself, I haven't been on a ward for two years, and I feel guilty.

Another participant echoed this sentiment, while also reflecting on how the 'essential workers' narrative was reductive in general:

> … this theory about people being 'essential workers'? We've learned that key workers aren't just those who have been hailed heroes – doctors, nurses or, before this, celebrities – but everyday people deserve the key to the city. Nobody on their own is essential but as a collective we all are.

Participant responses to this exercise highlighted the results of the contradictions presented by being an 'essential worker'. Clinical staff during the pandemic were under pressure to curtail their emotional responses, a process of minimisation that speaks to what Peter Phiri and colleagues have described as the 'silent under layer' of emotional stress brought on by clinical work during the pandemic.[25] They have also noted that these stresses are compounded by 'continuing to work whilst having suffered a loss without sufficient time available to grieve'.[26] Creative writing may provide a low-impact outlet for grief or any number of emotions that can be difficult to process while also being self-managed.

Conclusion

In bringing this chapter to its close, I return again to the words of Rick Snyder, whose work on hope has been so instrumental to my thinking on the forms and functions of bibliotherapy:

> People rhetorically ask, 'Surely you would much prefer to have a non-risk-taking pessimist flying your plane rather than a risk-taking optimist?' Ignoring the questionable assumption that the optimist is necessarily a risk taker, I would ask the readers to think about this question when it is posed differently: Do we really want the pessimistic pilot – filled with anxiety, tension, worry, sadness, rejection, anger, self-criticalness, and profound uncertainty – to be at the controls when our jet is landing during a thunderstorm? Not me. I want a high-hope pilot in that cockpit.[27]

Rarely has a metaphor felt as fitting as likening NHS clinical staff during the COVID-19 pandemic to a pilot navigating a plane through a storm. Snyder's observation – that we should wish for a 'high-hope pilot' – is all the more keenly observed with the understanding that hope is an emotional state that manifests intuitively when creative therapies are applied. Participants in my earlier shared reading work, who were routinely asked about their hopes in the context of my workshops, talked confidently and assuredly about their hopes for the future and those they had in the past, and this process ensured positive well-being outcomes when they were surveyed about their mental health. The process of imaginatively empathising with a character in a narrative was all the stimulus they required to begin the process of opening up about how they hoped, and for what. James Pennebaker, who has written extensively on the role of bibliotherapy in managing mental health outcomes, has suggested that writing about emotional experiences is an especially fruitful process in this regard, noting that 'the effects are found in both subjective and objective markers of health and well-being'.[28] I would contend that the prevalence of creative writing as a bibliotherapy technique is more easily evidenced due to the documentation of creative writing being more concrete than oral post-reading discussions and that shared reading models of bibliotherapy may yet produce extraordinary outcomes for a wider range of participants who may have barriers to accessing writing as a mode of self-expression. By its nature, much of the evidence is anecdotal. As a practitioner who has spent my career in bibliotherapy as a person reporting from a room, I can attest to the academic limitations of this position. However, I would also argue that any person who is interested in studying or practicing bibliotherapy should not allow academic limitations to limit the potential of bibliotherapy as a valuable process of self-discovery, self-expression, and even self-managed therapeutic practice. It necessarily deals with subjective experience, and it works best when practitioners inhabit a non-academic space, using everyday language and adapting the experiment – if one wants to consider it thus – to the participants, rather than defining experimental parameters and seeing how participants react to them.

With that being said, the work of Dr Campbell and my colleagues on the Open University 'Creative and Expressive Writing with Frontline Health Care Workers during and after COVID-19' project found its most definitive outcomes when participants enjoyed a blend of shared reading of selected poetry and directed writing exercises. The outcomes from this project were exemplary, with 100% of participants either agreeing or strongly agreeing with the statements 'I believe this workshop has been valuable to me', 'The exercises helped me to express myself', and 'The workshop helped me feel good about myself'. It is certainly true that the cohort who participated in these workshops – namely clinical NHS staff – have unique and often significant mental health needs, which they struggle to meet by the services available to them. This was true before the pandemic, which only served to exacerbate their situation.[29] We cannot claim that expressive therapies such as bibliotherapy can bridge this gap by themselves. We can show, however, that the outcomes suggested by this practice are positive. The work itself is easily self-managed, with participants benefiting from some direction and reassurance at the beginning of exercises but ultimately conducting the work without continuous oversight. We also have seen that hope is a thematic area that novice creative writers who participated in these workshops reached for intuitively and with sophistication. Hope is the impetus both for creativity and for care, two vocations that are clearly more integrated than one might expect. Blake Morrison has somewhat poetically described bibliotherapy as 'the reading cure'. My own hope for this work is that it can continue to produce positive outcomes for all, by non-invasively exploring our emotional narratives and giving us a permissive space to experiment, express ourselves, and hope out loud.

Notes

1 Liz Brewster, Barbara A. Sen, and Andrew Martin Cox, 'Legitimising Bibliotherapy: Evidence-based Discourses in Healthcare', *Journal of Documentation* 68 (2012): 185–205; Sarah McNicol and Liz Brewster, eds., *Bibliotherapy* (London: Facet Publishing, 2018).

2 Derry City and Strabane District Council, NIMDM 2017: Summary of those super output areas within the Derry City and Strabane District Council area (2018).

3 'About', *Reading Agency*, https://readingagency.org.uk/about (accessed 9 February 2021).

4 C. R. Snyder, et al., 'The Will and the Ways: Development and Validation of an Individual-Differences Measure of Hope', *Journal of Personality and Social Psychology* 60 (1991): 570–85.

5 Katelyn Long, et al., 'The Role of Hope in Subsequent Health and Well-Being for Older Adults: An Outcome-Wide Longitudinal Approach', *Global Epidemiology* 2 (2020): 100018.

6 James Joyce, 'Eveline', in *Dubliners* (London: Penguin Modern Classics, 1968), 34–9.

7 For example, Geoff Lowe has demonstrated that, in many settings, the implementation of a creative writing practice has been associated with an improved immune response. See Geoff Lowe, 'Health Related Effects of Creative and Expressive Writing', *Health Education* 106 (2006): 60–70.

8 See Jenny Secker, Helen Spandler, Suzanne Hacking, Lyn Kent, and Jo Shenton, 'Art for Mental Health's Sake', *Mental Health Today* 34 (2007): 34–6.

9 With thanks to Dr Siobhan Campbell as well as the other project staff: Dr Sally Blackburn-Daniels, Mr Mel McEvoy, and Dr. Donna Wakefield. I also wish to express my gratitude to Aoife Lyons, whose collaboration in the earliest stages of my career in bibliotherapy was absolutely instrumental and invaluable to me.

10 Siobhan Campbell and Meg Jensen, *The Expressive Writing Life Handbook* (London and Edinburgh: Beyond Borders Scotland, 2017).

11 S. J. Lepore, 'Expressive Writing Moderates the Relation between Intrusive Thoughts and Depressive Symptoms', *Journal of Personality and Social Psychology* 7 (1997): 1030–7.

12 Tait Shanafelt, Sonja Boone, Litjen Tan, Lotte N. Dyrbye, Wayne Sotile, Daniel Satele, et al., 'Burnout and Satisfaction with Work-Life Balance among US Physicians Relative to the General US Population', *Archives of Internal Medicine* 172 (2012): 1377–85.

13 Jianbo Lai, Siment Ma, Ying Wang, Zhongziang Cai, Jianbo Hu, Ning Wei, et al., 'Factors Associated with Mental Health Outcomes Among Health Care Workers Exposed to Coronavirus Disease 2019', *JAMA Network Open* 3(3) (2020): e203976. doi: 10.1001/jamanetworkopen.2020.3976. PMID: 32202646; PMCID: PMC7090843.

14 Peter Phiri, Shanaya Rathod, Kathryn Elliot, and Gayathri Delanerolle, 'The Impact of COVID-19 on the Mental Wellbeing of Healthcare Staff', *European Journal of Pharmaceutical and Medical Research* 7 (2020): 66–71.

15 Phiri et al., 'Impact of COVID-19', 2020.

16 Mary Oliver, 'Wild Geese', in *Staying Alive: Real Poems for Unreal Times*, edited by Neil Astley (Eastburn: Bloodaxe, 2002), 28.

17 Nicholas Mazza, 'No Place for Indifference: Poetry Therapy and Empowerment in Clinical, Educational and Community Practice', *Journal of Poetry Therapy* 31, no. 4 (2018): 203–8.

18 Rafael Campo, 'Why Should Medical Students Be Writing Poems?', *Journal of Medical Humanities* 27, no. 4 (2006): 253–4.

19 Jeanne Merkle Sorrell, 'Remembrance of Things Past through Writing: Esthetic Patterns of Knowing in Nursing', *Advances in Nursing Science* 17 (1994): 60–70; Vicki Holmes and David Gregory, 'Writing Poetry: A Way of Knowing Nursing', *Journal of Advanced Nursing* 28 (1998): 1191–4.

20 Holmes and Gregory, 'Writing Poetry'.

21 See Susan M. D. Carr and Susan Hancock, 'Healing the Inner Child through Portrait Therapy: Illness, Identity, and Childhood Trauma', *International Journal of Art Therapy* 22 (2017): 8–21.

22 Hosein Souri and Turaj Hasanirad, 'Relationship between Resilience, Optimism and Psychological Well Being in Students of Medicine', *Procedia - Social and Behavioural Sciences* 30 (2011): 1541–4.

23 Helen Wood and Beveley Skeggs, 'Clap for Carers? From Care Gratitude to Care Justice', *European Journal of Cultural Studies* 23 (2020): 641–7.

24 Kate Bahn, Jennifer Cohen, and Yana van der Meulen Rodgers, 'A Feminist Perspective on COVID-19 and the Value of Care Work Globally', *Feminist Frontiers* 27 (2020): 1–5.

25 Phiri et al., 'Impact of COVID-19'.

26 Phiri et al., 'Impact of COVID-19'.
27 C. R. Snyder, 'Hope Theory: Rainbows in the Mind', *Psychological Inquiry* 13 (2002): 249–75.
28 James W. Pennebaker, 'Writing about Emotional Experiences as a Therapeutic Process', *Psychological Science* 8 (1997): 162–6.
29 Phiri et al., 'Impact of COVID-19'.

References

Bahn, Kate, Jennifer Cohen, and Yana van der Meulen Rodgers. 'A Feminist Perspective on COVID-19 and the Value of Care Work Globally', *Feminist Frontiers* 27 (2020): 1–5.

Campbell, Siobhan, and Meg Jensen. *The Expressive Writing Life Handbook*. London and Edinburgh: Beyond Borders Scotland, 2017.

Campo, Rafael. 'Why Should Medical Students Be Writing Poems?', *Journal of Medical Humanities* 27, no. 4 (2006): 253–4.

Carr, Susan M.D., and Susan Hancock. 'Healing the Inner Child through Portrait Therapy: Illness, Identity, and Childhood Trauma', *International Journal of Art Therapy* 22 (2017): 8–21.

Holmes, Vicki, and David Gregory. 'Writing Poetry: A Way of Knowing Nursing', *Journal of Advanced Nursing* 28 (1998): 1191–4.

Joyce, James. 'Eveline', In *Dubliners*, 34–9. London: Penguin Modern Classics, 1968.

Lai, Jianbo, Siment Ma, Ying Wang, Zhongziang Cai, Jianbo Hu, Ning Wei, et al. 'Factors Associated with Mental Health Outcomes among Health Care Workers Exposed to Coronavirus Disease 2019', *JAMA Network Open* 3 (2020): e203976. http://dx.doi.org/doi:10.1001/jamanetworkopen.2020.3976.

Lepore, S. J. 'Expressive Writing Moderates the Relation between Intrusive Thoughts and Depressive Symptoms', *Journal of Personality and Social Psychology* 7 (1997): 1030–7.

Long, Katelyn, Eric S. Kim, Ying Chen, Matthew F. Wilson, Everett L. Worthington Jr., and Tyler J. VanderWeele. 'The Role of Hope in Subsequent Health and Well-Being for Older Adults: An Outcome-Wide Longitudinal Approach', *Global Epidemiology* 2 (2020): 100018.

Mazza, Nicholas. 'No Place for Indifference: Poetry Therapy and Empowerment in Clinical, Educational and Community Practice', *Journal of Poetry Therapy* 31, no. 4 (2018): 203–8.

Morrison, Blake. 'The Reading Cure', *The Guardian* (5 January 2008).

Oliver, Mary. 'Wild Geese'. In *Staying Alive: Real Poems for Unreal Times*, edited by Neil Astley, 28. Eastburn: Bloodaxe, 2002.

Pennebaker, James W. 'Writing about Emotional Experiences as a Therapeutic Process', *Psychological Science* 8 (1997): 162–6.

Phiri, Peter, Shanaya Rathod, Kathryn Elliot, and Gayathri Delanerolle. 'The Impact of COVID-19 on the Mental Wellbeing of Healthcare Staff', *European Journal of Pharmaceutical and Medical Research* 7 (2020): 66–71.

Secker, Jenny, Helen Spandler, Suzanne Hacking, Lyn Kent, and Jo Shenton. 'Art for Mental Health's Sake', *Mental Health Today* 34 (2007): 34–6.

Shanafelt, Tait, Sonja Boone, Litjen Tan, Lotte N. Dyrbye, Wayne Sotile, Daniel Satele, et al. 'Burnout and Satisfaction with Work-Life Balance among US Physicians Relative to the General US Population', *Archives of Internal Medicine* 172 (2012): 1377–85.

Snyder, C. R. 'Hope Theory: Rainbows in the Mind', *Psychological Inquiry* 13 (2002): 249–75.

Souri, Hosein, and Turaj Hasanirad. 'Relationship between Resilience, Optimism and Psychological Well Being in Students of Medicine', *Procedia – Social and Behavioural Sciences* 30 (2011): 1541–4.

Wakefield, Donna, Mel McEvoy, Sally Blackburn-Daniels, and Siobhan Campbell. 'Tackling the NHS Mental Health Crisis of Working through the COVID-19 Pandemic; Pilot Creative Writing Programme Has Potential to Support Wellbeing of Recovering Healthcare Workers', *Journal of the Royal College of Physicians of Edinburgh* 53, no. 1 (2023): 81–2.

Wood, Helen, and Beverly Skeggs. 'Clap for carers? From Care Gratitude to Care Justice', *European Journal of Cultural Studies* 23 (2020): 641–7.

Index

Note: Endnotes are indicated by the page number followed by 'n' and the endnote number e.g., 20n1 refers to endnote 1 on page 20.

FSC
www.fsc.org
MIX
Papier | Fördert gute Waldnutzung
FSC® C083411

Kolibri 360 GmbH
Ferdinand-Jühlke-Straße 7
99095 Erfurt, Deutschland
produktsicherheit@kolibri360.de